CITRUS ESSENTIAL OILS

CITRUS ESSENTIAL OILS
Flavor and Fragrance

Edited by
Masayoshi Sawamura
Kochi University, Japan

WILEY
A JOHN WILEY & SONS, INC., PUBLICATION

Published by John Wiley & Sons, Inc., Hoboken, New Jersey.
Published simultaneously in Canada.

Library of Congress Cataloging-in-Publication Data:

Citrus essential oils : flavor and fragrance / edited by Masayoshi Sawamura.
p. cm.
ISBN 978-0-470-37218-0 (cloth)
1. Citrus oils. I. Sawamura, Masayoshi.
TP959.C54C58 2010
661′.806—dc22

2009045874

MIX
Paper from responsible sources
FSC® C013604
FSC
www.fsc.org

CONTENTS

PREFACE

Masayoshi Sawamura

Today, citrus fruit is widely grown from temperate to tropical zones in the northern and southern hemispheres. Citrus fruit has been first ranked in the annual amount of world fruit production since 1992, meaning that it is the favorite type of fruit worldwide. It has pleasant taste and aroma, and is also an important source of vitamin C. Essential oil of citrus fruit is intensively accumulated in oil glands of the peel, accounting for approximately 1% of fruit weight on average. Citrus essential oil is also the most popular of natural essential oils. The oil is commercially used for food flavorings, toiletry products, cosmetics, perfumes, and so forth. Recently, citrus essential oil has been known not only for its aromatic functions, but also for its physiological properties, such as chemoprevention against cancer and aromatherapy effects. There are more than 10,000 varieties of citrus fruit. However, many citrus varieties are not familiar to us. Each aroma is unique and quite different even among those varieties. There has been lack of information on the overall characteristics of the *Citrus* genus. Citrus fruit is an important aromatic resource and its value will increase in the future. There is much useful information to be gleaned about the creative aromatic character and functional properties. This book provides an overview of citrus essential oils from various aspects covering basic and methodological application and recent topics of citrus essential oils research.

We hope that this book will provide inspiration and creative ideas for flavor and fragrance professionals and researchers. The book is intended for professionals as well as advanced students active in the food sciences, flavor chemistry, and aromatherapy. We believe our readers would benefit from a book that describes concepts, analytical methods, and diverse properties.

I owe a debt of gratitude to all the authors of this volume, who are leading specialists in their fields.

CONTRIBUTORS

Prof. Farid Chemat Université d'Avignon et des Pays de Vaucluse, UMR A 408 INRA-UPAV, 84000 Avignon, France

Hyang-Sook Choi, Ph.D. Asst. Prof., Department of Food Nutrition and Culinary Art, Kyungin Women's College, 101 Gyesangil Kyeyanggu, Inchon 407-740, Korea

Dr. Hisakatsu Iwabuchi San-Ei Gen F.F.I., Inc., 1-1-11 Sanwa-cho, Toyonaka, Osaka 561-8588, Japan

Dr. Takehiro Kashiwagi Assoc. Prof., Major of Food Science, Faculty of Agriculture, Kochi University, B-200 Monobe, Nankoku, Kochi 783-8502, Japan

Dr. Chizu Kumagai Palliative Care Unit, Municipal Ida Hospital, City of Kawasaki 2-27-1 Ida, Nakahara-ku, Kawasaki, Kanagawa, Japan 211-0035

Nguyen Thi Lan-Phi, Ph.D. Faculty of Chemical Engineering, Ho Chi Minh City University of Technology (HCMUT), 268 Ly Thuong Kiet Street, District 10, Ho Chi Minh City, Vietnam

Nguyen Thi Minh-Tu, Ph.D. Institute of Biological and Food Technology, Hanoi University of Technology, 1 Dai Co, Viet Road, Hanoi, Vietnam

Simon Muhoho Njoroge, Ph.D. Assoc. Prof., Department of Food Science and Technology, Jomo Kenyatta University of Agriculture and Technology, Nairobi, Kenya

Prof. Marco Poiana Dipartimento di Biotecnologie per il Monitoraggio Agroalimentare ed Ambientale, Facoltà di Agraria, Università Degli Studi di Reggio Calabria, 89124, Reggio Calabria, Italy

Dr. Atsushi Satake Research and Development Center, Nagaoka Perfumary Co. Ltd., 1-3-30, Itsukaichi, Ibaraki, Osaka 567-0005, Japan

Prof. Masayoshi Sawamura Tosa Food Business Creator Project Team, Kochi University, B-200 Monobe, Nankoku, Kochi 783-8502, Japan

Masaki Shimada, M.Eng. San-Ei Gen F.F.I., Inc., 1-1-11 Sanwa-cho, Toyonaka, Osaka 561-8588, Japan

U-Sun Son, M.Agr. Flavor Part/Scent Berry Perfume House, LG Household & Health Care Ltd., Seoul National University, San 56-1, Silim-dong, Gwanak-gu, Seoul 151-742, Korea

Hee-Sun Song, Ph.D. Assoc. Prof., Department of Food and Nutrition, Gwangju Health College, 688-3, Shinchang-dong, Gwangsan-gu, GwangJu, 506-701, Korea

Nguyen Thi Thao, Ph.D. Institute of Biological and Food Technology, Hanoi University of Technology, 1 Dai Co, Viet Road, Hanoi, Vietnam

Prof. C. Hanny Wijaya Department of Food Science and Technology, Faculty of Agricultural Technology, Bogor Agricultural University, Kampus IPB Damaga, Bogor 16002, Indonesia

Xiaolin Yu, M.Agr. Assoc. Prof., Department of Food Science, South China Agricultural University, Wushan, Guangzhou 510642, China

Dr. Chiyoki Yukawa San-Ei Gen F.F.I., Inc., 1-1-11 Sanwa-cho, Toyonaka, Osaka 561-8588, Japan

1

INTRODUCTION AND OVERVIEW

Masayoshi Sawamura

Kochi University
Kochi, Japan

There are a great number of *Citrus* varieties widely distributed in the world. It is said that the *Citrus* genus originated near Assam in India about 30 or 40 million years ago (Iwamasa, 1976). The *Citrus* fruits that spread to the West migrated to the Middle East and the Mediterranean, crossed the Atlantic Ocean, and finally reached America via the West Indies. Others, spreading to the East, migrated to Thailand, Malaysia, China and other Southeast Asian countries. Nowadays, most citrus fruits are grown extensively in the temperate and tropical zones of the northern and southern hemispheres.

Citrus can be propagated and new varieties can be produced by asexual nuclear or chance seedlings, by crossing, and by mutation. In addition to these natural forms of propagation, many new artificially crossed cultivars have been created by *Citrus* breeders. The classification of this expanding family is complex and is becoming confused. The best-known taxonomies of genus *Citrus* are those of Swingle (1943) and Tanaka (1969a,b). These two taxonomies differ greatly in the number of species admitted: Swingle identified 16 species, Tanaka 159. Although the basic concept underlying the two taxonomies is different, assignment is almost the same.

Citrus Essential Oils: Flavor and Fragrance, Edited by Masayoshi Sawamura

The four major fruit types commercially produced worldwide are citrus fruit, bananas, apples and grapes, followed by pears, peaches, and plums. Citrus fruit finally replaced grapes as the world's most-produced fruit in 1991. The recent production volume of major fruits is shown in Figure 1.1. The production of citrus

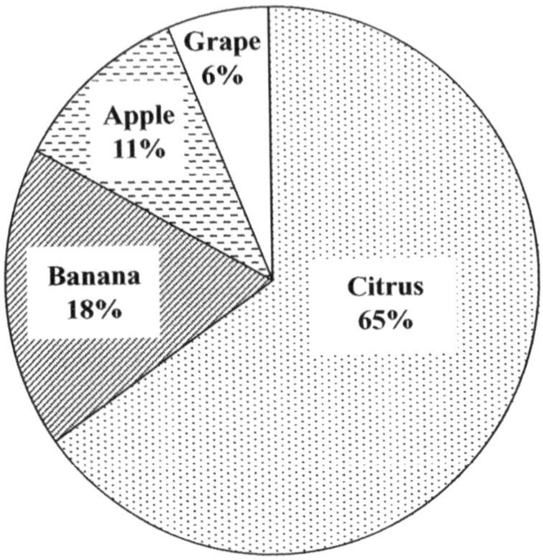

Figure 1.1. Worldwide production of major fruits.

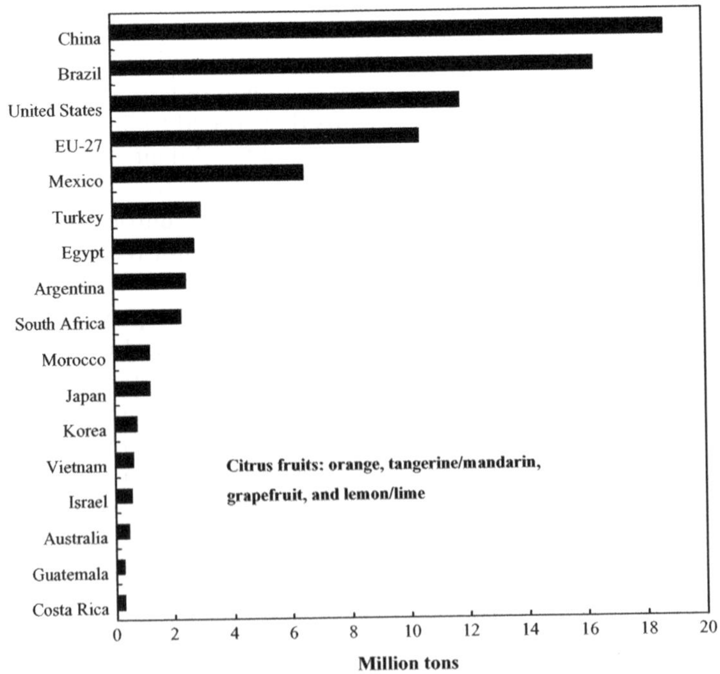

Figure 1.2. Major citrus fruits production in 2007.

fruit accounts for more than 65% of fruits produced. The total world production of citrus fruit in 2008 was about 79.6 million tons; major citrus-producing countries are shown in Figure 1.2. The greatest producer is China, followed by Brazil, the United States, the EU, Mexico, and Turkey. Citrus essential oils have also long been the most popular source of perfume and fragrance essences. There are four reasons why citrus fruit is the most popular fruit in the world: (1) good sour and sweet tastes; (2) pleasant, refreshing aroma; (3) good source of vitamin C; and (4) extensive growing areas worldwide. There are two categories of citrus fruit in terms of food chemistry: sweet citrus fruit, with a sugar/acid ratio of approximately 10, and sour citrus fruit, with a ratio of less than 1. Sweet citrus fruit such as orange, grapefruit, Satsuma mandarin, and pummelo are popular varieties. Sour citrus fruit, on the other hand, such as lemon, lime, bergamot, and yuzu, are less produced, but they are popular in culinary materials such as fruit juice vinegar, and their essential oils are also frequently used in flavoring, cosmetics, and perfume.

The aim of flavor or aroma research is to determine a fruit's composition, aroma characteristics, functionality, and industrial or commercial value. The concept of flavor research is outlined in Figure 1.3. First, essential oil is extracted from raw material such as citrus fruits. Then, aroma samples are analyzed using modern instruments, organoleptic procedures, and/or mechanical sensors. The resulting information can give a detailed understanding of the fruit and can be used in further studies of aroma or flavor.

The *Citrus* genus is said to have more than 10,000 varieties and to be produced more than any other kind of fruit in the world. Citrus essential oils account for the largest proportion of commercial natural flavors and fragrances. Essential oils from citrus peel are natural flavoring materials of commercial importance. They have been used in beverages, confectioneries, pharmaceuticals, cosmetics, and perfumes. The quality, freshness, and uniqueness of citrus oils are major factors contributing to their value and application. Citrus fruits, with their unique and attractive individual aromas, are popularly accepted worldwide, and citrus essential oils are a large and important aroma resource. Quantitative data concerning the volatile components of a number of citrus essential oils (Shaw, 1979; Sawamura, 2000) and their wide commercial use are presented in this book.

The twenty-first century has been referred to as "the era of fragrance." We live in an atmosphere greatly enriched by aromas and fragrances. Everyday items such as fresh and cooked foods, perfumes, cosmetic and toiletry goods, medicines, and insecticides contain natural or artificial fragrances. Aroma commonly gives us a strong impact in trace amounts. The characteristic odor of an individual substance is composed of roughly a thousand compounds. It is almost impossible to blend every compound of an odor in the exact proportion required to reconstruct the original. It has been determined, however, that there are usually one or two or a few key compounds that can accurately simulate the original odor. One goal of flavor research is to elucidate key aroma compounds by means of a combination of instrumental and organoleptic analyses. Many flavor researchers have tried to find the key aroma compounds of various kinds of citrus. *Gas*

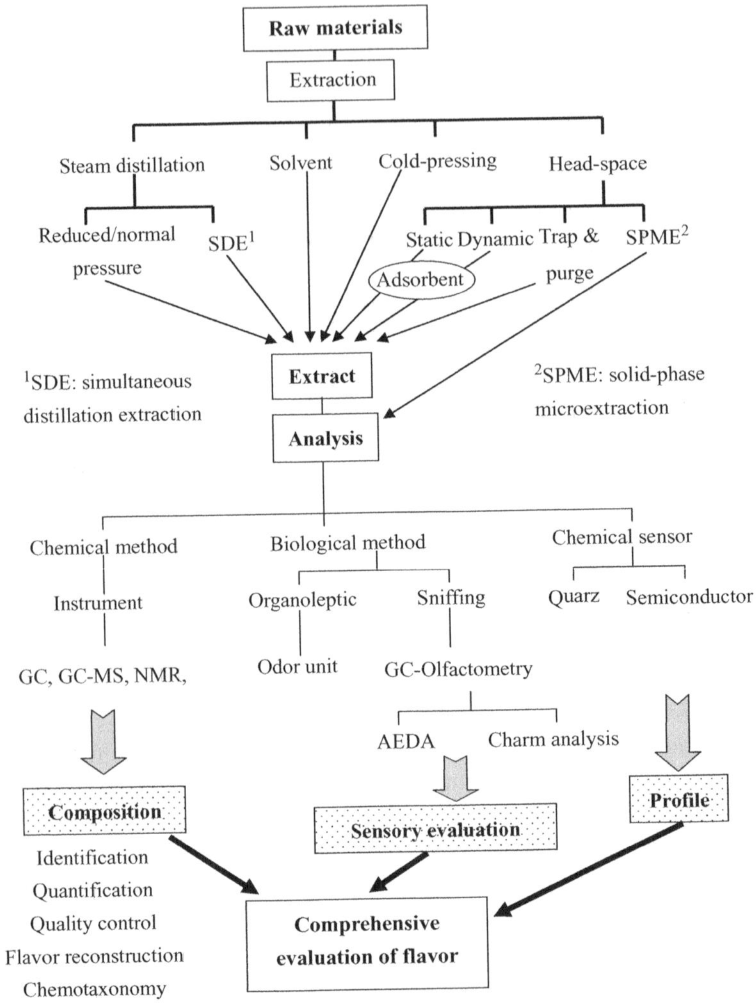

Figure 1.3. Flowchart of flavor research.

chromatography–olfactomery (GC-O) is a superior method for such studies (Acree, 1993).

Aroma is one of the functional properties of food because aroma compounds stimulate us physically and physiologically (this is referred to as *organoleptic effects*). A great number of aroma compounds have been identified in a variety of foods to date. Such studies have been a major theme in flavor research. Aroma compounds have a number of properties other than odor production, including antibiotic, deodorant, and blood vessel stimulation. *Aromatherapeutic effect* also falls into this category. Antioxidants have been investigated most intensively as constituents preventing diseases associated with oxidative damage, and decreasing lipid oxidation during the processing and storage of seafood (Pisano, 1986).

Synthetic antioxidants such as butylated hydroxytoluene (BHT), butylated hydroxyanisole (BHA), and propyl gallate (PG) are used as food additives to inhibit the actions of toxic and carcinogenic substances (Chang et al., 1977). Natural antioxidants from natural foods such as herbs (Boyd et al., 1993; Pizzocaro et al., 1994), vegetables (Tsushida et al., 1994; Vinson et al., 1998), fruits (Nogata et al., 1996), oilseeds (Medina et al., 1999), spices (Shahidi et al., 1994), green tea (Amarowicz and Shahidi, 1996), and cereals (Hendelman et al., 1999) have been studied, and some of them, such as ascorbate and tocopherols, are currently used in a variety of food products. In recent reports much attention has been given to citrus components, since they present various pharmaceutical activities including anticarcinogenicity, antimutagenicity, antioxidative activity, antiaging, and radical-scavenging (Nogata et al., 1996; Rapisarda et al., 1999; Choi et al., 2000; Sawamura et al., 1999, 2005). Grapefruit oil and lemon extracts have been suggested as effective natural antioxidative compounds (Tokoro, 1997). It has been recently discovered that some foods or foodstuffs serve to inhibit the formation of carcinogens. Essential oils containing terpenoids are well known to have some physiological and pharmaceutical effects, and it is known that citrus essential oils have antimicrobiological (Griffin et al., 1999) and chemopreventive properties (Crowell, 1997; Gould, 1997; Kawaii et al., 1999). The major component of citrus essential oils is *terpenes*, whose basic structure is isoprenoid (C_5H_8). The most typical terpenes are limonene, citrus-like odor; γ-terpinene, waxy; terpinolene, green; α-pinene and β-pinene, pine-like. These compounds have been reported to inhibit the growth of cancer cells. One carcinogen, nitrosodimethylamine, which is formed with dimethylamine and nitrite in an acidic condition, has been noted in this regard. Dimethylamine and nitrite are commonly present in meats and vegetables, respectively. It was suggested that some foods or foodstuffs might contain cancer-inhibitory and -preventive compounds as well as cancer-inducing substances (Sawamura et al., 1999, 2005).

Aromatherapy, a medical treatment intended to stimulate or calm the mind, is an applied therapy using the functional properties of essential oils. A variety of vegetable essential oils have been widely used in aromatherapy. Essential oils are extracted from the flowers, leaves, stems, roots, and fruits of various plants and purified for commercial use. Aromatherapy originated in Europe in the eighteenth century and has grown popular in many countries recently, but the most famous essential oil products are still produced in Europe. There are currently seven kinds of commercial citrus essential oils used in aromatherapy: orange, mandarin, lemon, lime, bergamot, grapefruit, and neroli. Yuzu (*Citrus junos* Sieb. ex Tanaka), a typical Japanese sour citrus fruit, has attracted the interest of aroma therapists over the past ten years. Recently, the effect of yuzu essential oil on the autonomic nervous system has been studied (Sawamura et al., 2009). It is expected that yuzu essential oil will soon be adopted for use in aromatherapy. One obstacle to such application for aromatherapy is that the composition of essential oils changes readily. It has been pointed out that the composition of yuzu (Njoroge et al., 1996) and lemon essential oils (Sawamura et al., 2004) can change considerably under different storage conditions. It is important to carefully consider quality change in commercial essential oil products intended for therapeutic use. This book presents a few attractive studies of functional citrus properties, including aromatherapy.

Recently, food safety or reliability has been a prominent concern, along with food quality. All Japanese foods and products, for example, are controlled under standards such as the European Union regulations regarding food safety and traceability, Japanese Agricultural Standard (JAS), and other regulations governing responsibility to consumers and manufacturers in the United States, Canada, Australia, and England. However, there are few methods for discriminating as to the quality and characteristics of crops from various producing districts. One of the most reliable methods is isotope analysis of food constituents by mass spectrometry. In nature, the isotopes of each element are distributed in a fixed ratio. Plants on the earth first convert solar energy into biochemical energy; the food chain begins with plants. Higher plants fix CO_2 by the Calvin-Benson cycle to biosynthesize various organic compounds for their constituents. It is known that the enzyme ribulose-1,5-diphosphate carboxylase differentiates a small mass difference between $^{12}CO_2$ and $^{13}CO_2$, when it fixes CO_2 in the atmosphere (O'Leary, 1981). This function is referred to as the *isotope effect*. It is thought that the isotope effect could occur in every enzyme involved in biosynthetic and metabolic pathways. Thus, we can see that this effect should also be applicable to the essential oils comprising terpene compounds. Every species, variety, or strain of a plant has some substantially distinct characteristics. Even among the same cultivars, different growing conditions such as annual atmosphere and moisture, or soil and fertilizers, can bring about small but appreciable differences in composition. Several researchers (Faber et al., 1995; Faulharber et al., 1997; Sawamura et al., 2001; Thao et al., 2007) have tried to distinguish these isotope differences of biological constituents. Some sections of this book discuss methods of verifying the genuineness of food.

Finally, fundamental and academic information about citrus essential oils have contributed to commercial development. In the references section on this chapter, several experts present the reader with attractive topics regarding the wide utilization of citrus essential oils.

REFERENCES

Acree, T.E. (1993). Bioassays for flavor. In: Acree, T.E., Teranishi, R. (eds.), Flavor science. Washington, DC: American Chemical Society, pp. 1–18.

Amarowicz, R., Shahidi, F. (1996). A rapid chromatographic method for separation of individual catechins from green tea. *Food Research International* **29**: 71–76.

Boyd, L.C., Green, D.P., Giesbrecht, F.B., King, M.F. (1993). Inhibition of oxidative rancidity in frozen cooked fish flakes by *tert*-butylhydroquinone and rosemary extract. *Journal of the Science of Food and Agriculture* **61**: 87–93.

Chang, S.S., Ostric-Matijasevic, B., Hsieh, O.A., Chang, C.L. (1977). Natural antioxidants from rosemary and sage. *Journal of Food Science* **42**: 1102–1106.

Choi, H.S., Song, H.S., Ukeda, H., Sawamura, M. (2000). Radical-scavenging activities of citrus essential oils and their components: Detection using 1,1-diphenyl-2-picrylhydrazyl. *Journal of Agricultural and Food Chemistry* **48**: 4156–4161.

Crowell, P.L. (1997). Monoterpenes in breast cancer chemoprevention. *Breast Cancer Research Treatment* **46**: 191–197.

Faber, B., Krause, B., Dietrich, A., Mosandl, A. (1995). Gas chromatography–isotope ratio mass spectrometry in the analysis of peppermint oil and its importance in the authenticity control. *Journal of Essential Oil Research* **7**: 123–131.

Faulharber, S., Hener, U., Mosandl, A. (1997). GC-IRMS analysis of mandarin essential oils. 2. $d^{13}C_{PDB}$ values of characteristic flavor components. *Journal of Agricultural and Food Chemistry* **45**: 4719–4725.

Gould, M.N. (1997). Cancer chemoprevention and therapy by monoterpenes. *Environmental Health Perspectives* **105**: 977–979.

Griffin, S.G., Wyllie, S.G., Markham, J.L., Leach, D.N. (1999). The role of structure and molecular properties of terpenoids in determining their antimicrobial activity. *Flavour Fragrance Journal* **14**: 322–332.

Hendelman, G.J., Cao, G., Walter, M.F., Nightingale, Z.D., Paul, G.L., Prior, R.L., Blumberg, J.B. (1999). Antioxidant capacity of oat (*Avena sativa* L.) extracts. 1. Inhibition of low-density lipoprotein oxidation and oxygen radical absorbance capacity. *Journal of Agricultural and Food Chemistry* **47**: 4888–4893.

Iwamasa, M. (1976). Citrus varieties. Shizuoka: Shizuoka Prefectural Citrus Agricultural Cooperative Association, p. 30.

Kawaii, S., Tomono, Y., Katase, E., Ogawa, K., Yano, M. (1999). Quantitation of flavonoid constituents in *Citrus* fruits. *Journal of Agricultural and Food Chemistry* **47**: 3565–3571.

Medina, I.M., Satué-Gracia, T., German, J.B., Frankel, E.N. (1999). Comparison of natural polyphenol antioxidants from extra virgin olive oil with synthetic antioxidants in tuna lipids during thermal oxidation. *Journal of Agricultural and Food Chemistry* **47**: 4873–4879.

Njoroge, S.M., Ukeda, H., Sawamura, M. (1996). Changes in the volatile composition of yuzu (*Citrus junos* Tanaka) cold-pressed oil during storage. *Journal of Agricultural and Food Chemistry* **44**: 550–556.

Nogata, Y., Yoza, K., Kusumoto, K., Kohyama, N., Sekiya, K., Ohta, H. (1996). Screening for inhibitory activity of citrus fruit extracts against platelet cyclooxigenase and lipoxigenase. *Journal of Agricultural and Food Chemistry* **44**: 725–729.

O'Leary, M.H. (1981). Carbon isotope fractionation in plants. *Phytochemistry* **20**: 553–567.

Pisano, R.C. (1986). The future of natural essential oils in the flavor and fragrance industry. *Perfumer and Flavorist* **11**: 35–41.

Pizzocaro, F., Senesi, E., Babbini, G. (1994). Protective effect of rosemary and sage on frozen beef hamburgers. *Industrie Alimentari* **33**: 289–294.

Rapisarda, P., Tomaino, A., Lo Cascio, C., Bonina, F., Saijo, A., De Pasquale, A. (1999). Antioxidant effectiveness as influenced by phenolic content of fresh orange juices. *Journal of Agricultural and Food Chemistry* **47**: 4718–4723.

Sawamura, M., Song, H.S., Ozaki, K., Ishikawa, J., Ukeda, H. (1999). Inhibitory effects of citrus essential oils and their components on the formation of *N*-nitrosodimethylamine. *Journal of Agricultural and Food Chemistry* **47**: 4868–4872.

Sawamura, M. (2000). Volatile components of essential oils of the *Citrus* genus. In: Pandalai, S.G. (ed.), Recent research developments in agricultural and food chemistry, Vol. 4. Trivandrum, India: Research Signpost, pp. 131–164.

Sawamura, M., Ito, T., Une, A., Ukeda, H., Yamasaki, Y. (2001). Isotope ratio by HRGC-MS of *Citrus junos* Tanaka (yuzu) essential oils: *m/z* 137/136 of terpene hydrocarbons. *Bioscience, Biotechnology, and Biochemistry* **65**: 2622–2629.

Sawamura, M., Son, U.S., Choi, H.S., Lee Kim, M.S., Lan Phi, N.T., Fears, M., Kumagai, C. (2004). Compositional changes in commercial lemon essential oil for aromatherapy. *International Journal of Aromatherapy* **14**: 27–36.

Sawamura, M., Wu, Y., Fujiwara, C., Urushibata, M. (2005). Inhibitory effects of yuzu essential oil on the formation of *N*-nitrosodimethylamine in vegetables. *Journal of Agricultural and Food Chemistry* **53**: 4281–4287.

Sawamura, M., Fukata, J., Kumagai, C., Lan Phi, N.T., Mizushima, N., Hori, N., Wada, M., Kamano, S. (2009). Functional activities of Japanese yuzu essential oil. *Japanese Journal of Aromatherapy* **9**: 1–11.

Shahidi, F., Wanasundara, U.N., Amarowicz, R. (1994). Natural antioxidants from low-pungency mustard flour. *Food Research International* **27**: 489–493.

Shaw, P.E. (1979). Review of quantitative analyses of citrus essential oils. *Journal of Agricultural and Food Chemistry* **27**: 246–257.

Swingle, W.T. (1943). The botany of *Citrus* and its wild relatives. In: Webber, H.J., Batchelor, L.D. (eds.), The citrus industry, Vol. 1. Berkeley, FL: University of California Press, pp. 190–430.

Tanaka, T. (1969a). Taxonomic problem of citrus fruits in the orient. *Bulletin of University of Osaka Prefecture* **B 21**: 133–138.

Tanaka, T. (1969b). Misunderstanding with regard to citrus classification and nomenclature. *Bulletin of University of Osaka Prefecture* **B 21**: 139–145.

Thao, N.T., Kashiwagi, T., Sawamura, M. (2007). Characterization by GC-MS of Vietnamese citrus species and hybrids based on the isotope ratio of monoterpene hydrocarbons. *Bioscience, Biotechnology, and Biochemistry* **71**: 2155–2161.

Tokoro, K. (1997). Antioxidants in grapefruit oil. *Aromatopia* **24**: 42–44.

Tsushida, T., Suzuki, M., Kurogi, M. (1994). Evaluation of antioxidant activity of vegetable extracts and determination of some active compounds. *Nippon Shokuhin Kogyo Gakkaishi* **41**: 611–618.

Vinson, J.A., Hao, Y., Su, X., Zubik, L. (1998). Phenol antioxidant quantity and quality in foods: Vegetables. *Journal of Agricultural and Food Chemistry* **46**: 3630–3634.

2

TECHNIQUES FOR OIL EXTRACTION

Farid Chemat

Université d'Avignon
Avignon, France

Essential oils have been used probably since the discovery of fire. Egyptians and Phoenicians, Jews, Arabs, Indians, Chinese, Greeks, Romans, and even Mayans and Aztecs all possessed a fragrance culture of great refinement. The Egyptian art of perfumery was preeminent in the civilized antique world, hence the use of aromatic fumigation in religious ceremonies and in mummification. The advent of Christianity and the fall of the Roman Empire caused the art and science of perfumery to move into the Arabic world, where it reached an unequalled level of refinement. During the Middle Ages, the Crusaders introduced the art of alchemy to Europe (Guenther, 1948). The process used by alchemists was the distillation technique using the alambic to produce *spirit* or *Quinta essentia*, precisely what we know today as *essential oils* (French, 1651). Essential oils are also known as *volatile oils* in contrast to fatty vegetable, animal, and mineral oils. Thus, a drop of essential oil on a piece of cloth or paper disappears within a few minutes or a few days at most, depending on the temperature, which is not the case for fatty oils.

The traditional way of isolating volatile compounds as essential oils from *Citrus* is performed mostly by cold pressing the *Citrus* peels. Steam distillation is also used to recover citrus essential oils but principally for production of

Citrus Essential Oils: Flavor and Fragrance, Edited by Masayoshi Sawamura

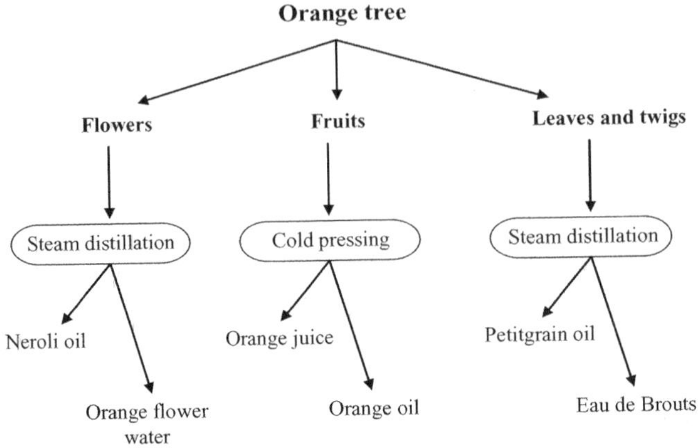

Figure 2.1. Complete valorization of citrus trees.

limonene used as green solvent. Not only are citrus fruits completely used but all of the citrus tree could be valorized, for example, by steam distillation of orange flowers to get neroli oil and the by-product orange flower water. With increasing energy prices, it was not economical to perform steam distillation of citrus leaves and twigs to get petitgrain oil and the by-product eau de brouts (Figure 2.1). Citrus essential oils have been applied in many products such as foods, beverages, cosmetics, and medicines, as flavoring agents as well as for aromatherapy. They are also used for their germicidal, antioxidant, and anticarcinogenic properties (Mukhopadhyay, 2000).

Essential oils and aromas are complex mixtures of volatile substances generally present at low concentrations. Before such substances can be used or analyzed, they have to be extracted from the plant matrix. Different methods can be used for this purpose (e.g., hydrodistillation, steam distillation, cold pressing, solvent extraction, and simultaneous distillation-extraction). Losses of some volatile compounds, low extraction efficiency, degradation of unsaturated or ester compounds through thermal or hydrolytic effects, and toxic solvent residue in the extract may be encountered using these extraction methods. Citrus essential oils are a mixture of volatile compounds and consist mainly of monoterpene hydrocarbons that possess high levels of unsaturation and are generally unstable due to many factors such as light, heat, oxidation, and hydration. These shortcomings have led to the consideration of the use of new "green" techniques in essential oil extraction, which typically use less solvent and energy, such as microwave extraction, supercritical fluid extraction, ultrasound extraction, and subcritical water extraction. Alternatives to conventional extraction procedures may increase production efficiency and contribute to environmental preservation by reducing the use of solvents and fossil energy and the generation of hazardous substances.

This chapter presents a complete picture of current knowledge on conventional and innovative techniques of extraction of citrus essential oils.

2.1 STEAM AND HYDRODISTILLATION

Farid Chemat

According to ISO and AFNOR standards, essential oils are defined as products obtained from raw plant material that must be isolated by physical means only. The physical methods used are distillation (steam, steam/water, and water), expression (also known as cold pressing for citrus peel oils), or dry distillation of natural materials. Following distillation, the essential oil is physically separated from the water phase (Figure 2.2) (Essentielle, 2000).

The traditional way of isolating volatile compounds as essential oils from plant material is distillation. During distillation, fragrant plants exposed to boiling water or steam release their essential oils through evaporation. Recovery of the essential oil is facilitated by distillation of two immiscible liquids, namely, water and essential oil, based on the principle that, at the boiling temperature, the combined vapor pressure equals the ambient pressure. Thus the essential oil ingredients, for which boiling points normally range from 100 to 300°C, are evaporated at a temperature close to that of water. The essential oil–laden steam rises and enters narrow tubing that is cooled by an outside source. As steam

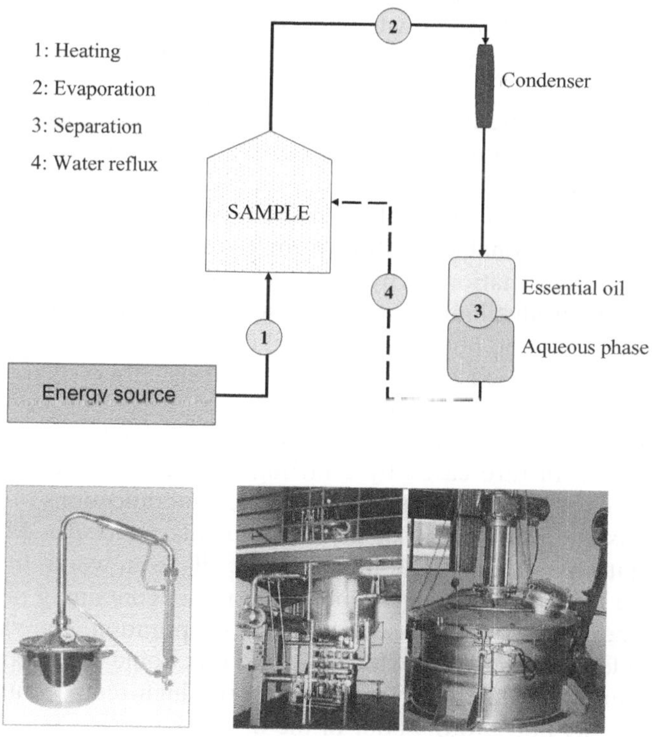

Figure 2.2. Laboratory and industrial conventional recovery of essential oils.

and essential oil vapors are condensed, both are collected and separated in a vessel traditionally called the "Florentine flask" (Guenther, 1948). The essential oil, being lighter than water, floats at the top while water goes to the bottom and can be easily separated. The amount of essential oil produced depends on four main criteria: the length of distillation time, the temperature, the operating pressure and, most importantly, the type and quality of the plant material. Typically, the yield of essential oils from plants is between 0.005 and 10% (Naves, 1974).

Historically, there have been three types of distillation: water distillation, water/steam distillation, and steam distillation. Water distillation is sometimes referred to as *indirect* steam distillation. In this method, plant material is soaked in water and heated until it boils. The resulting steam from boiling water carries the volatile oils with it. Cooling and condensation subsequently separate the oil from the water. Apart from its slowness, the disadvantage of this technique is that both materials and scent deteriorate from constant heat exposure. In the water/steam method, the leafy plant material is placed on a grill above the hot water, and the steam passes through the plant material. The leaves must be carefully distributed on the grill to allow for even steaming and thorough extraction. "Direct" steam distillation is the most common method for essential oil extraction. In this process, no water is placed inside the distillation tank itself. Instead, steam is directed into the tank from an outside source. The essential oils are released from the plant material when the steam bursts the sacs containing the oil molecules. From this stage, the process of condensation and separation is standard.

In addition to those mentioned previously, there are numerous other improved methods of producing natural fragrance materials and essential oils, including turbodistillation (Figure 2.3), hydrodiffusion, vacuum-distillation, continuous-distillation, dry-distillation, and molecular-distillation (Koedam, 1987).

All these conventional extraction techniques have important drawbacks, such as low yields, formation of by-products, and limited stability. For steam-distillation and hydrodistillation methods, the steam is percolated through the flask with plants from the bottom and the oil evaporates. The emerging mixture of vaporized water and oil moves through a coil usually cooled with running water, where the steam is condensed.

The mixture of condensed water and essential oil is collected and separated by decantation or, in rare cases, by centrifugation. The elevated temperatures and prolonged extraction time can cause chemical modifications of the essential oil components and often a loss of the most volatile molecules. Manufacturers use dry distillation to extract high-boiling-point oils from wood. In this process, heat is applied usually as a direct flame to the vessel containing plant material. The high temperatures release essential oils by evaporation. The vapor is piped away and condensed to give a mixture of liquid oils. Some of the components in the plant material get degraded (pyrolyze) at the high temperatures used and add burned, smoky notes to the odor of the oil.

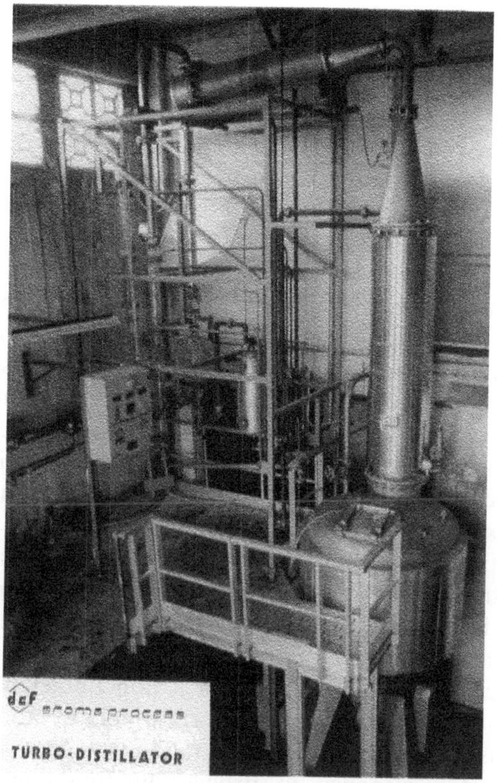

Figure 2.3. Turbodistillation of citrus essential oils.

With the increasing energy prices and the drive to reduce CO_2 emissions, chemical and food industries are challenged to find new technologies in order to reduce energy consumption, to meet legal requirements on emissions, product/process safety, and control, and for cost reduction and increased quality as well as functionality. Extraction and distillation technologies are the promising innovation themes that could contribute to sustainable growth of chemical and food industries. For example, existing extraction technologies have considerable technological and scientific bottlenecks to overcome—often requiring up to 50% of investments in a new plant and more than 70% of total process energy used in food, fine chemicals, and pharmaceutical industries. These shortcomings have led to the consideration of the use of new "green" techniques in separation, which typically use less solvent and energy, such as microwave extraction, supercritical fluid extraction, and ultrasound extraction. Separation under extreme or nonclassical conditions is currently a dynamically developing area in applied research and industry.

2.2 SOLVENT- AND WATER-FREE MICROWAVE EXTRACTION

Farid Chemat

Microwave energy is well known to have a significant effect on the rate of various processes in the chemical and food industries. Much attention has been given to the application of microwave dielectric heating for the extraction of natural products that typically need hours or days to reach completion with conventional methods. Using microwaves, fully reproducible extractions can now be completed in seconds or minutes with high reproducibility, reducing the consumption of solvent, simplifying manipulation and workup, giving higher purity of the final product, eliminating post-treatment of waste water, and consuming only a fraction of the energy normally needed for a conventional extraction method such as steam distillation or solvent extraction. Several classes of compounds such as essential oils, aromas, pigments, antioxidants, and other organic compounds have been extracted efficiently from a variety of matrices (mainly animal tissues, food, and plant materials) (Paré and Bélanger, 1997).

Microwave extraction is a research area that has an impact in several fields of modern chemistry. All the reported applications have shown that microwave-assisted extraction is an alternative to conventional techniques for such matrices. The main benefits are decrease of extraction time and solvents used. The advantages of using microwave energy, which is a noncontact heat source, for the extraction of essential oils from plant materials include more effective heating, faster energy transfer, reduced thermal gradients, selective heating, reduced equipment size, faster response to process heating control, faster startup, increased production, and elimination of process steps. Extraction processes performed under the action of microwave radiation are believed to be affected in part by polarization, and volumetric and selective heating (Metaxas and Meredith, 1983).

Microwave-assisted solvent extraction (MASE) was first used in the extraction of several compounds from food products (citrus, aromatic plants, cereals, etc.). Numerous classes of compounds such as aromas, antioxidants, colors, biophenols, and other secondary and primary metabolites have been extracted efficiently, in terms of rapidity and reproducibility, from a variety of matrices. The technique was patented in 1990 as Microwave Assisted Process (MAP) (Paré and Bélanger, 1990). Typically, plant material is immersed in a nonabsorbing microwave solvent such as hexane and irradiated by microwave energy. When the oil glands of the plant are subjected to severe thermal stresses and localized high pressures, as in the case of microwave heating, the pressure buildup within the glands exceeds their capacity for expansion, and causes their rupture more rapidly than in conventional extraction. Volatile oil dissolves in the organic solvent before being separated by liquid–liquid extraction. In all cases, yields and composition of microwave extracts are comparable to those obtained by a classical solvent extraction such as Soxhlet extraction but have been achieved with reduced extraction time (Paré and Bélanger, 1997).

Vacuum Microwave Hydro Distillation (VMHD) was elaborated and patented by Archimex in 1994 (Mompon and Mengal, 1994). This technique is based on selective heating by microwaves combined with application of sequential vacuum. The plant material is placed in a microwave cavity with water to refresh the dry material. The plant material is afterward exposed to microwave radiation to free the natural extract. Reducing the pressure to between 100 and 200 mbar allowed the evaporation of the azeotropic water-volatile oil mixture from the biological matrix. The procedure is repeated in a stepwise fashion in order to extract all the volatile oil from the plant. Up to 30 kilograms per hour of material can be treated (Figure 2.4).

Solvent Free Microwave Extraction (SFME) is a recent method of extraction patented in 2004 and specifically aimed at obtaining essential oil from plant material (Chemat et al., 2004). SFME apparatus is an original combination of microwave heating and distillation at atmospheric pressure (Figure 2.5). SFME was conceived for laboratory-scale applications in the extraction of essential oils from different kinds of aromatic plants and fruits. Based on a relatively simple principle, this method involves placing plant material in a microwave reactor, without any added solvent or water. The internal heating of the in-situ water within the plant material distends the plant cells and leads to rupture of the glands and oleiferous receptacles. Thus, this process frees essential oil that is evaporated by the in-situ water of the plant material. A cooling system outside the microwave oven condenses the distillate continuously. The water excess is refluxed to the extraction vessel in order to restore the in-situ water to the plant material. The effect of SFME on the kinetic of extraction is illustrated in Figure 2.6. Microwaving offered advantages such as less extraction time, less solvent consumption, high efficiency, and high yield and reproducibility; organoleptic properties of essential oil were also improved. Essential oils obtained by SFME from fresh orange peels were colorless with fresh, light, and sweet citrusy odor as compared to the pale-yellow oil with pungent smell extracted with traditional methods. Higher abundance of oxygenated compounds in essential oil is related to the rapid heating of polar substances by microwaves, and only in-situ water was used, which prevented the decomposition of principal oxygenated constituents by thermal and hydrolytic reactions. The SFME method also offers a reduced environmental burden as it rejects less CO_2 in atmosphere (200 g CO_2 per gram of essential oil compared to the traditional method, which was rejecting 3600 g CO_2 per gram of essential oil) (Ferhat et al., 2006, 2007; Lucchesi et al., 2004a, 2004b).

Microwave Hydrodiffusion and Gravity (MHG) (Chemat et al., 2008a) is a new and green technique for the extraction of essential oils discovered at the Laboratory of Green Extractions (Université d'Avignon–France) in 2008 (Figure 2.7). This green extraction technique is an original "upside-down" microwave alembic combining microwave heating and earth gravity at atmospheric pressure. MHG was conceived for laboratory and industrial-scale applications for the extraction of essential oils from different kinds of aromatic plants. Based on a relatively simple principle, this method involves placing plant material in a microwave reactor, without adding any solvent or water. The internal heating of the

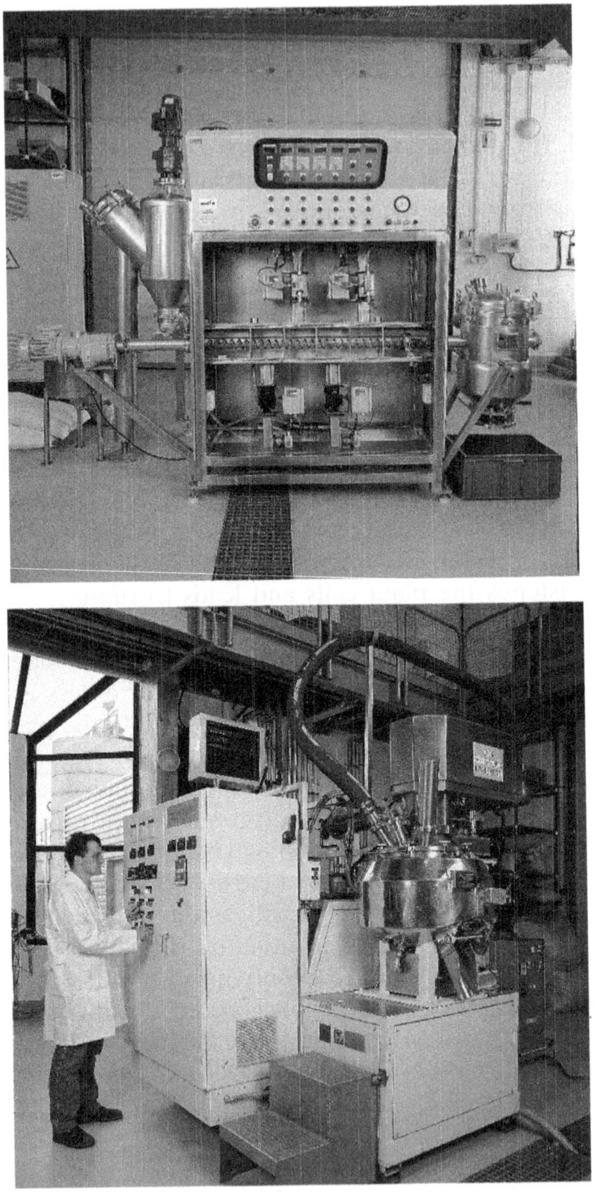

Figure 2.4. MASE (100 kg/h) and VMHD (100 liters).

in-situ water within the plant material distends the plant cells and leads to the rupture of glands and oleiferous receptacles. The heating action of microwaves thus frees essential oil and in-situ water, which are transferred from the inside to the outside of the plant material. This physical phenomenon, known as *hydrodiffusion*, allows the extract (water and essential oil), diffused outside the plant

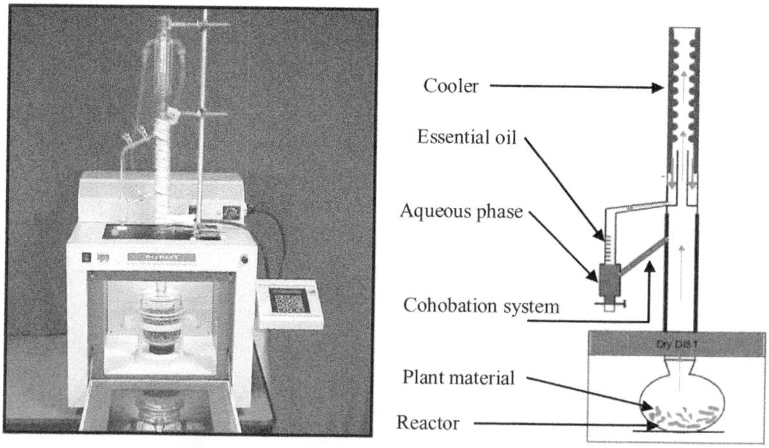

Figure 2.5. Solvent-free microwave extraction: "Microwave Clevenger."

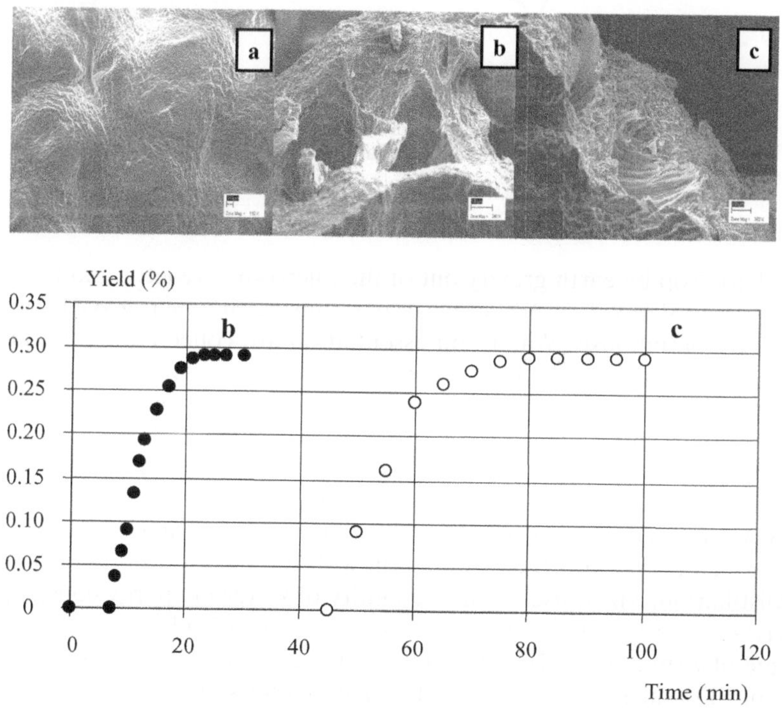

Figure 2.6. Microwave extraction (b) versus conventional hydrodistillation (c).

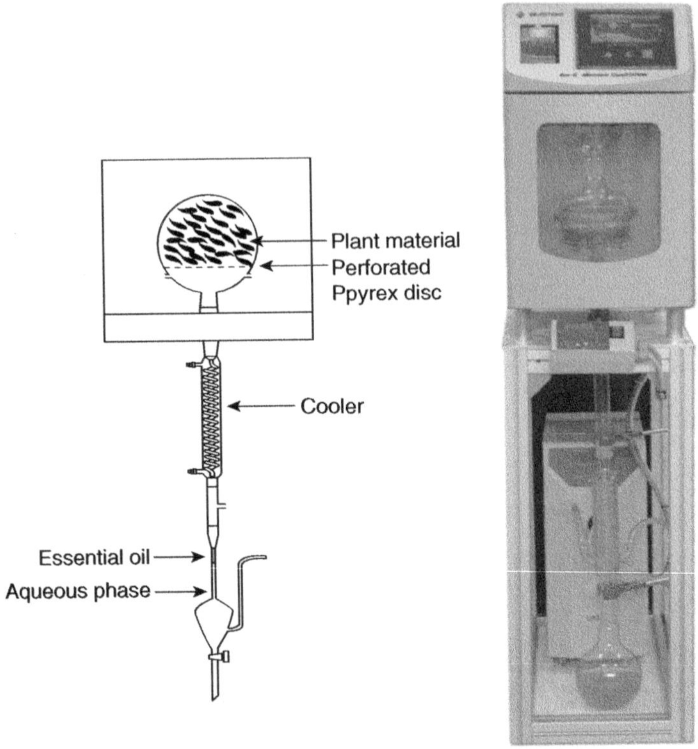

Figure 2.7. Microwave hydrodiffusion and gravity. "Upside-down" alembic.

material, to drop by earth gravity out of the microwave reactor and fall through the perforated Pyrex disc. A cooling system outside the microwave oven cooled the extract continuously. Water and essential oil are collected and separated in a vessel traditionally called the "Florentine flask." The essential oil, being lighter than water, floats at the top while water goes to the bottom and can be easily separated. It is important to note that this green method permits extracting essential oils without distillation and evaporation, which are the most energy-consuming processes between the unit operations. MHG is neither a modified microwave-assisted extraction (MAE), which uses organic solvents, nor an SFME, which evaporates the essential oil with the in-situ water, nor a modified hydrodistillation, which uses a large quantity of water in energy consumption.

MHG is clearly quicker than conventional steam distillation (SD); an extraction time of 15 min with MHG provides yields comparable to those obtained by means of SD, which is one of the reference methods in essential oil extraction. The essential oils of lime peels extracted either by MHG or conventional methods are rather similar in their composition and contain the same dominant components. In this application, microwave irradiation highly accelerated the extraction

TABLE 2.1. Chemical composition of citrus essential oils obtained by MHG, HD, and CP

No.	Compounds	Lemon			Lime		
		MHG[1]	HD[2]	CP[3]	MHG	HD	CP
	Monoterpenes						
1	α-pinene	1.60	1.75	1.62	1.86	1.94	1.62
2	β-pinene	10.20	15.35	14.00	11.60	13.09	14.00
5	limonene	69.65	65.25	68.81	60.56	63.44	68.81
	Oxygenated Monoterpenes						
7	linalool	0.20	0.18	0.10	0.25	0.36	0.22
8	citronellal	0.10	0.05	0.08	0.05	0.05	0.08
14	geranial	1.08	0.89	1.30	2.23	2.05	1.82
	Sesquterpenes						
16	(*E*)-caryophyllene	0.13	0.18	0.24	0.56	0.31	0.35
18	α-humulene	0.03	0.04	0.06	0.13	0.06	0.09
23	β-bisabolene	0.38	0.44	0.75	1.51	0.81	0.87
	Oxygenated Sesquiterpenes						
25	(*E*)-neroridol	*[4]	*	*	*	*	*
26	α-bisablol	0.01	0.03	0.03	0.02	0.02	0.03
27	nootkatone	0.01	*	0.01	*	*	*
	Other Oxygenated Compounds						
28	nonanal	0.08	0.09	0.06	*	*	*
29	citronellyl acetate	0.02	0.03	0.04	0.04	0.02	0.04
30	neryl acetate	0.30	0.26	0.19	0.87	0.60	0.19
	Extraction time (min)	15	180	60	15	180	60
	Yield (%)	0.7	0.8	0.1	0.8	0.8	0.2

[1] Microwave hydrodiffusion and gravity.
[2] Hydrodistillation.
[3] Cold pressing.
[4] Trace.

process, but without causing considerable changes in the volatile oil composition, a phenomenon that was already described (Table 2.1).

The organoleptic properties of essential oils extracted by MHG have been done according to sensory evaluation. For MHG and cold pressing (CP), the extracted essential oils have the same odor of terpenes hydrocarbons with fresh, light, flora woody and sweet citrusy odor. The MHG method offers the possibility of better reproduction of natural aroma of the fruit essential oil, comparable to

CP but more than the hydrodistilled (HD) essential oil. This sensory evaluation has been confirmed by the statistical analysis done on eight varieties of citrus extracted by MHG and other conventional extraction methods. This statistical analysis confirms the sensory analysis and that essential oil extracted by MHG has an odor relatively comparable to CP essential oil (Bousbia et al., 2009a, 2009b). The reduced cost of extraction is clearly advantageous for the proposed MHG method in terms of time and energy. The energy required to perform the two extraction methods is, respectively, 3 kW·h for HD, and 0.2 kW·h for MHG. Regarding environmental impact, the calculated quantity of carbon dioxide rejected in the atmosphere is much higher with HD (2400 g) than with MHG (160 g). These calculations have been made according to literature considering that recovering 1 kW·h from coal or fuel combustion is associated with 800 g of CO_2 being rejected.

2.3 ULTRASOUND-ACCELERATED SOLVENT EXTRACTION

Farid Chemat

Power ultrasound, having frequencies between 20 kHz and 1 MHz, is now well known to have significant effects on the rate of various physical and chemical processes. Cleaning and solubilization are the more developed applications and a large variety of ultrasound baths exist for chemical laboratory use. The effect of ultrasonic waves on solid samples is widely used for the extraction of aromas from plant materials. Degassing and stripping are widely used in flavor analysis. Other interesting ultrasound applications involve homogenization, emulsification, sieving, filtration, and crystallization. The most interesting effect of ultrasound-based operational units is a reduction of processing time and increase of product quality. All these effects are attributed to acoustic cavitation: When a liquid is irradiated by ultrasound, microbubbles form, grow, and oscillate extremely fast, and eventually collapse powerfully if the acoustic pressure is high enough. These collapses, occurring near a solid surface, generate microjets and shockwaves that result in cleaning, erosion, and fragmentation of the surface. Power ultrasound involves the mechanical and chemical effects of cavitation. The mechanism can be explained by two competing theories. The hotspot theory assumes that high pressures and temperatures generated in the bubbles during the last nearly adiabatic compression, just before collapse, are responsible for the breakage of molecular bonds and formation of radicals. On the other hand, the electrical theory involves microdischarges due to high electrical fields generated by deformation and fragmentation of the bubbles (Mason, 1990).

Citrus peel tissues consist of cells surrounded by walls. Some cells exist in the form of glands (external or internal) that are filled with the target products (generally secondary metabolites). A characteristic of such glands (when external) is that their skin is very thin and can be very easily destroyed. For internal glands, it is the degree of milling of the plant material that plays an important role.

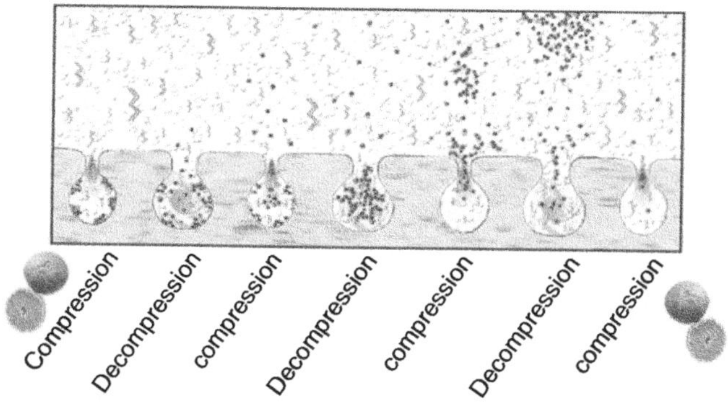

Figure 2.8. Ultrasound cavitation accelerated extraction of aromas from orange peels.

Conventional solvent extraction may be thought of as a transfer of solutes from one phase (e.g., a solid phase) into another (the solvent). The food matrix can be compared to a grain constituted of an impermeable core covered by a solvent boundary layer. Secondary metabolites are extracted in three steps: desorption from the matrix surface or release from internal glands, diffusion through the boundary layer to the boiling solvent, and solubilization in the solvent. The extraction recovery can be limited by one or several steps.

The phenomena at play in *ultrasound-accelerated extraction (UAE)* could be visualized by referring to our investigations where we designed a series of solid–liquid extraction steps using various extraction procedures (Figure 2.8). The effects of such extraction processes on the physical microstructure of the material being extracted were closely monitored using scanning electron microscopy. Ultrasound focused its power, at the beginning of extraction, on cuticular layer destruction and oil exudation. Then, it deflected this power against cell wall perforation mainly due to the high resistance of the particles in the medium toward ultrasound energy.

When the glands were subjected to more severe stresses and localized high pressures induced by cavitation, as in the case of ultrasound-accelerated extraction, the pressure buildup within the glands could have exceeded their capacity for expansion and caused their rupture more rapidly than in the control experiment. In general, microscopy observations pointed to two distinct extraction mechanisms for conventional and ultrasound procedures, respectively. The first involves diffusion of the plant extract components across the unbroken gland wall due to the temperature increase in the medium, and the other one, exudation of oil from damaged cell walls and even cells, due to a strong ultrasonic mechanical effect, which generally triggers an instantaneous release of the plant extract components into the surrounding solvent.

Proper selection of the solvent is the key to successful UAE. Solvent choice is dictated by the solubility of the analytes of interest, the interactions between the solvent and matrix, and the intensity of ultrasound cavitation phenomena

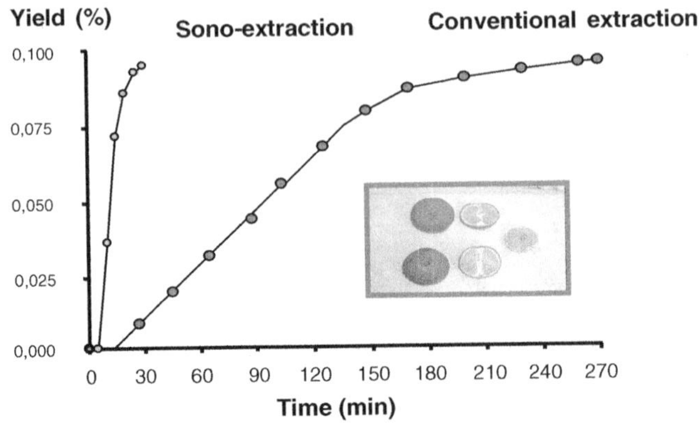

Figure 2.9. Rapid sono-extraction of orange peels in alcoholic beverages.

in the solvent. Important physical parameters related to UAE are presented in this section.

Ultrasound power, temperature, and extraction time affect not only the extraction yield but also the composition of the extract. A higher temperature for UAE means a higher efficiency in the extraction process due to the increase of the number of cavitation bubbles and a larger solid–solvent contact area. However, this effect is decreased when the temperature is near the solvent's boiling point. Generally, the highest efficiency of UAE, in terms of yield and composition of the extracts, can be achieved by increasing the ultrasound power, reducing the moisture of food matrices to enhance solvent–solid contact, and optimizing the temperature to allow a shorter extraction time (Figure 2.9).

The two most common pieces of ultrasound equipment used for extraction are the ultrasonic cleaning bath and the more powerful probe system (Figure 2.10). For small extraction volumes, an ultrasound horn with the tip submerged in the fluid can be sufficient. Large volumes of fluids have to be sonicated in an ultrasound bath or in continuous or recycled-flow sono-reactors. There are special ultrasonic reactors conceived for solvent extraction at laboratory (3 liters), pilot plant (30 liters), and industrial scale (250–1000 liters).

Ultrasound-accelerated extraction (UAE) is a clean method that avoids the use of large quantities of solvent and voluminous extraction vessels as with maceration. The reduced environmental impact of UAE is clearly advantageous in terms of energy and time. The energy required to perform the three extraction methods is, respectively, 6 kW·h for maceration at the solvent's boiling point (electrical energy for mechanical mixing and for heating), 8 kW·h for Soxhlet (electrical energy for heating), and 0.25 kW·h for UAE (electrical energy for ultrasound supply). The power consumption was determined with a Wattmeter at the ultrasound generator supply and the electrical heater power supply.

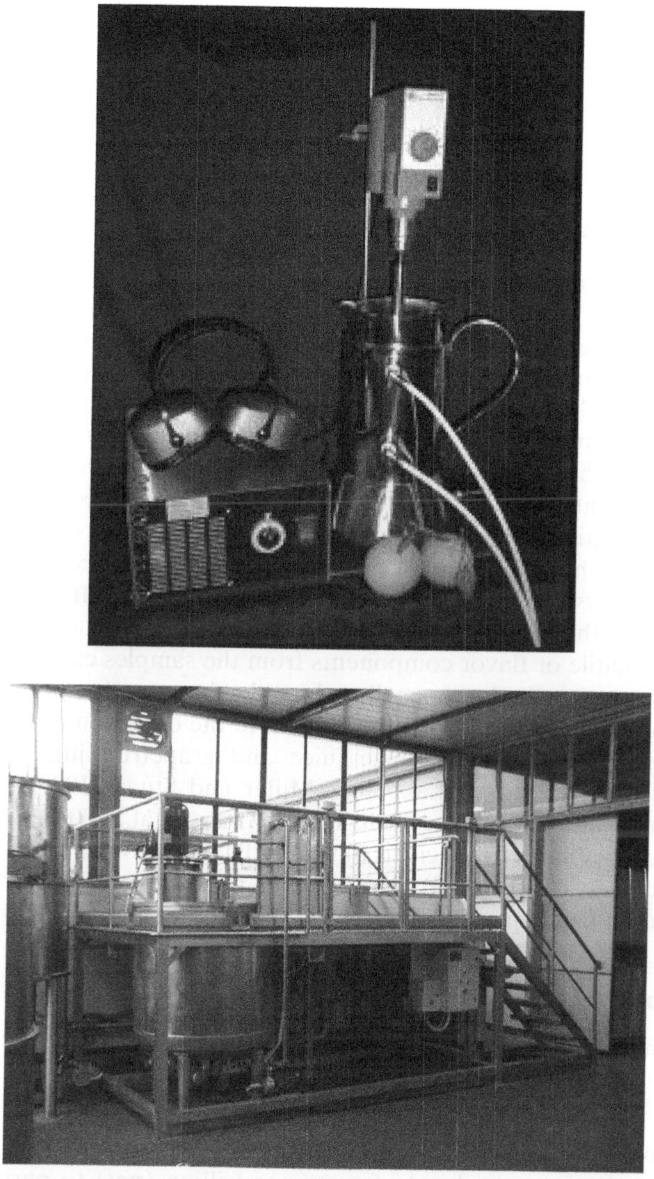

Figure 2.10. Laboratory (3 liters) and industrial (1000 liters) ultrasound reactors.

Regarding environmental impact, the calculated quantity of carbon dioxide rejected in the atmosphere is higher in the case of Soxhlet (6400 g CO_2/100 g of extracted solid material) and maceration (3600 g CO_2/100 g of extracted solid material) than for UAE (200 g CO_2/100 g of extracted solid material). These calculations have been carried out based on the following assumptions: To obtain

1 kW·h from coal or fuel, 800 g of CO_2 will be rejected in the atmosphere during combustion of fossil fuel. UAE is thus proposed as an environmentally friendly extraction method suitable for extraction of citrus peels in alcoholic beverages (Chemat et al., 2008b).

2.4 SOLID-PHASE MICROEXTRACTION

Masayoshi Sawamura

Solid-phase microextraction (SPME) is a new analytical technique that is a solvent-free method of extracting analytes from a variety of matrices by partitioning them from a liquid or gaseous sample into an immobilized stationary phase. The recent trend in sample preparation processes focuses on how to miniaturize the process and which medium to use for the extraction and preconcentration for sample components (Kataoka, 2005). SPME eliminates preconcentration steps by directly extracting the analytes into a coated fiber. It has been shown to be a very sensitive method for headspace analysis and has been recommended for the quantitative analysis of flavor and fragrance compounds (Steffen and Pawliszyn, 1996). SPME method is applicable for various samples of liquid, solid, and atmosphere. The volatile or flavor components from the samples can be conveniently extracted or concentrated at a small scale and subsequently determined by gas chromatography or GC-MS. It can be applied to the detection of flavor volatiles in citrus beverages such as orange juice and grapefruit juice (Steffen and Pawliszyn, 1996; Bazemore et al., 1999; Miller and Stuart, 1999; August et al., 2000; Coleman and Lawrence, 2000; Dharmawan et al., 2007). SPME is also applied to sensory analysis for citrus flavor study linked to GC (Rega et al., 2003) and electric nose (Choi, 2003). This section presents a brief introduction of microextraction techniques.

2.4.1 Features of SPME

There are many convenient features for flavor analysts, such as:

- No use of solvent for extraction.
- Application is for any sample form of solid, liquid, and gas.
- Microanalysis at the level of parts per trillion (ppt) to parts per billion (ppb) because of administration of the whole amount extracted into gas chromatography (GC).
- The necessary sample volume is as small as 100 μL.
- The total analytical time for extraction and determination of the components can be minimized. The term SPME *extraction* implies not merely extraction but also concentration, purification, and preparation.
- Autosystem line can be constructed.

2.4.2 Principle of SPME

Extraction of headspace gas by SPME fiber is subjected to partition equilibrium among the three phases: gaseous phase in the headspace and liquid phase in the test sample and the fiber, as shown in Figure 2.11. Its equilibrium theory and kinetic theory can be better understood by examining a three-phase system in which a liquid polymeric coating, a headspace, and an aqueous solution are involved. The basic study was carried out by Zhang and Pawliszyn (1993). The time to reach an equilibrium accounts for an extraction time in the SPME. Thus, in the SPME method, the whole amount in the sample is not extracted, but a proportional amount corresponding to the partition coefficient is done. An internal standard is essential to the quantitative determination by SPME. The apparatus for SPME is composed of two assemblies, holder and fiber. As shown in Figure 2.12, holder is an assembly for keeping a fiber inside, and a fiber is composed of a needle and a wire on which the stationary liquid phase is coated. The

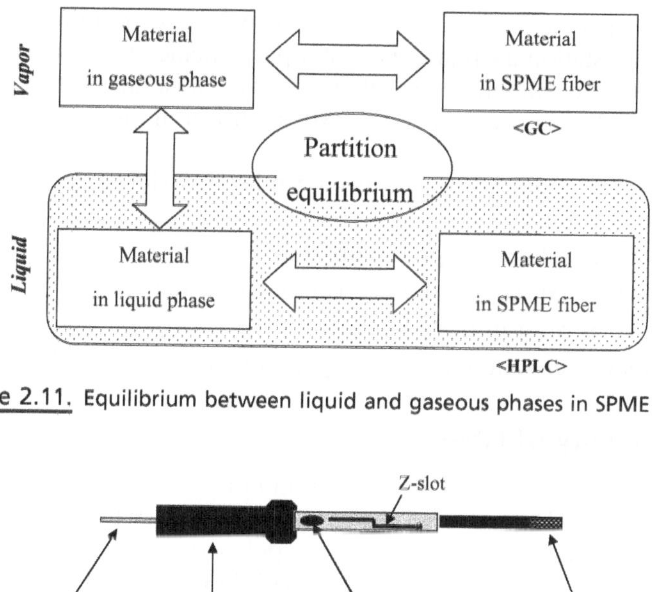

Figure 2.11. Equilibrium between liquid and gaseous phases in SPME assay.

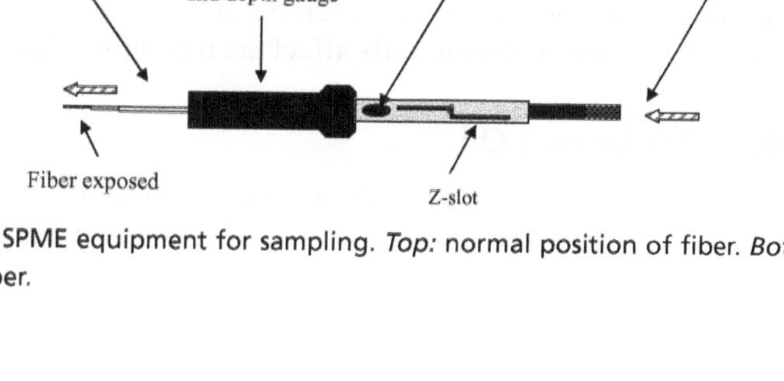

Figure 2.12. SPME equipment for sampling. *Top:* normal position of fiber. *Bottom:* exposed position of fiber.

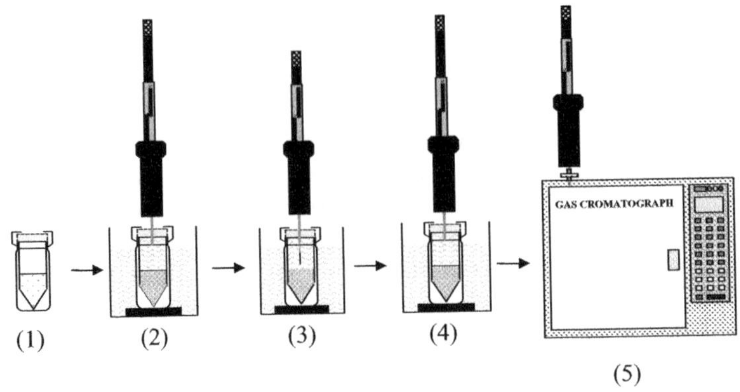

Figure 2.13. Procedure for SPME assay. (1) Sample solution in a vial; (2) a syringe inserted through septum; (3) a fiber exposed into headspace; (4) the fiber returned into a holder after absorption; (4) GC analysis.

wire inside the needle is exposed in the headspace gas for a given period to be adsorbed in the stationary phase. For high-performance liquid chromatography (HPLC), the wire is immersed directly in the sample solution.

The GC analytical procedure of SPME is shown in Figure 2.13.

1. The sample material is put into a 5-mL glass vial sealed with a silicone rubber septum.
2. The sample solution is pre-incubated.
3. The fiber is exposed in the headspace gas in the vial.
4. The fiber is reset in the holder.
5. The fiber after sampling is deployed directly to GC or GC-MS.

2.4.3 Selectivity of Fiber

In the preliminary experiment, we should find the most suitable type of fiber for the sample desired. There are several types of stationary phase on the fiber, for example, polydimethylsiloxane (PDMS), polyacrylate (PAC), PDMS/divinyl benzene (PDMS/DVB), and Carboxen™/PDMS (CAR/PDMS). Figure 2.14 shows gas chromatograms using different type of fibers for the same sample (Sawamura et al., 2003). Each type of fiber has the characteristics of compounds. Extraction factors such as incubation time, temperature, and the volume of the container are also significant, as they greatly affect the reproducibility of the result.

2.4.4 Analysis for Lemon Oil

As an example of SPME assay, consider the lemon essential oil analysis using a 100-μm PDMS fiber linked to GC. The gas chromatogram and analytical conditions are shown in Figure 2.15 (SUPELCO, 1996). Even at 1-min headspace

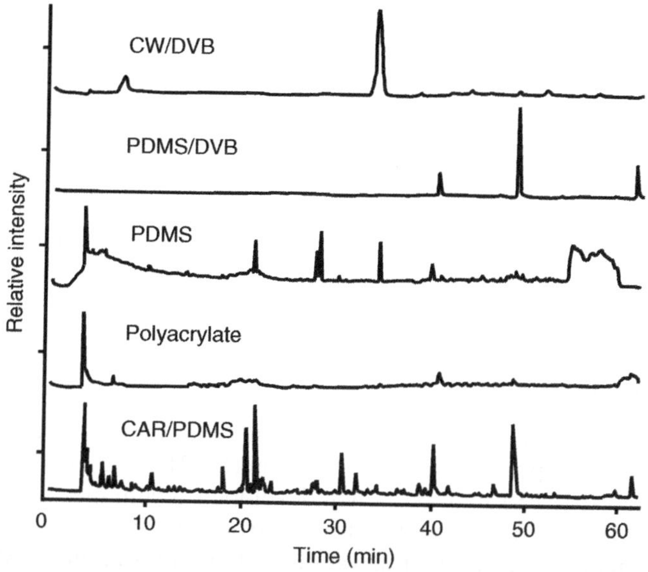

Figure 2.14. Gas chromatograms of the extract by different types of stationary phase from a test sample.

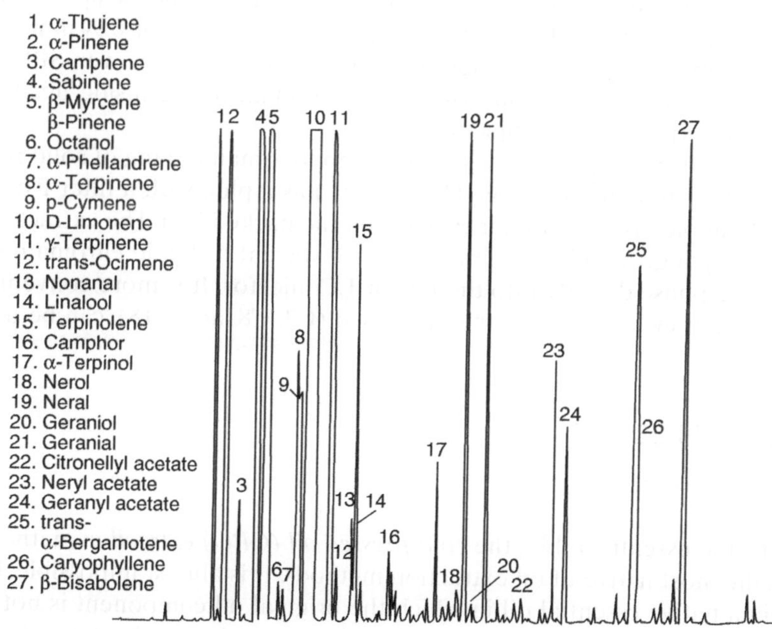

Figure 2.15. Gas chromatogram of lemon essential oil by SPME assay. Sample: 0.5 g lemon oil; fiber: PDMS; sampling: 1 min headspace at 30°C. GC conditions: column, SPB-1 (100 m × 0.25 mm I.D., 1 μm film); column oven, 40°C to 220°C at 4°C/min; injection port, 250°C; detector port, 300°C.

sampling at 30°C, sesquiterpenoids possessing high-boiling point compounds such as bergamotene, caryophyllene, and bisabolene were extracted. The profile of monoterpene hydrocarbons such as limonene, terpinenes, and pinenes seems to be comparable to an ordinary analysis. Neral and greranial, which are characteristic lemon-flavor compounds, are extracted at their reasonable ratio. SPME analysis is more effective for convenient analysis, especially for quality control analysis.

2.4.5 Other Techniques

The defect of SPME is that the loading volume of a sample is very small and the fiber is fragile. Solid-phase dynamic extraction (SPDE) and microextraction in a packed syringe (MEPS) may be newly developed techniques to overcome the defects of SPME. The following details are introduced by Kataoka (2005). SPDE is an inside-needle technique for vapor and liquid sampling. Stainless-steel needles coated with a 50-mm film of PDMS and 10% activated carbon are used. Dynamic sampling is performed by passing the headspace through the tube using a syringe. The analytes are concentrated onto PDMS and activated carbon coated onto the inside wall of the stainless-steel needle of a 2.5-mL gas-tight syringe. The volume of the stationary phase of the SPDE needle is approximately 5.99 mm^3, while a 100-μm PDMS SPME fiber has a volume of 0.94 mm^3. SPDE sampling permits keeping the headspace volume constant. However, SPDE may have carryover, because the analytes tend to remain in the inside needle wall after heat desorption in GC injection port.

In MEPS, according to Kataoka (2005), approximately 1 mg of solid packing material is inserted into a syringe (100–250 μL) as a plug with a filter from both sides, and sample preparation takes place on the packed bed. The extracted analytes in the syringe are eluted with an organic solvent or liquid chromatography (LC) mobile phase directly into the GC or LC injector. It is more convenient as any absorption materials, such as silica based (C2, C8, and C18), can be used.

2.5 COLD PRESSING

Masayoshi Sawamura

Preparing the essential oil by the *cold-pressed oil (CPO) extraction* method is, in a sense, the most native of oil extraction methods. It is almost impossible, in fact, to obtain a native essential oil in which the original oil component is not modified, though we wish to get the native oil without any change. As shown in Figure 2.16, we cannot avoid some loss, chemical changes in the constituents, and formation of artifacts during any process of essential oil extraction. Aroma or flavor components are commonly volatile and convertible and isomerism. In order to minimize these changes, there are better or milder extraction conditions, such as steam-distillation under reduced pressure and lower temperature, utilization of

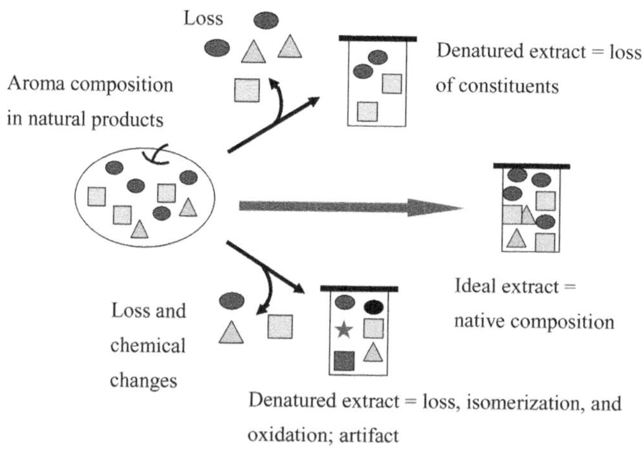

Figure 2.16. Problems occurring during extraction of volatile components from natural materials.

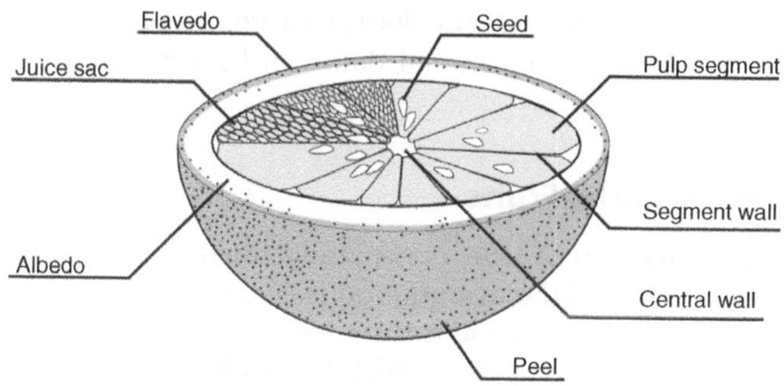

Figure 2.17. Structure of citrus fruit.

lower boiling-point solvent for solvent extraction, and extraction line using chemically and physically stable materials such as glasswares, Teflon,® and stainless steel. Among the various methods of extracting essential oils from citrus fruits, cold pressing includes minimum extraction steps, because this technique is not substantially accompanied with concentration, distillation, and removal of solvent. This section deals with the cold pressing method for extraction of essential oils from citrus materials.

2.5.1 Occurrence of Essential Oil

Citrus fruit is segmented into two sections, peel and flesh, as illustrated in Figure 2.17. The peel consists of flavedo and albedo. The flavedo is the outer peel, in which there are a number of oil glands. The albedo is located next to the flavedo, and is rich in pectic substances. Essential oil of citrus fruit is accumulated in flavedo. When the oil gland of the flavedo is disrupted, the essential oil comes out easily.

2.5.2 Laboratory CPO

For native aroma or flavor component analysis, the hand-pressing technique under cold temperature is convenient and reliable. The procedure for laboratory CPO extraction is shown in Figure 2.18 (Sawamura and Kuriyama, 1988). First, the fruit is sliced into 6 to 8 pieces lengthwise, and the mesocarp and albedo layers are peeled off from the flavedo and discarded. The flavedo is pressed by hand to express the oil, which is collected in brine solution on ice. After centrifugation at 4000 × *g* for 15 min at 5°C, the oils are decanted or taken carefully with a Pasteur pipette. Then, the crude oil is dried with anhydrous Na_2SO_4 for 24 h at 5°C to remove wax and other nonvolatile manterials. The CPO is stored at −21°C until analysis. This procedure does not include any process of warming or heating, vacuum, or evaporation and solvent extraction; the CPO is close to the oil in nature. This method is reliable and important for comparative study of various kinds of citrus essential oils. We have carried out citrus flavor research using the CPO by this method (Sawamura, 2001; Lan Phi and Sawamura, 2007). It is advantageous that these compositional data can be compared directly among citrus fruits.

2.5.3 CPO from Citrus Fruits

Common citrus fruits: Citrus fruit is generally squeezed for commercial juice products. In this technique, the essential oil is considered by-product. The most popular juice extractor in the world is the FMC (Food Machinery and Chemical Corporation) In-line juice extractor, which is widely used in citrus juice industries. Figure 2.19 illustrates the assembly of the squeezer. As soon as the fruit is

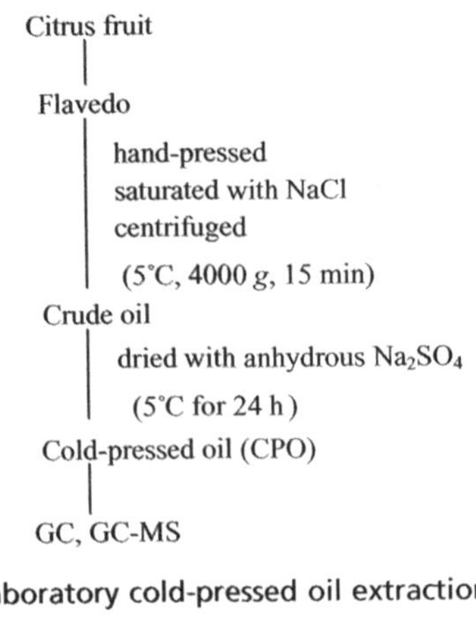

Figure 2.18. Laboratory cold-pressed oil extraction from citrus fruit.

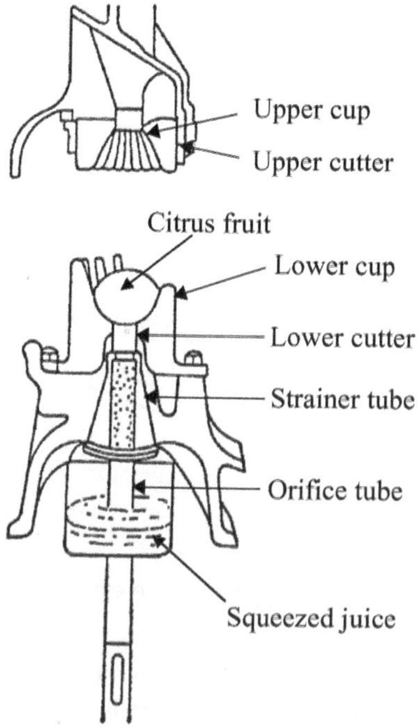

Figure 2.19. Squeezer assembly of FMC In-line juice extractor.

placed onto the lower cup, the upper cup goes down and the fruit is compressed into the strainer tube. When the next fruit is set on the lower cup, the orifice tube goes up to express the fruit. The juice is collected in a tank downside and the wasted peel, juice sacs, and seeds are discarded from an exit in the orifice tube. The In-line juice extractor is applicable to a wide variety of citrus fruits, such as orange, grapefruit, lemon, Satsuma mandarin, natsudaidai, and hassaku. The essential oil content in the juice is approximately 0.03–0.04%. The extraction capacity of this system is about 800 fruits per minute. During this squeezing process, essential oil can be also obtained. The wasted peel is cut into small pieces with showering. The emulsion containing peel oil and water is centrifuged to obtain cold-pressed oil. Among other types of citrus juice extractors, the Brown juice extractor equipped with the function of oil extraction is also used for CPO production.

Yuzu Fruit Juice Extractor. Yuzu (*Citrus junos* Tanaka) is a traditional Japanese sour citrus fruit (see Figure 8.5). In Japan, sour citrus juice and its products mixed with soy sauce are preferred for culinary purposes. Yuzu fruit is squeezed by a unique juice extractor developed for yuzu fruit. It is difficult to employ common juice extractors such as the In-line or Brown juice extractors, because yuzu juice is much more viscous than any other citrus juice and it causes many problems in common extractors.

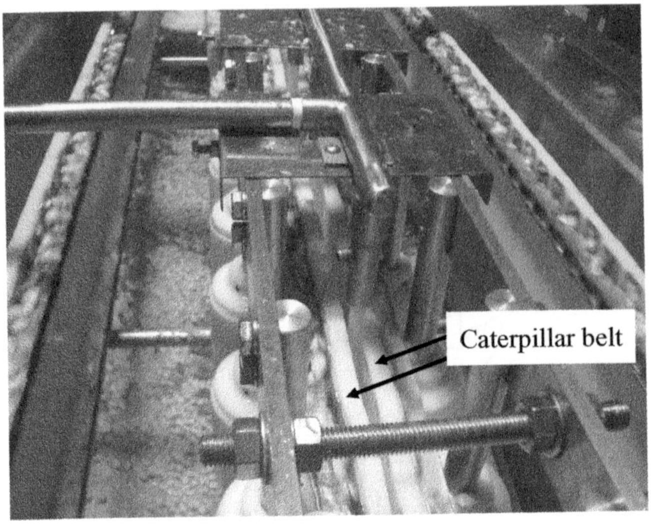

Figure 2.20. Yuzu juice extractor.

As shown in Figure 2.20, this extractor is equipped with a pair of moving caterpillar belts between which the yuzu fruit is compressed. This type of juice extractor was first developed in Kochi. Nowadays, it is popular throughout Japan and Korea. It is an open juice extraction system. Yuzu CPO is, on the other hand, obtained by centrifuging the juice. Yuzu is comparatively rich in essential oil, accounting for about 2%. The yuzu juice obtained by this method contains 0.4–0.6% essential oil. In order to enhance the essential oil content in the juice, we have developed a revised version of the yuzu juice squeezer in which the juice is circulated under computer-system control. The oil content accounted for 1% at maximum (Sawamura et al., 2008). On the other hand, there still remains essential oil in the wasted yuzu peel, which is almost thrown away. We have also developed an innovative technology to more effectively recover yuzu oil from the waste than is possible with conventional technology (Sawamura et al., 2006). The details will be described in Chapter 8. Yuzu essential oil is commercially useful for flavor and fragrance essences and aromatherapeutic oil.

Bergamot Oil Extractor. The origin of bergamot (*Citrus bergamia* Risso) is uncertain, although Italy, China, the Barbados, Greece, Spain, and the Canary Islands are suggested. Today, the essential oil of bergamot produced in Italy has been evaluated as having the highest commercial quality in the world market. Likewise, the bergamot produced in Reggio Calabria, Southern Italy, has the highest quality in the world, and is cultivated only in an extremely narrow band of land stretching about 100 km from Gioiosa Ionica, a town on the coast of the Ionian Sea, to Villa San Giovanni, a town on the coast of the Tyrrhenian Sea. The Ivory Coast, Brazil, Argentina, and China also produce a considerable quantity of bergamot, but these oils are considered to be of lower quality (Sawamura

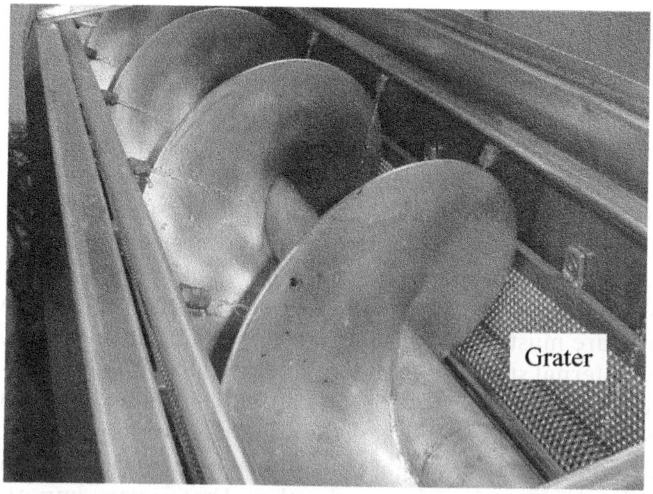

Figure 2.21. Pelatrice-type bergamot oil extractor.

et al., 1999). Regarding bergamot, its essential oil is a main product that is an important aroma source for perfumes, toilet-waters, deodorants, face-powders, blushers, lotions, pharmaceutical products (due to high antiseptic and antibacterial power), and tea and liquor flavorings. According to the Consorzio Del Bergamotto (1989), the first known bergamot orchard was planted near Reggio Calabria by Nicola Parisi in the Giunchi Feudal estate in 1750. In those days, the essence was extracted by hand, from the skin of the fruit, and absorbed by natural sponges placed on special containers. Today, it is extracted by abrasion through a system of "graters" in the peelers of the outside of the fruits. In 1844, the first real industrial form of the extraction invention by Nicola Barilla' was an extracting mechanism called "The Calabrian Mchine," which was capable of guaranteeing not only high output in a short time, but also an essence of excellent quality. Today's bergamot oil extractor is a rasping method by the Pelatrice system. The peel of bergamot is rasped on the rolling graters in the extractor (Figure 2.21) and the showering water carries the oil to the centrifuge. The average yield of peel oil from the variety called "Fantastico" is 0.5–0.6%. Further information on bergamot oil extractors is given by Dugo and Giacomo (2002).

2.5.4 Quantitative Determination of CPO

The chemical composition of cold-pressed oil (CPO) is determined quantitatively by GC. Use of relative-peak-area percent is more acceptable than relative-peak-height percent. All cold-pressed citrus oils contain a significant amount of non-volatile material that will not be eluted from a gas chromatographic column. Shaw (1979) pointed out and reviewed that unless some preliminary separation step is used to remove these materials, they need to be taken into account when the percentage of each GC volatile compound present in the oil is determined. The percentage of nonvolatiles present in an oil sample depends on the species and the amount of winterizing (storage at cool temperature) it has undergone. Any type of GC detector used in quantitating oils is a significant source of error unless response correction factors are determined. Response factors are easily determined from a mixture of pure compounds shown to be present in the citrus oil. Known amounts of the components are mixed in the proportion in which they have been determined to be present in the oil, from peak-area percentages, and the mixture is chromatographed under the same conditions used for the citrus oil sample. When a pure chemical of a compound in the oil is not available, one of similar structure must be substituted. For this quantitative determination, they should use an internal standard that does not overlap with any peak of the citrus oil. Thus, the weight percent for the oil can be calculated from GC peak-area percent. Sawamura and his co-workers (Sawamura, 2000; Lan Phi and Sawamura, 2003) have demonstrated the weight percent of a number of citrus oils. Therefore, our data can be compared against each other. That is very important in flavor analysis.

REFERENCES

Augusto, F., Valente, A.L.P., Tada, E.D., Rivellino, S.R. (2000). Screening of Brazilian fruit aromas using solid-phase microextraction–gas chromatography–mass spectrometry. *Journal of Chromatography A* **873**: 117–127.

Bazemore, R., Goodner, K., Rouseff, R. (1999). Volatiles from umpasteurized and excessively heated orange juice analyzed with solid phase microextraction and GC-Olfactometry. *Journal of Food Science* **64**: 800–803.

Bousbia, N., Abert-Vian, M., Ferhat, M.A., Meklati, B.Y., Chemat, F. (2009a). A new process for extraction of essential oil from Citrus peels: Microwave hydrodiffusion and gravity. *Journal of Food Engineering* **90**: 409–413.

Bousbia, N., Abert-Vian, M., Ferhat, M.A., Meklati, B.Y., Chemat, F. (2009b). Comparison of two isolation methods for essential oil from rosemary leaves: Hydrodistillation and MHG. *Food Chemistry* **114**: 355–362.

Chemat, F., Lucchesi, M., Smadja, J. (2004). Solvent free microwave extraction of volatile natural substances. *United States Patent*, USP 2004/0187340A1.

Chemat, F., Abert-Vian, M., Visinoni, F. (2008a). Microwave hydro-diffusion for isolation of natural products. *European Patent*, EP 1 955 749 A1.

Chemat, F., Tomao, V., Virot, M. (2008b). Ultrasound assisted extraction in food analysis. In: Otles, S. (ed.), *Handbook of food analysis instruments*. New York: Taylor & Francis.

Choi, H.S. (2003). Characterization of *Citrus unshiu* (*C. unshiu* Marcov. forma *Miyagawa-wase*) blossom aroma by solid-phase microextraction in conjugation with an electronic nose. *Journal of Agricultural and Food Chemistry* **51**: 418–423.

Coleman, W.M., Lawrence, B.M. (2000). Examination of the enantiomeric distribution of certain monoterpene hydrocarbons in selected essential oils by automated solid-phase microextraction–chiral gas chromatography–mass selective detection. *Journal of Chromatographic Science* **38**: 95–99.

Consorzio Del Bergamotto. (1989). Il Bergamotto di Reggio Calabria. Reggio Calabria: Domenico Laruffa Editore.

Dharmawan, J., Kasapis, S., Curran, P., Johnson, J.R. (2007). Characterization of volatile compounds in selected citrus fruits from Asia. Part I: freshly squeezed juice. *Flavour and Fragrance Journal* **22**: 228–232.

Essentielle, H. (2000). Echantillonnage et méthodes d'analyse (Tome 1). Monographie relative aux huiles essentielles (Tome 2). AFNOR, Paris.

Ferhat, M.A., Meklati, B.Y., Smadja, J., Chemat, F. (2006). An improved microwave Clevenger apparatus for distillation of essential oils from orange peel. *Journal of Chromatography A* **1112**: 121–126.

Ferhat, M.A., Meklati, B.Y., Chemat, F. (2007). Comparison of different isolation methods of essential oil from Citrus fruits: Cold pressing, hydrodistillation and microwave "dry" distillation. *Flavour and Fragrance Journal* **22**: 494–504.

French, J. (1651). *The art of distillation*. London: Richard Cotes.

Giacomo, A.D., Giacomo, G.D. (2002). Essential oil production. In: Dugo, G., Giacomo, A.G. (eds.), *Citrus*. London: Taylor & Francis, pp. 114–147.

Guenther, E. (1948). *The essential oils*. New York: Van Nostrand Reinhold.

Kataoka, H. (2005). Recent advances in solid-phase microextraction and related techniques for pharmaceutical and biochemical analysis. *Current Pharmaceutical Analysis* **1**: 65–68.

Koedam, A. (1987). Capillary gas chromatography. In: Sandra, P., Bicchi, C. (eds.), *Essential oil analysis*. New York: Huethig.

Lan Phi, N.T., Sawamura, M. (2007). Recent studies on citrus essential oils from East Asia. In: Jirovetz, L., Dung, N.X., Varshney, V.K. (eds.). *Aromatic plants from Asia, their chemistry and application in food and therapy*. Dehradun, India: Har Krishan Bhalla & Sons, pp. 127–153.

Lucchesi, M.E., Chemat, F., Smadja, J. (2004a). Solvent-free microwave extraction of essential oil from aromatic herbs: Comparison with conventional hydro-distillation. *Journal of Chromatography A* **1043**: 323–327.

Lucchesi, M.E., Chemat, F., Smadja, J. (2004b). An original solvent free microwave extraction of essential oils from spices. *Flavour and Fragrance Journal* **19**: 134–138.

Mason, T.J. (1990). *Chemistry with ultrasound*. New York: Elsevier Applied Science.

Metaxas, A.C., Meredith, R.J. (1983). *Industrial microwave heating*. London: Peregrinus.

Miller, M.E., Stuart, J.D. (1999). Comparison of gas-sampled and SPME-sampled static headspace for the determination of volatile flavor components. *Analytical Chemistry* **71**: 23–27.

Mompon, B., Mengal, B. (1994). Procédé et installation d'extraction sans solvant de produits naturels par micro-ondes. *International Patent*, WO 94/26853.

Mukhopadhyay, M. (2000). *Natural extracts using supercritical carbon dioxide*. New York: CRC Press.

Naves, Y.R. (1974). *Technologie et Chimie des Parfums Naturels*. Paris: Masson.

Paré, J.R.J., Bélanger, J.M.R. (1990). Extraction de produits naturels assistée par micro-ondes. *European Patent*, EP 398798.

Paré, J.R.J., Bélanger, J.M.R. (1997). *Instrumental methods in food analysis*. Amsterdam: Elsevier.

Rega, B., Fournier, N., Guichard, E. (2003). Solid phase microextraction (SPME) of orange juice flavour: Odor representativeness by direct gas chromatography olfactometry (D-GC-O). *Journal of Agricultural and Food Chemistry* **51**: 7092–7099.

Sawamura, M., Kuriyama, T. (1988). Quantitative determination of volatile constituents in the pummel (*Citrus grandis* Osbeck forma Tosa-buntan). *Journal of Agricultural and Food Chemistry* **36**: 567–569.

Sawamura, M., Poiana, M., Kawamura, A., Itoh, T., Song, H.S., Ukeda, H., Mincione, B. (1999). Volatile components of peel oils of Italian and Japanese lemon and bergamot. *Italian Journal of Food Science* **11**: 121–130.

Sawamura, M. (2001). Citrus fruits and their aroma and functional properties. *Koryo* **211**: 81–92.

Sawamura, M., Imae, N., Fazian, A.K., Ukeda, H., Fukami, K. (2003). Cooked flavor created by amino acid–glucose models in Muroto deep seawater. *Bulletin of the Society of Sea Water Science, Japan* **57**: 113–121.

Sawamura, M., Kashiwagi, T., Sakamoto, H., Kiji, M. (2006). Eco-conscious system for utilization of post-squeezing citrus wastes. Abstract for *Regional Symposium on Chemical Engineering 2006* (*RSCE 2006*), Singapore, pp. 158–159.

Sawamura, M., Asano, K., Toutani, M. (2008). Development of yuzu (*Citrus junos*) juice squeezing system. Abstract for *fourteenth World Congress of Food Science and Technology*, Shanghai, p. 536.

Shaw, P.E. (1979). Review of quantitative analyses of citrus essential oils. *Journal of Agricultural and Food Chemistry* **27**: 246–257.

Steffen, A., Pawliszyn, J. (1996). Analysis of flavour volatiles using headspace solid-phase microextraction. *Journal of Agricultural and Food Chemistry* **44**: 2187–2193.

SUPELCO. (1996). Solid phase microextraction/capillary GC analysis of drugs, alcohols, and organic solvents in biological fluids. *Bulletin 901*, pp. 1–8.

Zhang, Z., Pawliszyn, J. (1993). Headspace solid-phase microextraction. *Analytical Chemistry* **65**: 1843–1852.

3

COMPOSITIONAL ANALYSIS

Masayoshi Sawamura

Kochi University
Kochi, Japan

Citrus fruits slowly spread for a long time from Assam in India to East Asia and the Mediterranean region, where a great number of varieties were born by numerous mutations. Today, major citrus fruits are sweet oranges, mandarins, grapefruit, and lemons. The most popular citrus fruit has been sweet orange, with production amounting to 51 million tons in 2007. When we intend to know something about a food, the primary approach is to analyze its composition. The aroma of a food, in general, is composed of more than a thousand aromas. Aroma compounds must be volatile; the molecular weight should be as low as 300. Moreover, the concentration of aroma compounds in a food is very low—as little as one-to-one-hundred-millionth. Aroma can, however, give food a strong impact; therefore we can recognize the characteristics of food. The composition of essential oil is the most basic information needed to understand the character, quality, or profile of aroma and/or flavor. We encounter the importance of the composition of citrus essential oil in many fields, such as horticulture, postharvest, ripening process, food additives, cosmetics, perfume, and medicine.

Nowadays, citrus fruits are grown in many countries between the temperate and tropical zones. A number of reports on citrus essential oils have been published. These does not seem to be as much information on Asian and African

Citrus Essential Oils: Flavor and Fragrance, Edited by Masayoshi Sawamura

citrus essential oils compared to American and European oils. The composition of a citrus essential oil depends, in general, on growing area, maturity, and storage condition. Moreover, methods for extraction of essential oils will affect their original composition. However, within the specified condition the information will make sense. On the other hand, the number of familiar citrus fruits is only a few tens of varieties among tens of thousands of varieties in the world. Every citrus fruit as far as we know has its own characteristic aroma. It is easy to assume that every other citrus fruit would have its specific aroma. Therefore, the genus *Citrus* is noted as one of the aroma-resource plants.

A great number of analytical studies on volatile compounds have been presented, since A.J.P. Martin (who was awarded the Nobel Prize in 1952) and A. T. James developed a gas–liquid chromatograph (GC). After half a century, GC and its combined apparatus, such as GC-MS, GC-IR, and GC-GC, has been surprisingly improved to become more sensitive, accurate, and convenient. Today, GC and GC-MS is a common instrument in most laboratories. Shaw (1979) presented a compositional review including several kinds of citrus essential oils including sweet oranges, bitter oranges, mandarins, and so on. Recently, compositions of a number of citrus essential oils were reviewed (Sawamura, 2000; Lan Phi et al., 2006). This chapter deals with compositional information on citrus essential oils from worldwide regions.

3.1 ANALYTICAL METHOD: GC-FID, GC-MS, AND GC × GC

Nguyen Thi Minh-Tu

The use of essential oils as functional ingredients in foods, drink, cosmetics, toiletries, and so on is increasing in folk medicine, classical medicine, food, perfumery, and cosmetics because of their relatively safe status, their wide acceptance by consumers, and their exploitation for potential multipurpose functional use.

Chromatography is a technique for separating chemical substances that relies on differences in partitioning behavior between a flowing mobile phase and a stationary phase to separate the components in a mixture. Gas chromatography (GC) is the state-of-the-art method to analyze the constituents of an aroma system; a genuine product like plant, plant extract, and essential oils; and synthetic and artificial composition. Without the use of GC, the analysis of essential oil would be extremely difficult. Prior to the technique being developed, only the major components of the oils could be separated, achieved by distillation with high-efficiency columns. Even so, such columns rarely contained more than 100 theoretical plates (distillation plates), were very slow in operation, and took many days to complete an analysis. Due to the limited separation efficiency of the distillation column, even the major components were contaminated with trace materials, many of which had strong olfactory intensity and thus confused the olfactory character of the major component. The first separations of essential oil were carried out on packed columns that provided limited efficiency but nevertheless represented a tremendous advance on distillation. However, it was not until the capillary column, with its many thousands of theoretical plates, became commercially available that the true complex nature of many of the essential oils has been revealed. The introduction of the technique of temperature programming improved the separation even more. Because of its simplicity, sensitivity, and effectiveness in separating components of mixtures, gas chromatography is one of the most important tools in chemistry. It is widely used for quantitative and qualitative analysis of mixtures, for the purification of compounds, and for the determination of such thermochemical constants as heats of solution and vaporization, vapor pressure, and activity coefficients. Gas chromatography is also used to monitor industrial processes automatically: Gas streams are analyzed periodically and manual or automatic responses made to counteract undesirable variations. The gas chromatograph had a startling impact on the essential oil industry. Not only was the complex nature of the raw material disclosed for the first time, but the character of each pure individual component could be accurately ascertained by olfactory assessment of the eluted peaks using a nondestructive detector. In GC, the sample is carried by a moving gas stream through a tube packed with a finely divided solid or may be coated with a film of a liquid. The method consists of, first, introducing the test mixture or sample into a stream of an inert gas that acts as carrier, commonly helium or argon as well as nitrogen if cost effectiveness is concerned. Liquid samples are vaporized before injection into the carrier stream. The gas stream is passed through a column, through which the components of the sample move at velocities that are influenced by the degree of interaction of each constituent with the stationary nonvolatile phase. The substances having the greater interaction with the stationary phase are retarded to a greater extent and consequently separate from those with smaller interaction. As the components elute from the column they can be quantified by a detector and/or collected for further analysis. Figure 3.1 represents the scheme of gas chromatography.

To be introduced on the chromatography system, gas samples are injected through a gas sampling valve or injected with a syringe. In the case of essential oil, it can be injected in the form of a liquid, and if the column is capillary it goes through an injection chamber from which only a small part of the vaporized sample is transferred to the column, called *split injection*. This is necessary in order not to overload the column in regard to the sample volume. When a trace amount is subjected to gas chromatography, *on-column injection* can be used. The liquid sample is injected directly into the column with a syringe; the solvent is thereafter allowed to evaporate in order to leave a concentration of the sample. If the sample is gaseous, the concentration is achieved by cryo-focusing.

3.1.1 Column in Citrus Essential Oil Analysis

There are two primary types of columns used in GC; traditional packed columns and open tubular capillary columns (Raymond and Scott, 2003a; Agilent, 2004).

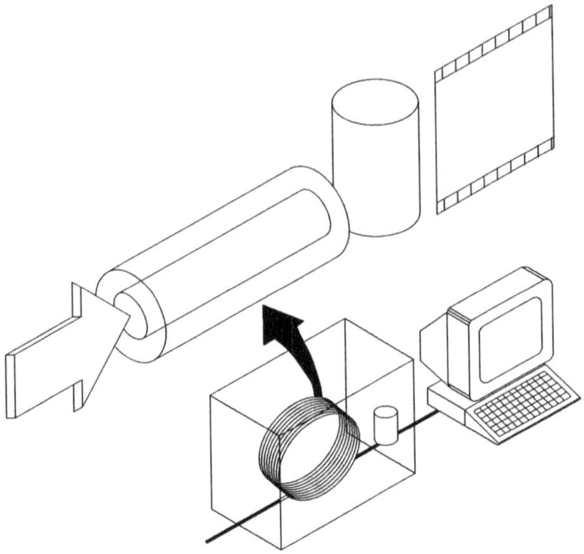

Figure 3.1. Gas chromatography scheme.

Packed columns are literally packed with a material for adsorption or absorption and capillary columns have inside walls coated with an adsorbing of absorbing material. Most applications today utilize capillary-type columns; however, there are some specific applications, especially fixed gas analyses, where packed columns are still used. Some ideas for column selection in citrus essential oil analysis by GC would be column diameter, column length, film thickness or loading percentage, and stationary phase. The column diameter ranges from 0.530 mm (mega-bore), 0.320 mm (wide bore) to 0.250 mm (narrow bore) and 0.100 mm (high speed), where 0.250 mm is the most common diameter found in citrus essential oil analysis. The length of the capillary column depends on its type; for Wall Coated Open Tube, 30-m and 60-m lengths are the most commercially available.

The main stationary phases are as followings, in order of increasing polarity: hydrocarbon C_{30}, methyl silicon (MeSi), methyl phenyl silicon (MePhSi), cyanopropyl silicon (CPSi), methyl tetra fluoro silicon (MTFSi), high-molecular-mass polyethylene glycol (PEGHMW). Based on five main stationary phases, ten principal groups of columns are classified:

Group 1: This is 100% bonded and cross-linked dimethylpolysiloxane, which is nonpolar and solvent rinseable. This type of phase has high temperature limit, wide range of column dimensions, and stationary phase film thicknesses. The column is characterized by low column bleed, inert surface, and high efficiency. It is popular in general applications; commercially available types are: AB-1, SE-30, OP-1, DB-1, HP-1, Ultra-1, SPB-1, RTX-1, CP-Sil 5CB, BP-1, ZB-1, AT-1, MDN-1, OV-1, OV101.

Group 2: This group contains 5% phenyl added to 95% methylpolysiloxane, which is bonded and cross-linked, nonpolar, and solvent cleaning. It has high temperature limit, wide range of column dimensions, and stationary phase film thicknesses. The column has low column bleed, inert surface with neutral surface, and high efficiency. These are popular for general applications: AB-5, DB-5, HP-5, Ultra-5, SPB-5, RTX-5, CP-Sil 8CB, BP-5, ZB-5, AT-5, MDN-5, OV-5, SE-52, SE-54.

Group 3: This group is bonded and cross-linked, with 6% cyanopropyl-phenyl plus 94% dimethyl siloxane phase. It is characterized from low- to mid-polarity and inert to many active compounds. This type of stationary phase is widely found in applications such as pesticide, herbicide, and halogenate analyses: DB-1301, BP-10, RTX-1301, AB 1301.

Group 4: The stationary phase contains 50% methyl–50% phenyl polysiloxane, and the most popular are RTX-50, DB-17, DB-17ht, DB-608, SP-2250, SPB-50, HP-17, HP-50+, AT-50, OV-17, EP-17.

Group 5: The stationary phase is 50% trifluoropropyl-methylpolysiloxane, which is high-polarity, bonded and cross-linked, and solvent cleaning. The DB-210 and HP-210 are the most commercially available.

Group 6: This column group is made from bonded and cross-linked 14% cyanopropyl-phenyl, 86% dimethylsiloxane phase, which is low- to mid-polarity, and inert to many active compounds. It is used in analyzing pesticides, herbicides, and halogenates, namely DB-1701, ZB-1701, BP-10, RTX-1701, CP-Sil 19 CB, AB-1701.

Group 7: This group is bonded and cross-linked, mid-polarity, and inert to many active compounds, such as DB-624, ZB-624, AT-624, RTX-624, CP-624.

Group 8: The stationary phase is bonded and cross-linked with mid-polarity and improved separations, namely DB-VRX, HP-VOC, RTX-VRX, HP-624.

Group 9: This group is characterized by bonded and cross-linked polyethylene glycol (PEG), which is solvent cleaning. It has wide applications of polar-solvent analysis in the food, pharmacy, cosmetics, and petrochemical industries. DB-WAX, AT-WAX, RTX-WAX, and ZB-WAX are the most popular.

Group 10: The stationary phase is nitroterephthalic acid modified polyethylene glycol (PEG), bonded and cross-linked, which is non-alcohol/aqueous solvent cleaning with high temperature limit. These columns are designed for the analysis of volatile fatty acids and phenols HP-FFAP, DB-FFAP: CB-WAX 58 (FFAP) CB, Stabilwax-DA, BP-21, 007-CW, AT-100.

The composition of citrus essential oils comprises mainly monoterpenes and their oxygenated compounds. Therefore, for the analysis of their composition, a column from both the polar and nonpolar stationary phase is needed. A column with stationary phase as complex of 5% diphenyl and 95% dimethylsiloxan as stationary phase (i.e., DB-5) has been used for separation of lime oil. The diphenyl group presenting in a complex of stationary phase contributes some induced polarizability capability to interact with polar solutes. It is largely a dispersive stationary phase, and thus substances are eluted roughly in order of their boiling points (excepting very polar solutes). The introduction of the diphenyl groups contributes more to phase temperature stability than it does to solute selectivity. On the other hand, the strong field from the hydroxyl group of PEG stationary phase made DB-WAX strongly polar corresponding to a bonded polyethylene glycol. Retention was affected largely by polar interactions between the permanent and induced dipoles of the stationary phase and solute molecules, respectively. For that reason, when citrus essential oil composition is required, the results should be read out not merely on one kind of stationary phase.

Nowadays, when a special composition of a complex matrix is being analyzed, more special column with a particular stationary phase is recommended. In aqueous injection, as in the case of alcoholic beverage analysis, an AQUAWAX column would be introduced to the GC system, while chiral composition required a column consisting of a (2,3-*di-O*-acetyl-6-*tert*-butyldimethylsilyl)-β-CD stationary phase instead.

3.1.2 GC-FID

A GC detector is a device that senses the presence of a component different from the carrier gas, and converts that information to an electrical signal. Detector types are selected by the user depending on the particular application, detection limit required, matrix interferences, and/or regulatory guidelines (Raymond and Scott, 2003b,c; Minh Tu, 2003). There are several principal detectors:

Thermal Conductivity Detector (TCD): Filament temperature increases as analytes present in the carrier gas pass over while causing the resistance to increase.

Flame Ionization Detector (FID): Components burn in a flame, producing ions, which are collected and converted into a current. It responds to any molecule with a carbon–hydrogen bond, but not at all, or poorly, to compounds such as H_2S, CCl_4, or NH_3.

Electron Capture Detector (ECD): As electronegative species pass through the detector, they capture low-energy thermal electrons, causing a decrease in cell current.

Nitrogen Phosphorus Detector (NPD): Nitrogen and phosphorous compounds produce increased currents in a flame enriched with vaporized alkali metal salt.

Flame Photometric Detector (FPD): Sulfur and phosphorous compounds burn in a flame, producing chemiluminescent species, which are monitored at selective wavelengths.

Electrolytic Conductivity Detector (ELCD): Halogens, sulfur, or nitrogen compounds are mixed with a reaction gas in a reaction tube. The products are mixed with a suitable liquid, which produces a conductive solution.

Photoionization Detector (PID): Molecules are ionized by excitation with photons from a UV lamp. The charged particles are then collected, producing a current.

Mass Selective Detector (MSD): Molecules are bombarded with electrons, producing ion fragments, which pass into the spectrometer's mass filter. The ions are filtered based on their mass/charge ratio.

Infrared Detector (IRD): Molecules absorb infrared energy, the frequencies of which are characteristic of the bonds within that molecule.

Atomic Emission Detector (AED): Molecules are energized by a plasma source and separated into excited atoms. As electrons return to their stable state, they emit light, which is specific to that element.

Detector response is characterized by sensitivity selectivity and dynamic range, which are the response per amount of sample (the slope of the response/amount curve); the minimum amount on the curve is defined as the minimum detectable level (MDL) and the range of sample concentrations for which the detector can provide accurate quantitation, respectively. For the FID, the typical samples are hydrocarbons, the sensitivity ranges from 10 to 100 pg. For the usual condition of FID, gas flow rates for carrier gas, hydrogen, and air are 20–60 ml/min, 30–40 ml/min, and 200–500 ml/min, respectively.

As shown in Figure 3.2, the carrier gas effluent from the GC column is mixed with hydrogen and then routed through an unbreakable stainless-steel jet; then the hydrogen supports a flame at the tip of the jet, ionizing the molecules. A collector electrode attracts the negative ions to the electrometer amplifier, producing an analog signal that is connected to the data system input. For organic components in general and for citrus essential oil analysis in particular, FID is the only choice for the best separation and resolution and extreme sensitivity with a large dynamic range; therefore, the carrier gas is helium, which is the best, or nitrogen, as an alternative, where their purity must be the highest. To remove hazardous impurities, the carrier gas system must contain traps to remove these impurities. For FID, the sample to be analyzed is eluted from the GC column; then it is mixed with a special burner fuel, hydrogen plus helium or hydrogen plus nitrogen. Ions and electrons formed in the flame enter the electron gap, decrease the gap resistance, and thus permit a current, which is proportional to the rate of ion formation depending on the hydrocarbon concentration in the gas.

For Vietnamese citrus essential oil composition analysis, a DB-Wax column (60 m × 0.25 mm i.d., film thickness of 0.25 μm; J&W Scientific, Folsom, CA), a

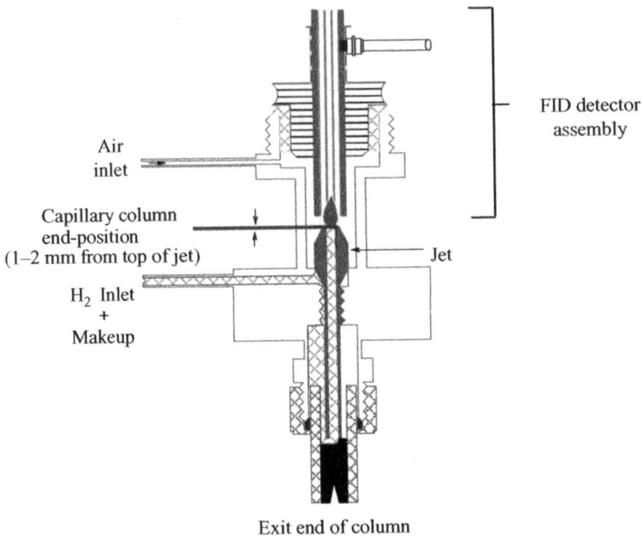

Figure 3.2. Flame ionization detector scheme.

DB-5 column (60 m × 0.25 mm i.d., film thickness of 0.25 μm; J&W Scientific, Folsom, CA), and an FID were used. The column temperature was programmed from 70°C (2 min) to 230°C (20 min) at the program rate of 2°C/min. The injector and detector temperatures were 250°C. Nitrogen was the carrier gas at a flow rate of 2 ml/min. An oil sample of 1 μl was injected, the split ratio of the injector being 1:50.

3.1.3 GC-MS

The combination of two individual techniques—gas chromatography and mass spectrometry (GC-MS)—has undoubtedly had wide application in studying the quality and quantity of volatile components of many essential oils for the past few decades (Raymond and Scott, 2003b,c; Minh Tu, 2003). It is becoming a standard tool in the protocols for analysis in many national pharmacopoeias, for example. While GC-FID is the traditional method for essential oil quantification, GC-MS is the most common analytical method for component identification. The presence of numerous isomers (terpenes and oxygenated terpene structures) as well as the wide concentration range of analytes from ppm to ppb add an additional challenge in solving the puzzle created by these mixtures. For this MS detector, while analyzing Vietnamese citrus essential oil, 70 eV and 250°C were set as ionization voltage and ion source temperature, respectively.

Recently selective detection using GC-MS is limited when the mass spectrum of interesting compounds resembles other spectra, especially those of terpenes and terpenoids. In this case, a particular example is β-damascenone, intense fragments of which delivered from MS are not specific to the compound (*m/z*: 69, 77, 91, 105, and 121), whereas the high mass ions 190 and 175 are more characteristic, but present in low abundance. In the MS-MS mode, the signal-to-noise ratio for these smaller ions can be enhanced due to its selectivity, which removes the background noise contributed by the matrix. The technique has been used to evaluate the origin of citrus essential oils, where the isotope ratio of fragment peaks on GC-MS of the volatile compounds from various citrus oils was measured. The MS fragment ratio was found by the ratio of fragment peak intensity, $m + 1/m$ (*m/z*). This ratio reflects the isotope effect of volatile compounds; that is, it provides information about locality, quality, and species of essential oils. Multivariate analysis based on the MS fragment ratio of monoterpene hydrocarbons clearly distinguished three citrus species, yuzu, lemon, and lime. The method was successful because the ratio of isotope $^{13}C/^{12}C$ is abundant in citrus oil.

3.1.4 GC × GC

Comprehensive two-dimensional GC (GC × GC) needs two gas chromatographs, a thermoregulated transfer line, and a system with mechanical valves to regulate the flux and pressure of the carrier gas. This design enhances peak capacity for a chromatographic run, allowing better separation in complex sample analysis (Raymond and Scott, 2003c; Agilent, 2004).

Nowadays, where information on provenance, quality, botanical origin, and authenticity of an oil sample is concerned, gas chromatographic analysis of the enantiomeric distribution of the component is preferred. For this purpose, the chiral modified cyclodextrin columns are frequently used to determine the enantiomeric ratios between the different volatile compounds present in the essential oil. The single GC is often difficult because of the possible overlapping of peaks of different components, but the GC multidimensional techniques permit the fractionation of the mixture into a pre-column and then allow the chiral analysis of the single component or of a simple fraction in that multidimensional system. This very complex and expensive method produces good results and so has been adopted in many research laboratories.

Figure 3.3 shows the basic components of Agilent's simplified two-dimensional GC system. A sample is injected into column 1 and the chromatogram is observed on FID detector 1. The retention time of the peak of interest is determined from the FID1 signal. The Deans switch is then time-programmed to turn on at the beginning of elution of the peak from column 1 and then to turn off at the end of the peak. The box labeled "cut" in the figure shows the time range where the Deans switch is turned on. The peak of interest and any interfering peaks are directed onto column 2 for further separation. Because column 2 was chosen to have a stationary phase of different selectivity than

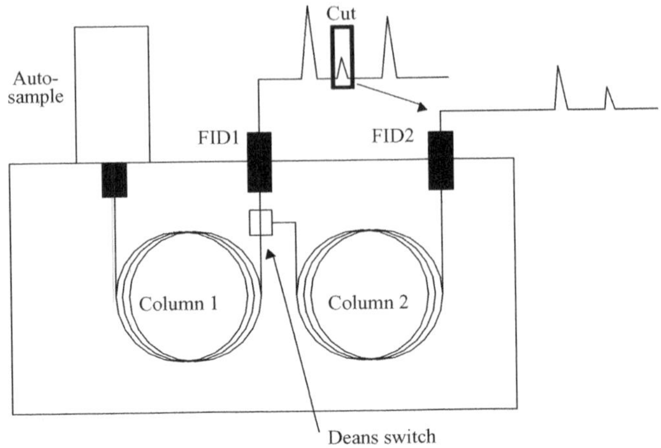

Figure 3.3. Basic component of simplified 2-dimensional GC system.

column 1, the peak of interest should be completely resolved from the interferences with which it co-eluted on column 1.

For separating chiral isomers of citronellal, a simple online coupled DB-5 fused silica capillary column, 30 m × 0.25 mm i.d., film thickness of 0.25 μm (J&W Scientific Inc.), and a main column consisting of a (2,3-*di-O*-acetyl-6-*tert*-butyldimethylsilyl)-β-CD stationary phase, 30 m × 0.25 mm i.d., film thickness of 0.25 μm (Supelco, USA), was used for enantioselective GC analysis. The column temperature was programmed from 70°C (2 min) to 100°C (60 min) at the rate of 2°C/min.

For determination of some popular monoterpene hydrocarbon and monoterpene alcohol in citrus essential oil, such as α-pinene, β-pinene, sabinene, limonene; linalool, terpinen-4-ol, and α-terpineol, respectively, a dual column has been used: Column 1 (pre-column): Megadexdettbsbeta (diethyl-*tert*-butylsilyl-β-cyclodextrin), 25 m × 0.25 mm, 0.25 μm film thickness (Mega, Legnano, Italy); and Column 2 (main-column): Megadexdmtbsbeta (2,3-*di-O*-methyl-6-*tert*-butyldimethyl-silyl-β-cyclodextrin) 30 m × 0.25 mm, 0.25 μm film thickness (Mega, Legnano, Italy). The oven temperature is 50°C (10 min) to 180°C at 2°C/min; injector and detector temperatures are 250°C. Beside gas chromatography, with its various detector and configuration mentioned above, multidimensional high-performance liquid chromatography HPLC/GC has also been mentioned. An HPLC is online coupled with a GC, which has been recognized as being a separation technique whereby much information concerning the samples can be obtained in a single run. Therefore, multidimensional HPLC/GC is useful for the analysis of complex samples, such as natural products. Various applications are reported, including a type of analysis for citrus essential oils. One of the problems in the HPLC/GC system is removing a large volume of HPLC eluent when introduced into the GC injector. Although various types of interfaces for HPLC/GC have been proposed, they are complicated.

3.2 AFRICA

Simon Muhoho Njoroge and Masayoshi Sawamura

The African continent produces appreciable quantities of *Citrus* fruits. The countries where production was more than 6.3 million tons in 2008 are Egypt, South Africa, and Morocco. The most popular citrus fruit in Africa is the sweet orange. Egypt produces the greatest volume of this species in Africa with an amount of 3.5 million tons, followed by South Africa with 1.5 million tons. Mediterranean countries of Africa such as Morocco, Algeria, Tunisia, Libya, and Egypt produce good-quality citrus fruits. Tunisian neroli essential oil from bitter orange flowers is of the best quality in the world. The major varieties in Africa are orange, mandarin, grapefruit, lemon, and lime. As seen in the postage stamps in Figure 3.4, citrus fruits are popular in many African countries. In the East and Central African countries, different types of citrus fruits are produced. However, there are few publications on the essential oils of the cultivated varieties. In this chapter, we provide some information on the composition of citrus essential oils from Kenya, Uganda, Rwanda, Burundi, and Ethiopia.

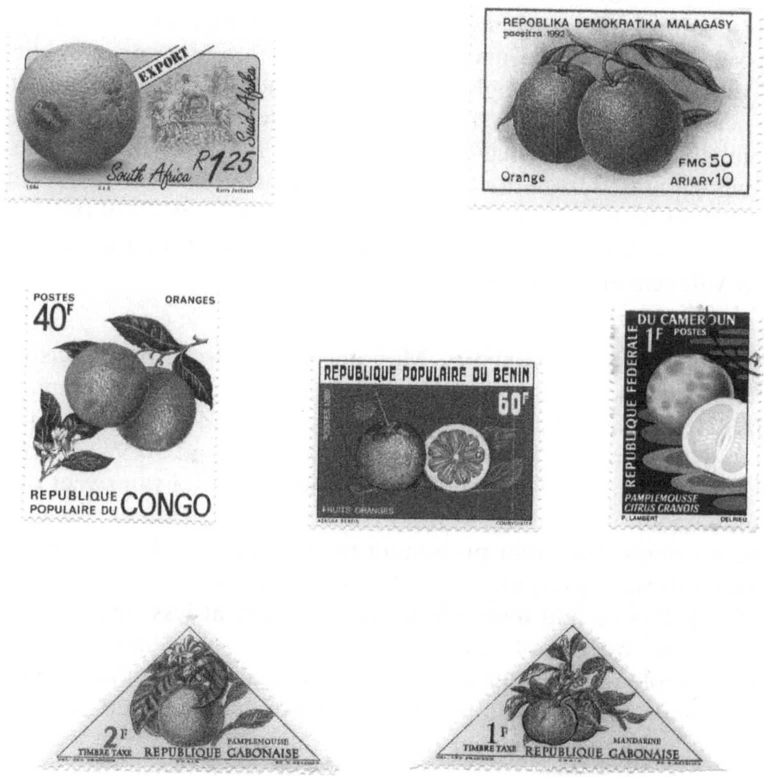

Figure 3.4. Postage stamps illustrated with citrus fruits from several African countries.

3.2.1 Kenya

Orange. Sweet oranges are the major *Citrus* fruits produced in Kenya (Mwasaru et al., 1998). Commercial production of the fruits is done at the Coast, Central, and Rift Valley provinces. The fruits are popular in the local markets and are widely consumed when fresh or as processed juices and preserves. The production levels are increasing (2007 annual production was 0.2 million tons). Volatile chemical compounds of *Citrus* essential oils are among the most distinctive components for identification and evaluation of varieties. The qualitative and quantitative compositions of the *Citrus* essential oils vary according to environmental origins, varieties, and preparation methods. Several studies on the volatile components of peel essential oils of sweet oranges of different origins have been reported (Shaw, 1979; Mitiku et al., 2000; Sawamura, 2000; Minh Tu et al., 2002a). Reports on the volatile components of citrus fruits grown in Kenya are scarce. Here we provide information on the volatile flavor components of the peel essential oils of Salustiana, Valencia, and Washington navel sweet orange varieties grown in Kenya (Njoroge et al., 2005a).

The Salustiana, Valencia, and Washington navel fruits at their best harvest maturity were obtained from the Boarstal farm of the Kenya Prisons Department at Shimo la Tewa, Mombasa District, Coast Province. They were kept at 2°C prior to isolation of the peel oils, which was done within a week of harvest. The Kenyan Salustiana, Valencia, and Washington navel oranges were medium-sized *Citrus* fruits with average weights of 211, 200, and 250g, respectively. The peel flavedo accounted for 13.2, 12.1, and 14.5% (w/w) of the whole fruits, respectively. The yield of cold-pressed oil (w/w) was 0.1% from each fruit. The volatile compounds separated from the essential oils are listed in Table 3.1. A total of 85 different volatile compounds were separated from the peel oils of the three sweet orange varieties. Among them, 56 were found and identified in the Salustiana and 73 in Valencia and 72 in Washington navel oils.

Monoterpene Hydrocarbons. Monoterpene hydrocarbons constituted the most dominant chemical group among the volatiles of Salustiana (96.9%), Valencia (94.5%), and Washington navel (92.7%) peel oils. Limonene was the most abundant compound, constituting 94.6%, 92.5, and 90.5% of each of the oils, respectively. The high content of limonene in the Kenyan sweet orange oils was in agreement with published reports on varieties of sweet orange peel oils of different origins. The other prominent monoterpene hydrocarbons in each of the Kenyan oils were γ-terpinene (1.5–1.7%), α-pinene (0.3–0.5%), and sabinene (0.1–0.2%). β-Pinene and terpinolene were present at less than 0.05% in each oil, in accordance with reports of other sweet orange oils (Shaw, 1979; Sawamura, 2000). 1,8-Cineole was present at trace levels in each oil. The Salustiana oil contained γ-terpinene and α-phellandrene, which were not detected in the other two oils. γ-Terpinene is rarely present in sweet orange oils. The compound could be used as a basis to distinguish the Salustiana oil from other sweet orange oils. Myrcene has been reported as a prominent component of several types of sweet orange oils (Shaw, 1979; Sawamura, 2000). It constituted a minor quantity (less than 0.05%) in the Kenyan Salustiana and Washington navel oils, and was absent from the Valencia oil. The variations in quantitative levels of the minor volatile compounds among different types of sweet orange oils could be attributed to differences of varieties and environmental factors. Moreover, as previously indicated, the influences of fruit maturity and sample preparation methods may contribute significantly to variations of volatile compositions. The Valencia oil was distinguished from the other two oils by its unique possession of β-phellandrene and (*Z*)-β-ocimene. These compounds have been reported in trace quantities in some sweet orange peel oils of different origins (Sawamura, 2000). *p*-Cymene was found only in the Washington navel oil as a minor constituent.

Sesquiterpene Hydrocarbons. A total of 5 sesquiterpene hydrocarbon compounds were found in each of the Salustiana and Washington navel oils, and 7 in the Valencia oil. The relative amounts of these components were less than 0.05% in Salustiana and 0.1% in each of the Valencia and Washington navel oils. Among the constituents, (*E*,*E*)-α-farnesene was relatively notable. The others present in the three oils were δ-elemene, α-cubebene, α-cedrene, and β-caryophyllene at minor levels, as reported for most sweet orange oils of different origins. (*E*)-β-Farnesene, reported as a prominent component of Ethiopian Valencia and Hamlin peel oils (Mitiku et al., 2000), and valencene, reported in sweet orange oils from Florida (Shaw, 1979), were not found in the Kenyan samples. Germacrene D and aromadendrene were present at trace levels in the Valencia oil. The former compound was also found in Washington navel oil and neither compound was present in the Salustiana oil. The variations in occurrence of these sesquiterpenes could be used to differentiate the respective oils.

Oxygenated Compounds. A total of 40 oxygenated compounds were found in Salustiana, 55 in Valencia, and 56 in the Washington navel oils, amounting to 1.7, 3.4, and 4.5%, respectively. The compounds were categorized into carbonyl compounds, alcohols and ethers, esters, oxides/epoxides, and acids. Carbonyl (aldehydes and ketones) volatile compounds were relatively prominent, constituting 0.9, 1.1, and 1.7% of Salustiana, Valencia, and Washington navel oils, respectively. The aliphatic aldehydes, octanal, nonanal, decanal, undecanal, dodecanal, and octadecanal were present in each oil. Among them, octanal and decanal, constituting 0.2–0.3%, were the most prominent. Tetradecanal was relatively prominent in Washington navel oil, and was not detected in Salustiana oil. Among the oils, Washington navel had the highest amounts of octanal and tetradecanal, while Salustiana oil had comparatively the highest content of undecanal. The occurrence of the aliphatic aldehydes in the Kenyan samples was in agreement with reports on other sweet orange oils. Octanal and decanal are usually the dominant aldehydes of sweet orange peel oils. Hexanal and heptanol, reported as minor constituents of some orange oils (Chamblee et al., 1991), were not found in the samples. Octadecanal has not been previously reported as a component of sweet orange peel oils. The compositional variations of the

TABLE 3.1. Volatile components of several African citrus essential oils[a]

Compounds	Kenya					
	Orange			Mandarin		
	Salustiana	*Valencia*	*Washington navel*	*Kara*	*Sabine*	*Minneola*
ethyl acetate	nd	nd	nd	nd	nd	nd
methyl isobutyrate	nd	nd	nd	nd	nd	nd
α-pinene	0.5	0.3	0.5	0.1	0.4	0.2
camphene	nd	nd	nd	nd	nd	nd
β-pinene	*	*	*	0.3	0.2	0.1
sabinene	0.1	0.2	0.2	0.1	0.1	*
δ-3-carene	nd	nd	nd	nd	0.1	nd
myrcene	*	nd	*	1.8	1.5	1.5
α-phellandrene	tr	nd	nd	*	nd	*
α-terpinene	1.7	1.5	1.5	nd	3.4	nd
limonene	94.6	92.5	90.5	90.7	87.1	90.1
isoamyl acetate	nd	nd	nd	nd	nd	nd
β-phellandrene	nd	tr	nd	tr	tr	tr
1,8-cineole	tr	tr	tr	nd	nd	nd
(*Z*)-β-ocimene	nd	tr	nd	nd	0.1	tr
(*E*)-β-ocimene	nd	nd	nd	nd	nd	nd
γ-terpinene	*	nd	nd	2.7	1.5	2.9
p-cymene	nd	nd	*	0.1	0.1	0.2
terpinolene	*	*	*	1.4	2.2	1.7
octanal	0.2	0.2	0.3	0.2	0.3	0.2
heptyl acetate	nd	nd	nd	nd	0.1	nd
isoamyl isovalerate	nd	nd	nd	nd	nd	nd
2-nonenal	nd	nd	nd	nd	nd	nd
nonanal	*	*	*	*	*	*
myrcene epoxide	nd	tr	*	nd	nd	nd
(*E*,*Z*)-2,6-nonadien-1-ol	tr	*	*	nd	nd	nd
perillene	tr	tr	tr	nd	nd	nd
(*Z*)-linalool oxide	nd	tr	tr	tr	tr	nd
(*Z*)-limonene oxide	nd	tr	tr	0.1	*	*
(*E*)-limonene oxide	0.1	0.3	0.4	*	0.1	*
(*E*)-sabinene hydrate	*	tr	*	nd	nd	nd
(*E*)-linalool oxide	0.1	0.2	0.2	nd	nd	nd
menthone	nd	nd	nd	nd	nd	nd
heptanol	nd	tr	tr	nd	nd	nd
δ-elemene	tr	tr	tr	*	*	*
α-copaene	nd	nd	nd	nd	nd	nd
2,3-butanediol	nd	nd	nd	nd	nd	nd
octyl acetate	nd	nd	nd	nd	nd	nd
citronellal	*	tr	*	*	*	0.1
2-isononenal	nd	nd	nd	nd	nd	nd
decanal	0.2	0.2	0.2	0.2	0.3	0.2
α-copaene	nd	nd	nd	nd	nd	nd
α-cubebene	*	*	*	0.1	tr	0.1

		Burundi	Uganda		Rwanda		Ethiopia	
Grapefruit	Pummelo	Mandarin	Mandarin		Orange-1	Orange-2	Mandarin Hybrids	
Redblush	*C. grandis*	*C. reticulata*	*Jinja*	*Mbarara*	*C. sinensis*		Temple	Orlando
nd	nd	nd	nd	nd	0.1	0.1	nd	nd
nd	nd	nd	nd	nd	nd	tr	nd	nd
0.5	0.5	1.1	1.1	1.2	0.5	2.4	0.4	0.3
nd	nd	nd	nd	nd	nd	nd	tr	tr
*	*	0.4	0.3	0.5	nd	nd	<0.1	nd
0.4	0.4	0.3	0.4	0.3	1.6	0.2	0.4	0.1
nd	nd	nd	nd	nd	nd	*	nd	nd
nd	nd	2.2	2.2	2.5	2.4	2.2	1.8	1.7
nd	nd	*	*	*	*	*	tr	tr
1.3	1.8	0.1	*	0.1	nd	nd	tr	tr
91.1	94.8	84.8	85.3	86.9	89.7	92.5	9.36	96.8
nd	nd	nd	nd	nd	tr	nd	nd	nd
nd	nd	*	*	tr	nd	nd	tr	tr
nd	nd	0.4	nd	nd	nd	nd	nd	nd
nd	nd	nd	*	*	tr	tr	tr	tr
nd	nd	nd	nd	nd	nd	nd	<0.1	<0.1
*	*	5.4	6	5.4	0.1	*	tr	t
nd	nd	0.1	0.2	0.2	nd	nd	tr	tr
*	nd	0.3	0.3	0.3	tr	*	tr	tr
0.3	0.4	0.5	0.2	0.4	1.3	0.6	0.4	0.1
nd	nd	nd	nd	nd	nd	nd	nd	nd
nd	nd	nd	nd	nd	tr	nd	nd	nd
nd	nd	nd	nd	nd	tr	tr	nd	nd
0.1	*	*	*	*	0.1	*	tr	tr
*	nd	nd	nd	nd	nd	nd	nd	nd
*	nd	nd	nd	nd	nd	nd	nd	nd
*	nd	nd	nd	nd	nd	nd	nd	nd
0.5	0.3	tr	nd	nd	tr	nd	tr	tr
*	nd	nd	nd	nd	tr	tr	tr	tr
0.2	0.1	nd	*	tr	*	*	tr	tr
nd	nd	tr	*	*	tr	nd	tr	nd
nd	nd	nd	nd	nd	nd	nd	nd	nd
nd	nd	nd	nd	nd	nd	tr	nd	nd
nd	nd	nd	nd	nd	nd	nd	nd	nd
*	tr	*	0.1	0.1	nd	nd	nd	<0.1
*	*	nd	nd	nd	nd	tr	<0.1	<0.1
nd	nd	nd	nd	nd	tr	tr	nd	nd
nd	nd	0.1	nd	nd	nd	nd	<0.1	tr
nd	nd	*	*	0.1	*	*	—	0.1
nd	nd	nd	nd	nd	tr	tr	nd	nd
0.3	0.3	0.2	0.1	0.2	0.2	0.2	0.2	<0.1
nd	nd	nd	nd	nd	nd	tr	<0.1	<0.1
0.1	0.1	nd	nd	nd	nd	nd	nd	nd

TABLE 3.1. *Continued*

Compounds	Kenya					
	Orange			Mandarin		
	Salustiana	*Valencia*	*Washington navel*	*Kara*	*Sabine*	*Minneola*
linalool	0.4	0.5	0.5	0.2	0.3	0.6
1-octanol	nd	nd	nd	nd	nd	nd
menthyl acetate	nd	nd	nd	nd	nd	nd
β-cubebene	nd	nd	nd	nd	nd	nd
octanol	tr	tr	tr	nd	nd	nd
p-menth-8-en-1-ol	nd	nd	nd	tr	0.1	0.1
(*Z*)-verbenol	nd	nd	nd	—	*	*
linalyl acetate	*	0.1	0.1	tr	0.1	0.1
nonyl acetate	nd	nd	nd	nd	nd	nd
bornyl acetate	nd	nd	nd	nd	nd	nd
thymol methyl ether	nd	nd	nd	nd	nd	nd
α-cedrene	*	tr	tr	nd	nd	nd
isothujol	nd	nd	nd	nd	nd	nd
p-mentha-1(7), 8(10)-dien-9-ol	*	*	0.1	tr	0.1	0.1
terpinyl acetate	nd	nd	nd	nd	nd	nd
terpinen-4-ol	*	*	tr	tr	*	0.1
β-caryophyllene	tr	*	tr	0.1	0.2	0.1
(*Z*)-farnesene	nd	nd	nd	nd	nd	nd
myrcenol	nd	nd	nd	nd	nd	nd
l-menthol	nd	nd	nd	nd	nd	nd
(*E*)-2-decenal	nd	nd	nd	nd	nd	nd
β-elemene	nd	nd	nd	nd	nd	nd
methyl caprate	nd	nd	nd	nd	nd	nd
citronellyl acetate	nd	nd	nd	nd	nd	nd
thujol	nd	nd	nd	nd	nd	nd
pulegone	nd	nd	nd	nd	nd	nd
isoborneol	nd	nd	nd	nd	nd	nd
undecanal	0.1	tr	tr	tr	0.1	0.1
(*E*)-*p*-mentha-2,8-dienol	nd	nd	nd	nd	*	*
aromadendrene	nd	tr	nd	nd	nd	nd
dihydrocarveol	*	*	*	nd	nd	nd
(*E*)-*p*-2,8-menthadien-1-ol	*	*	*	nd	nd	nd
sabina ketone	0.1	0.2	0.2	nd	nd	nd
neral	*	*	*	*	0.1	0.1
(*Z*)-2-decenal	nd	nd	nd	tr	tr	*
isopropenyl 5-methylhex-4-enal	nd	nd	nd	nd	tr	tr
(*Z*)-piperitol	*	*	*	nd	nd	nd
α-terpineol	0.1	0.1	0.1	0.1	0.1	0.1
decylacetate	nd	nd	nd	nd	nd	nd
dodecanal	*	*	*	*	*	0.2

		Burundi	Uganda		Rwanda		Ethiopia	
Grapefruit	Pummelo	Mandarin	Mandarin		Orange-1	Orange-2	Mandarin Hybrids	
Redblush	*C. grandis*	*C. reticulata*	*Jinja*	*Mbarara*	*C. sinensis*		Temple	Orlando
0.1	0.1	0.7	1	0.7	1.2	0.9	1.8	0.3
nd	nd	nd	nd	nd	0.1	0.1	nd	nd
nd	nd	nd	nd	nd	tr	nd	nd	nd
nd	nd	*	nd	nd	nd	tr	<0.1	tr
nd	nd	*	nd	nd	nd	nd	0.4	0.1
nd	nd	nd	nd	nd	nd	nd	nd	nd
nd	nd	nd	nd	nd	nd	nd	nd	nd
0.1	0.1	nd	nd	nd	nd	nd	nd	nd
nd	nd	nd	nd	nd	*	*	nd	nd
nd	nd	*	nd	nd	*	*	nd	nd
nd	nd	0.1	nd	nd	nd	*	nd	nd
0.1	tr	*	nd	nd	nd	nd	nd	nd
tr	*	nd	nd	nd	nd	nd	nd	nd
nd	nd	nd	nd	nd	nd	nd	nd	nd
nd	nd	*	nd	nd	*	*	nd	nd
nd	nd	*	nd	nd	tr	tr	tr	tr
0.1	0.1	tr	0.1	*	*	nd	tr	tr
nd	nd	tr	nd	nd	nd	*	nd	nd
nd	nd	nd	nd	nd	tr	nd	nd	nd
nd	nd	tr	tr	*	nd	nd	nd	nd
nd	nd	nd	nd	nd	*	*	nd	nd
nd	nd	*	nd	nd	nd	*	tr	tr
nd	nd	nd	nd	nd	tr	nd	nd	nd
nd	nd	*	nd	nd	0.2	0.1	<0.1	tr
nd	nd	nd	nd	nd	*	tr	nd	nd
nd	nd	nd	tr	tr	*	tr	nd	tr
nd	nd	*	0.1	0.1	nd	tr	nd	nd
nd	nd	nd	nd	nd	nd	nd	nd	nd
0.2	0.1	nd	nd	nd	nd	nd	nd	nd
nd	nd	nd	nd	nd	nd	nd	nd	nd
*	tr	nd	nd	nd	nd	nd	nd	nd
*	tr	nd	nd	nd	nd	nd	nd	nd
0.2	0.1	nd	nd	nd	nd	nd	nd	nd
*	tr	nd	nd	nd	nd	nd	nd	nd
nd	nd	nd	nd	nd	nd	nd	nd	nd
nd	nd	nd	nd	nd	nd	nd	nd	nd
*	*	nd	nd	nd	nd	nd	nd	nd
0.1	0.1	nd	nd	nd	0.2	0.1	0.1	0.1
nd	nd	nd	nd	nd	0.1	0.1	tr	tr
*	0.1	tr	nd	nd	nd	nd	nd	nd

TABLE 3.1. *Continued*

Compounds	Kenya					
	Orange			Mandarin		
	Salustiana	*Valencia*	*Washington navel*	*Kara*	*Sabine*	*Minneola*
germacrene D	nd	*	*	nd	nd	nd
linalyl 2-methylpropanoate	nd	nd	nd	nd	*	*
geranial	0.1	*	0.1	0.1	0.1	0.1
(*Z*)-carvone	nd	nd	nd	0.1	*	0.1
(*E*,*E*)-α-farnesene	*	0.1	0.1	*	0.1	0.1
geranyl acetate	*	tr	*	nd	nd	nd
cumin aldehyde	*	*	0.1	nd	nd	nd
borneol	nd	nd	nd	nd	nd	nd
neryl acetate	nd	nd	nd	0.1	tr	—
valencene	nd	nd	nd	nd	nd	nd
β-bisabolene	nd	nd	nd	nd	nd	nd
bicyclogermacrene	nd	nd	nd	nd	nd	nd
germacrene B	nd	nd	nd	nd	nd	nd
citronellol	nd	nd	nd	tr	tr	nd
geranyl propionate	nd	nd	nd	nd	0.1	0.1
perillyl aldehyde	*	*	0.1	*	0.1	0.1
carvone oxide	*	*	*	nd	nd	nd
(*E*)-2-undecenal	nd	nd	nd	nd	nd	nd
decanol	nd	nd	nd	nd	nd	nd
nerol	nd	nd	nd	nd	tr	nd
methoxy citronellal	nd	nd	nd	tr	*	*
(*Z*)-carveol	0.1	0.3	0.5	tr	0.1	tr
(*E*)-carvone	*	0.1	0.1	tr	tr	tr
(*E*)-pinocarvyl acetate	nd	nd	nd	nd	tr	nd
(*E*)-carveol	0.1	0.2	0.3	tr	0.1	tr
dodecyl acetate	nd	nd	nd	tr	tr	tr
perillyl acetate	tr	*	*	nd	tr	nd
5-methylen-9-decen-2-one	nd	nd	nd	nd	tr	nd
tetradecanal	nd	*	0.1	nd	tr	tr
p-mentha-1-en-9-ol	nd	nd	nd	nd	nd	nd
tetradecenal	nd	nd	nd	tr	0.1	tr
globulol	nd	nd	nd	nd	nd	nd
limonen-10-ol	nd	nd	nd	nd	nd	nd
dihydrocarveol	nd	nd	nd	nd	nd	nd
caryophyllene oxide	nd	nd	nd	nd	nd	nd
(*Z*)-nerolidol	nd	*	nd	nd	tr	nd
(*E*)-caryophyllene epoxide	tr	0.1	0.2	nd	nd	nd
perillyl alcohol	*	0.1	0.1	nd	nd	nd
n-nonanoic acid	nd	0.1	0.1	nd	nd	nd
cinnamic aldehyde	nd	nd	nd	nd	nd	nd

		Burundi	Uganda		Rwanda		Ethiopia	
Grapefruit	Pummelo	Mandarin	Mandarin		Orange-1	Orange-2	Mandarin Hybrids	
Redblush	*C. grandis*	*C. reticulata*	*Jinja*	*Mbarara*	*C. sinensis*		Temple	Orlando
nd	nd	0.1	tr	0.1	nd	nd	<0.1	<0.1
nd	nd	nd	nd	nd	nd	nd	nd	nd
*	0.1	*	*	*	tr	*	nd	0.1
0.4	0.1	nd	nd	nd	nd	nd	tr	tr
0.1	0.1		nd	nd	nd	nd	nd	nd
nd	nd	*	nd	nd	*	*	<0.1	<0.1
0.1	*	nd	nd	nd	*	*	<0.1	<0.1
nd	nd	nd	nd	nd	nd	nd	nd	nd
nd	nd	*	tr	*	—	*	<0.1	—
nd	nd	0.1	nd	nd	nd	nd	nd	nd
nd	nd	*	*	tr	0.3	0.1	nd	nd
nd	nd	*	nd	nd	nd	nd	nd	nd
nd	nd	*	*	*	nd	nd	nd	nd
nd	nd	*	nd	nd	nd	tr	tr	<0.1
tr	tr	nd	nd	nd	—	tr	nd	nd
*	tr	0.1	*	*	0.1	*	<0.1	<0.1
nd	nd	nd	nd	nd	nd	nd	nd	nd
nd	nd	*	tr	*	nd	*	nd	nd
nd	nd	0.1	nd	nd	nd	*	nd	nd
*	tr	*	*	*	*	0.1	nd	nd
nd	nd	nd	nd	nd	nd	nd	nd	nd
0.3	*	nd	nd	nd	nd	nd	nd	nd
0.1	*	nd	nd	nd	tr	nd	tr	tr
nd	nd	nd	nd	nd	nd	nd	nd	nd
0.2	nd	nd	tr	tr	*	*	nd	nd
0.1	nd	nd	nd	nd	nd	nd	nd	nd
tr	nd	nd	nd	nd	nd	nd	nd	nd
nd	nd	nd	nd	nd	nd	nd	nd	nd
tr	nd	nd	nd	nd	nd	nd	nd	nd
0.1	tr	nd	nd	nd	nd	nd	nd	nd
tr	tr	nd	nd	nd	nd	nd	nd	nd
tr	nd	nd	nd	nd	nd	nd	nd	nd
tr	tr	nd	nd	nd	nd	nd	nd	nd
0.1	tr	nd	nd	nd	nd	nd	nd	nd
0.1	tr	nd	nd	nd	nd	nd	nd	nd
0.1	nd	tr	nd	nd	*	*	nd	nd
tr	tr	tr	nd	nd	nd	nd	nd	nd
tr	*	nd	nd	nd	nd	tr	nd	nd
*	tr	nd	nd	nd	nd	nd	nd	nd
0.1	nd	nd	nd	nd	nd	tr	nd	nd

TABLE 3.1. *Continued*

Compounds	Orange			Kenya Mandarin		
	Salustiana	*Valencia*	*Washington navel*	*Kara*	*Sabine*	*Minneola*
isosafrole	nd	nd	nd	nd	nd	nd
methyl *N*-methylanthranilate	nd	nd	nd	nd	nd	nd
decanoic acid	nd	nd	nd	tr	tr	tr
β-elemol	nd	*	*	tr	tr	tr
globulol	nd	tr	tr	nd	nd	nd
viridiflorol	nd	*	tr	tr	tr	tr
cedrol	nd	tr	*	nd	nd	nd
eugenol	nd	tr	tr	nd	nd	nd
thymol	nd	nd	nd	nd	0.1	0.2
α-cadinol	nd	nd	nd	nd	tr	tr
β-sinensal	nd	nd	*	tr	tr	0.1
dodecanoic acid	nd	nd	nd	nd	nd	nd
nerolidyl acetate	*	0.1	0.2	nd	nd	nd
cinnamyl alcohol	nd	nd	nd	tr	tr	0.1
(*Z*,*E*)-farnesol	tr	*	tr	nd	nd	nd
α-sinensal	nd	tr	tr	nd	0.1	nd
undecanoic acid	tr	tr	tr	nd	0.1	tr
octadecanal	tr	tr	tr	nd	nd	nd
nootkatone	*	0.1	*	nd	*	nd
monoterpene hydrocarbons	96.9	94.5	92.7	98.1	96.9	96.7
sesquiterpene hydrocarbons	*	0.1	0.1	0.2	0.3	0.3
oxygenated compounds	1.7	3.4	4.5	1.1	2.6	2.8

[a]Relative concentration (%), mean of triplicate determinations.
*Peak area was more than 0.005% but less than 0.05%.
tr: Trace, not quantified.
nd: Not detected.

aliphatic aldehydes among the three oils could be used to distinguish the oils. The monoterpene aldehydes, geranial, neral, cumin aldehyde, perilla aldehyde, and citronellal were present at relatively low levels (0.1% or less) in each oil, as in other sweet orange oils of various origins. Both α-sinensal and β-sinensal were present in the Washington navel oil. Valencia oil contained α-sinensal while both compounds were absent from the Salustiana oil. α-Sinensal, a farnesene-type sesquiterpenoid, has been reported in many sweet orange peel oils, and tangerine oil (Moshonas and Shaw, 1974), at concentrations less than 0.1% and contributes significantly to the aroma of the fruits (Herout, 1971; Moshonas and Shaw, 1974; Sawamura, 2000). (*Z*)-Carvone was the most prominent ketone in each of the Salustiana (0.2%), Valencia (0.3%), and Washington navel (0.5%) oils. The

		Burundi	Uganda		Rwanda		Ethiopia	
Grapefruit	Pummelo	Mandarin	Mandarin		Orange-1	Orange-2	Mandarin Hybrids	
Redblush	*C. grandis*	*C. reticulata*	*Jinja*	*Mbarara*	*C. sinensis*		Temple	Orlando
nd	nd	nd	nd	nd	tr	nd	nd	nd
tr	*	nd	nd	nd	tr	*	nd	nd
nd	nd	tr	nd	nd	tr	nd	nd	nd
0.1	tr	nd	nd	nd	nd	nd	nd	nd
nd	nd	nd	nd	nd	nd	nd	nd	nd
nd	nd	nd	nd	nd	nd	nd	nd	nd
0.1	tr	nd	nd	nd	nd	nd	nd	nd
nd	nd	nd	nd	nd	nd	nd	nd	nd
nd	nd	*	0.1	*	*	nd	nd	nd
nd	nd	nd	nd	nd	nd	nd	nd	nd
*	tr	*	*	*	nd	tr	nd	nd
nd	nd	nd	nd	nd	nd	nd	nd	nd
*	tr	nd	nd	nd	nd	nd	nd	nd
nd	nd	0.1	nd	nd	nd	nd	nd	nd
*	*	nd	nd	nd	nd	nd	nd	nd
*	tr	nd	*	*	*	*	<0.1	<0.1
tr	nd	nd	nd	nd	nd	nd	nd	nd
nd	nd	nd	nd	nd	nd	nd	nd	nd
0.2	0.1	nd	nd	nd	nd	nd	nd	tr
93.3	97.5	94.7	95.8	97.4	94.4	97.3	96.3	99.2
0.4	0.3	0.2	0.2	0.3	0.3	0.1	0.1	0.1
4.2	2.0	2.4	1.6	1.6	3.7	2.3	2.8	0.7

observed levels were higher than reported for sweet oranges of other origins (less than 0.1%). The other ketones present in each oil at minor levels (0.1% or less) were (*E*)-carvone, nootkatone, and sabina ketone. Alcohols and ethers amounted to 0.7, 1.3, and 1.6% of the Salustiana, Valencia, and Washington navel oils, respectively. Those relatively prominent in each oil were linalool (0.4–0.5%), (*Z*)-carveol (0.1–0.5%), (*E*)-carveol (0.1–0.3%), perillyl alcohol (0.1%), and α-terpineol (0.1%). Linalool has usually been reported as the most prominent alcohol of orange oils. The other alcohols present in the Kenyan samples were (*E*,*Z*)-2,6-nonadien-1-ol, octanol, isothujol, terpinen-4-ol, (*E*)-*p*-2,8-menthadien-1-ol, (*Z*)-piperitol, (*E*)-sabinene hydrate, (*E*,*E*)-farnesol, and dihydrocarveol at concentration levels less than 0.05%. Among the oil samples, Washington navel had the highest content of (*Z*)-carveol, (*E*)-carveol, and isothujol, while the Valencia oil contained (*Z*)-nerolidol, a rarely reported sesquiterpene alcohol in sweet orange oils. Salustiana oil was devoid of the sesquiterpene alcohols, globulol, β-elemol, and viridiflorol, which were found in the other oils at concentrations less than 0.05%. The terpene ether, 3-(4-methyl-3-pentenyl)-furan (perillene) was found in each of the oils in trace quantities. A total of four esters, linalyl acetate, nerolidyl acetate, geranyl acetate, and perillyl acetate, constituting less than 0.05%, 0.2%, and 0.3% in the Salustiana, Valencia, and Washington navel oils, respectively, were found. Reports on the peel oils of several types of sweet oranges have indicated esters to be either lacking or constituting a minor quantity (less than 0.1%). Nerolidyl acetate has not been previously reported in sweet orange oils. The oxides and epoxides identified in the oils were (*E*)-limonene oxide, (*E*)-linalool oxide, (*E*)-caryophyllene epoxide, α-pinene oxide, myrcene epoxide, (*Z*)-linalool oxide, (*Z*)-limonene oxide, and α-limonene diepoxide. They constituted 0.2%, 0.7%, and 0.8% of the Salustiana, Valencia, and Washington navel oils. Although oxides and epoxides may occur naturally in sweet orange oils, they could also be formed readily by oxidation of the respective hydrocarbons and alcohols under influence of heat or acids during sample preparation, storage, or analysis.

The volatile components of the Kenyan sweet orange peel oils are reported for the first time in this study. Several new compounds not previously reported in sweet orange peel oils of other origins were found. The results could explain the perceived differences of the characteristic aroma of each of the fruits and provide useful chemical quality information applicable for the improvement and utilization of various varieties of sweet orange fruits, based on the essential oil compositions.

Mandarin. It is popular for its rich flavor. Sabine is a local mandarin cultivar (*C. reticulata*) in Kenya, and possesses a sharp characteristic aroma. Minneola tangelo is a hybrid between Dancy tangerine (*C. tangerina* Tanaka) and Duncan grapefruit (*C. paradisi* Macfadyen). It is a specialty tangelo with high consumer acceptance. Mandarins are popular *Citrus* fruits in Kenya and are mainly consumed when fresh. New plantings and research on improved cultivars are ongoing and aimed at increased production and improved quality of the fruits (Mwasaru et al., 1998). These fruits at maturity were obtained from the Boarstal farm of the Kenya Prisons Department, Mombasa. The average fruit weights of the Kara, Sabine, and Minneola were 140, 71, and 211 g, respectively. The flavedo of each fruit constituted 18, 25, and 15% of the whole fruit (w/w), respectively. The yields of essential oils (w/w of whole fruit) were 0.03, 0.13, and 0.15%, respectively. The peel oils had fresh aromas characteristic of the respective fruits. The volatile components found in the oils and their distributions into chemical group classes are presented in Table 3.1. A total of 48, 72, and 58 compounds amounting to 99.4, 98.8, and another 99.8% were found in Kara, Sabine, and Minneola oils, respectively. Two unidentified compounds were found in Minneola oil at trace quantities (Njoroge et al., 2005b).

Hydrocarbons. In Kara, the main monoterpene hydrocarbons were limonene (90.7%), γ-terpinene (2.7%), and myrcene (1.8%). In Sabine oil, limonene (87.1%), α-terpinene (3.4%), and terpinolene (2.2%) were the most prominent. Those most prominent in Minneola oil were limonene (90.1%), γ-terpinene (2.9%), and terpinolene (1.7%). The Sabine oil also contained β-pinene (0.3%) and myrcene (1.8%) at higher quantities than the other two oils. The relative quantities of the major monoterpene hydrocarbons were closely similar to those reported for most mandarin oils (Shaw, 1979; Sawamura, 2000). The major monoterpene hydrocarbons of mandarin oils vary greatly among different varieties, where limonene ranges from 57 to 97%. Those oils reported to contain limonene at quantities less than 80%, such as Kunenbo, Tardivo di Ciaculli, Clementine, and Tachibana (*C. tachibana* Tanaka), possess high levels of either γ-terpinene or myrcene (Shaw, 1979; Sawamura, 2000). It is notable that varietal differences would impart a strong influence on volatile composition of mandarin oils. α-Phellandrene occurred in Kara and Minneola oils at minor quantities (less than 0.05%), but was not found in Sabine oil. β-Phellandrene, sabinene, and *p*-cymene were present in each oil at minor quantities (trace to 0.2%).

Four sesquiterpene hydrocarbons, (*E*,*E*)-α-farnesene, δ-elemene, α-cubebene, and β-caryophyllene, were found in each oil, constituting minor quantities (0.2–0.3%), as reported for other mandarin oils (Sawamura, 2000; Choi and Sawamura, 2002; Minh Tu et al., 2002a). Some sesquiterpene hydrocarbons reported in few mandarin oils at trace quantities, such as germacrene D, α-copaene, β-elemene, germacrene B, bicyclogermacrene, and α-humulene, were not found in the Kenyan samples.

Oxygenated Compounds. A total of 34, 52, and 41 oxygenated volatile compounds amounting to 1.1, 2.6, and 2.8% were found in the Kara, Sabine, and Minneola oils, respectively. The aliphatic aldehydes, octanal, nonanal, decanal, undecanal, (*E*)-2-decenal, dodecanal, and tetradecenal, were present in each oil. Octanal and decanal were the most prominent (0.2–0.3%), as reported for other mandarin oils (Ashoor and Bernhard, 1967; Moshonas, 1971; Shaw, 1979; Sawamura, 2000; Choi and Sawamura, 2002; Mitiku et al., 2002; Minh Tu et al., 2002a). Sabine oil contained relatively higher amounts of the two aldehydes, tetradecanal and undecanal, and tetradecenal as compared to the other two oils. The notably wide variations in the composition of aliphatic aldehydes could be useful to differentiate the oils. The terpene aldehydes present in the oils were neral, citronellal, geranial, perilla aldehyde, methoxy citronellal, and β-sinensal. α-Sinensal was present in Sabine oil (0.1%), unlike in the other samples. This compound has not been reported in most mandarin oils. 3-Cyclohexene-1-carboxaldehyde and isopropenyl 5-methylhex-4-enal were found in Sabine and Minneola oils at trace quantities, but were absent from the Kara oil. These aldehydes have not been previously reported in mandarin peel oils. The structural configurations of some of the newly identified components of mandarin oils are illustrated in Figure 3.5. Aldehydes have been reported as important contributors to mandarin flavor. (*Z*)-Carvone and (*E*)-carvone were present in the oils at

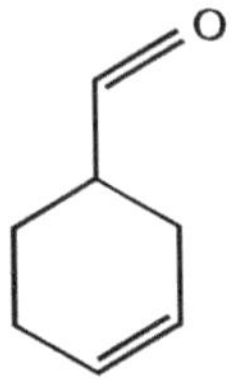

3-Cyclohexene-1-carboxal dehyde

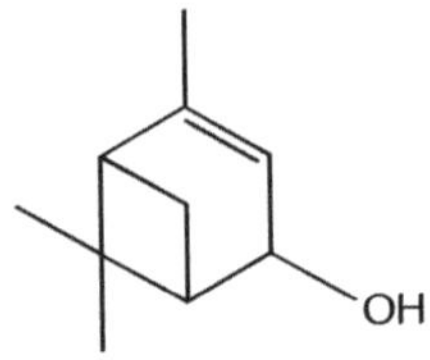

(*Z*)-Verbenol

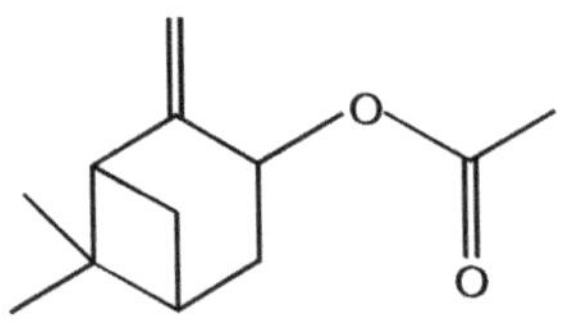

(*E*)-Pinocarvyl acetate

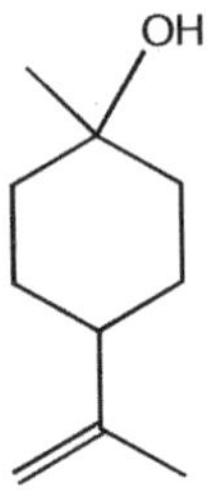

p-Menth-8-en-1-ol

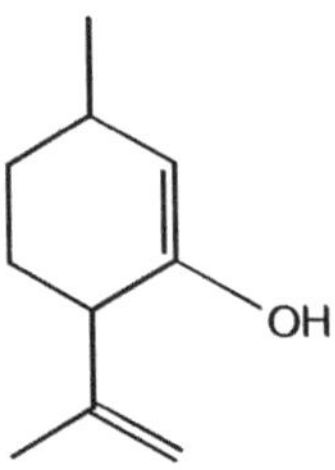

(*E*)-*p*-Mentha-2, 8-dienol

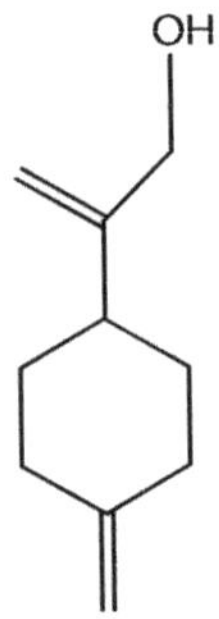

p-Mentha-1(7), 8(10)-dien-9-ol

Figure 3.5. Structural configurations of some volatile compounds of mandarin and tangelo peel oils.

minor quantities, as reported for other mandarin oils. Nootkatone and 5-methylene-9-decen-2-one were found in Sabine oil at minor quantities (less than 0.05%), but were absent from the Kara and Minneola oils. Nootkatone is a characteristic component of pummelos and grapefruits, and its content in the fruits increases with maturation and storage (Sawamura et al., 1990). The compound has not been reported in most mandarin oils.

The numbers of alcohols found in the oils were 12, 18, and 15, constituting 0.3, 0.9, and 1.3% of the Kara, Sabine, and Minneola oils, respectively. Linalool was the most abundant in each oil (0.2–0.6%). α-Terpineol constituted 0.1% of each oil. The oils exhibited variable and complex compositions of the alcohols present in trace or minor quantities, including cinnamyl alcohol, terpinene-4-ol, (*Z*, *Z*)-4,6-octadienol, (*Z*)-carveol, (*E*)-carveol, and elemol. *p*-Menth-8-en-1-ol

(*Z*)-β-terpineol) and *p*-mentha-1(7), 8(10)-dien-9-ol were present in each oil at low quantities (trace to 0.1%). The two alcohols have not been previously reported in mandarin peel oils. Thymol was a prominent component of the Minneola (0.2%) and Sabine (0.1%) oils but was absent from Kara oil. The alcohol is an important contributor to mandarin flavor. (*E*)-*p*-Mentha-2,8-dienol and (*Z*)-verbenol were present in Sabine and Minneola oils at minor quantities (less than 0.05%), but absent from Kara oil. The two alcohols have not been previously reported in mandarin oils. Sabine oil contained (*Z*)-nerolidol and nerol, which were absent from Kara and Minneola oils. The Sabine oil contained higher amounts of (*Z*)-carveol and (*E*)-carveol as compared to the other samples. Citronellol was present in Kara and Sabine oils, but absent from Minneola oil.

The esters, 4 in Kara, 8 in Sabine, and 4 in Minneola oils amounted to 0.1, 0.3, and 0.2%, respectively. Linalyl acetate and dodecyl acetate were present in each of the oils at minor quantities (trace to 0.1%). Neryl acetate was present in Kara (0.1%) and Sabine (trace) oils, but absent from the Minneola oil. Geranyl propionate was present in Sabine (0.1%) and Minneola (0.1%) oils, but absent from Kara oil. The Sabine oil contained (*E*)-pinocarvyl acetate at a trace amount. This ester has not been previously reported in mandarin oils. Sabine oil contained heptyl acetate (0.1%) and perillyl acetate (trace), which were absent from Kara and Minneola oils. Linalyl 2-methylpropionate was present in Sabine and Minneola oils, but absent from Kara oil. The compound has not been previously reported in mandarin peel oils. (*Z*)-Limonene oxide and (*E*)-limonene oxide were present in each oil at minor quantities (not more than 0.1%). (*Z*)-Linalool oxide was present in Kara and Sabine oils at trace quantities. Two acids, decanoic and undecanoic acids, amounting to less than 0.05% were found among the oils. Decanoic acid was present in each oil, while undecanoic acid was absent from the Kara oil. Two compounds at trace quantities in Minneola oil remained unidentified. Although the quantitative variations of some components among the oils were minor, they could be valuable in distinguishing the *Citrus* fruits studied based on varietal differences, and could also serve for quality assurance of the products made with the essential oils.

Grapefruit. In Kenya, grapefruit and pummelo are the second major group of cultivated *Citrus* fruits, after sweet oranges, with annual production of about 17,000 metric tons (Mwasaru et al., 1998). The fruits are mostly produced on the Indian Ocean coastal belt, at an altitude less than 30 m above sea level. The region is hot and humid, with average annual temperatures of 22 to 30°C and average annual rainfall of about 1100 mm. The production and utilization of *Citrus* fruits in the country are increasing rapidly (Njoroge et al., 2005a). The peel essential oils could be utilized in flavor and fragrance industries, but have not been commercially exploited. To our knowledge, there are no previous publications on the essential oils of redblush grapefruit and pummelo grown in Kenya. The understanding of the functional chemical constituents of valuable natural products is important for their utilization and quality standards. The aim of this study was to identify the volatile components of the peel essential oils of redblush grapefruit and pummelo from the Kenyan coast, and make comparisons with other *Citrus* oils.

The redblush grapefruit and pummelo fruits were obtained at harvest maturity in August 2004, from the same locality in Kilifi District, about 50 km north of Mombasa City on the Indian Ocean coastal region of Kenya. The whole fruits had average weights of 278 and 633 g, respectively. The yields of essential oils relative to the whole fruits were 0.06 and 0.12% (w/w), respectively. The identified volatile constituents in the two oils and their relative concentrations are shown in the Table 3.1 (Njoroge et al., 2005c).

Redblush Grapefruit. The oil contained 8 monoterpene hydrocarbons, amounting to a relative 93.3% of the total volatiles. Limonene was the most abundant (91.1%), followed by α-terpinene (1.3%), α-pinene (0.5%), and sabinene (0.4%). α-Thujene, α-pinene, γ-terpinene, and terpinolene occurred at <0.05%. The oil was notably devoid of myrcene, a compound that occurs widely among several grapefruit varieties in Japan (1.7–1.8%). In a study on the chemotaxonomic value of essential oil compounds in *Citrus* species produced in Venezuela (Gonzalez et al., 2002), limonene was the most dominant component of the essential oils from red and white varieties of *Citrus paradisi*. The limonene content of the Kenyan redblush grapefruit oil was also closely similar to that reported for Sweetie peel oils from Israel (Feger et al., 2001). The sabinene content of the Kenyan redblush grapefruit oil was comparatively less than reported for the Sweetie oil (0.8–1.0%). The aliphatic hydrocarbon, 4-methyl-1-octene, was detected at <0.05%. Sesquiterpene hydrocarbons amounted to 0.4% of the total volatiles. Among the six constituents detected in the oil, α–cubebene, α-cedrene, β-caryophyllene, and (*E*,*E*)-α-farnesene each occurred at 0.1%. δ-Elemene and α-copaene were found at <0.05%. According to reported studies, the peel oils of grapefruits, oranges, and mandarins generally contain low amounts of sesquiterpene hydrocarbons (<1.0%). Oxygenated compounds constituted 4.2% of the total oil volatiles, where carbonyl compounds (2.0%) were the major group. Aliphatic aldehydes accounted for 0.7%, with octanal (0.3%), decanal (0.3%), and nonanal (0.1%) as the main constituents. The level of octanal was much less than reported for Venezuelan grapefruit oils (2.2–3.6%) by Gonzalez et al. (2002). Dodecanal, tetradecanal, and tetradecenal occurred at trace levels. Terpene aldehydes constituted 0.4%, where citronellal (0.2%), cumin, and cinnamic aldehydes, at 0.1% each, were the relatively prominent. Neral, geranial, perilla aldehyde, and α- and β-sinensal occurred at <0.05%. Ketones accounted for 0.9%, where the main constituents included (*Z*)-carvone (0.4%), nootkatone (0.2%), sabina ketone (0.2%), and (*E*)-carvone (0.1%). The Kenyan redblush grapefruit oil had a higher level of nootkatone than reported for Sweetie oil (Feger et al., 2001). Sabina ketone, a bicyclic monoterpene ketone (El-Shazly et al., 2002), was a prominent component of the oil. Nootkatone is the characteristic aroma compound of grapefruit oil and has been thoroughly studied (Sawamura and Kuriyama, 1988). Alcohols amounted to 1.4%. The main constituents were (*Z*)-carveol (0.3%), (*E*)-*p*-mentha-2,8-dienol (0.2%), and (*E*)-carveol (0.2%).

Linalool, α-terpineol, *p*-mentha-1-en-9-ol, (*Z*)-nerolidol, elemol, and cedrol occurred at 0.1% levels. The other alcohols, including (*E*)-sabinene hydrate, isothujol, (*E,Z*)-2,6-nonadien-1-ol, (*Z,E*)-farnesol, dihydrocarveol, and (*E*)-*p*-2,8-menthadien-1-ol, occurred at <0.05%. (*E*)-Sabinene hydrate occurs widely among *Citrus* species (Sawamura, 2000). Esters accounted for 0.7%, where the main constituents were heptyl acetate (0.5%), linalyl acetate (0.1%), and dodecyl acetate (0.1%). Perillyl acetate, nerolidyl acetate, and geranyl propionate occurred at <0.05%. Except for linalyl acetate, reported at appreciable levels in bergamot (*C. bergamia* Risso) oil (30–36%) (Sawamura, 2000), the other esters are usually absent, or at low levels in most *Citrus* oils. Octyl formate, reported at appreciable levels in Venezuelan *Citrus paradisi* peel oils, was not found in the Kenyan redblush grapefruit. Perillene was detected at <0.05%. The compound has been reported in sweet orange oils (Njoroge et al., 2005a). Methyl *N*-methylanthranilate, a nitrogen-containing compound, was detected at a trace quantity. It is known to be the character-impact aroma compound of concord grapes, and is a major contributor to tangerine aroma (Nursten, 1977). Oxides and epoxides amounted to 0.1%, comprised of caryophyllene oxide (0.1%), caryophyllene epoxide, and myrcene epoxide. Studies on the inheritance mechanisms with regard to leaf and peel volatile compounds of an interspecific *Citrus* somatic hybrid from Mexican lime [*Citrus aurantifolia* (Christm.) Swingle] + Star Ruby grapefruit (*Citrus paradisi* Macfadyen), showed that the hybrid retained the parents' capacity to produce β-sinensal in the leaves and nootkatone in the peel (Gancel et al., 2002). Such knowledge would be valuable for the improvement of *Citrus* cultivars and aroma quality of *Citrus* essential oils.

PUMMELO. A total of six monoterpene hydrocarbons amounting to 97.5% of the oil volatiles were identified. Limonene was the most abundant (94.8%), as reported for other pummelo oils (5), followed by α-terpinene (1.8%), α-pinene (0.5%), and sabinene (0.4%). β-Pinene and γ-terpinene occurred at <0.05%. α-Thujene and terpinolene were not detected, unlike in the redblush grapefruit oil. Myrcene was virtually absent, as in most other pummelo oils. The limonene content of the Kenyan pummelo peel oil was closely similar to that of an Italian pummelo cultivar (cv. *Chandler*), extracted by cold-pressing manual pressure and analyzed by GC/MS using a fused silica capillary column (Mondello et al., 1996). Sesquiterpene hydrocarbons constituted 0.3%. The main constituents were α-cubebene, β-caryophyllene, and (*E,E*)-α-farnesene, each at 0.1%. The others were δ-elemene, α-cedrene, and α-copaene at <0.05% levels. Several oxygenated compounds amounting to 2.0% occurred in the oil, as indicated in Table 3.1. The main groups were carbonyl compounds (1.3%), alcohols (0.3%), and esters (0.4%). Aliphatic aldehydes (0.7%) consisted of octanal (0.4%), decanal (0.3%), dodecanal (0.1%) and tetradecenal (trace). Tetradecanal was not detected in the pummelo oil, unlike in the redblush grapefruit oil. The other aliphatic aldehydes present in the pummelo oil were nonanal, dodecanal, and tetradecanal. The main terpene aldehydes were citronellal and geranial. Neral, cumin aldehyde, perilla aldehyde, and α- and β-sinensal occurred at trace levels. Cinnamic aldehyde was not detected, unlike in the redblush grapefruit oil. Nootkatone, sabina ketone, and (*Z*)-carvone occurred at 0.1% each. Nootkatone has been reported in all types of pummelos and grapefruits growing in the Orient, at <0.05%. Alcohols constituted 0.3% of the oil volatiles. The prominent constituents were linalool, (*E*)-*p*-menthadien-1-ol, and α-terpineol at 0.1% each. The linalool content of the Kenyan pummelo oil was much less than reported for *Citrus grandis* grown in Venezuela (50.3%) (Gonzalez et al., 2002). The other alcohols in Kenyan pummelo oil occurred at <0.05%, and were similar to those in the redblush grapefruit oil, except for (*Z*)-nerolidol, globulol, (*E*)-carveol, and sabinene hydrate, which were absent in the former but present in the latter oil. Perillene was not detected, unlike in the redblush grapefruit oil. Methyl *N*-methylanthranilate occurred at <0.05%. Esters amounted to 0.4%, out of which heptyl acetate (0.3%) and linalyl acetate were the main constituents. The level of heptyl acetate was higher than reported for other pummelo oils (Sawamura, 2000; Minh Tu et al., 2002a). Geranyl acetate and nerolidyl acetate occurred at trace quantities. Perillyl and dodecyl acetates were not detected in the oil, unlike in the redblush grapefruit oil.

3.2.2 Uganda

Uganda is located in the East African region bordering with Kenya, Tanzania, Rwanda, Democratic Republic of Congo, and Sudan. The country has a moderate temperature through out the year (15–30°C) and a bimodal rainfall pattern (1380 mm per year). It grows a wide range of tropical fruits, the outstanding ones being pineapples, passion fruits, bananas, mangoes, and pawpaws. Several varieties of *Citrus* fruits, including oranges, lemons, and mandarins, are produced in low quantities. The demand for these fruits on the local market is high and the sector is bound to grow as the government continues its plan for modernization of agriculture.

Mandarin. Mandarin is among the most popular *Citrus* fruits in Uganda for fresh consumption. Few studies have reported on the chemical composition of Ugandan mandarin essential oil (Njoroge et al., 2008). The mandarin fruits were obtained from Jinja town in the Lake Victoria basin and Mbarara district to the west of the country. The average weights of the mandarin fresh fruit from Jinja and Mbarara were each 78 g, and the yields of essential oil (weight of oil/weight of fruit) was 0.10%. The aroma components of the essential oils of the mandarins from the two areas are listed in Table 3.1 (Njoroge et al., 2008).

MONOTERPENE HYDROCARBONS. Monoterpene hydrocarbons constituted 95.8% in the oil from Jinja and 97.4 % in that from Mbarara. In the respective oils, limonene (85.3 and 86.9%), γ-terpinene (6.0 and 5.4%), myrcene (2.2 and 2.5%), α-pinene (0.3 and 0.5%), and sabinene (0.4 and 0.3%) were the major components. Limonene is known to be the main aroma component of most mandarin species, at concentration levels of more than 85%. However, in some varieties of *C. nobilis* Loureiro and *C. deliciosa* Tenore, the levels of this compound are much less (56.7 to 69.3%) (Sawamura, 2000). Conversely, such oils contain appreciable levels of other monoterpene hydrocarbons, such as myrcene (32.2%) and γ-terpinene (19.6%).

The relative quantities of the major monoterpene hydrocarbons present in the Ugandan samples were closely similar to those reported for most mandarin oils of other origins (Sawamura, 2000; Mitiku et al., 2002). In view of the high content of limonene in the Ugandan oils, the corresponding levels of γ-terpinene and myrcene were much lower than those reported in the oils of some mandarin varieties, which contain about 19.6 and 32.2% of the two compounds, respectively. The other monoterpene hydrocarbons present in the oils were α-fenchene, *cis*-β-ocimene, α- and β-phellandrene, and α-terpinene at minor quantities. As has been widely reported, varietal differences and geographical origin of citrus fruits impart strong influences on the aroma profiles. The Ugandan mandarin oils possessed α-terpinene and *cis*-β-ocimene, which have not been commonly reported in mandarin oils of other origins (Ashoor and Bernhard, 1967; Sawamura, 2000; Choi and Sawamura, 2002; Mitiku et al., 2002).

Sesquiterpene Hydrocarbons. The Ugandan oils were notably deficient in sesquiterpene hydrocarbons, with that from Jinja showing 0.2% and that from Mbarara 0.3%. The compounds present in each oil were β-elemene, δ-elemene, β-caryophyllene, germacrene D, and β-bisabolene, at minor quantities (trace to 0.1%). Some sesquiterpene hydrocarbons reported in other mandarin oils at trace quantities, such as α-copaene, germacrene B, bicyclogermacrene, and α-humulene, were not detected in the Ugandan samples.

Oxygenated Compounds. A total of 24 oxygenated compounds amounting to 1.6% of the total aroma profile were found in the oils. As shown in Table 3.1, the aliphatic aldehydes, octanal, nonanal, decanal, and dodecanal, were detected at levels ranging from trace to 0.4%. Among them, octanal and decanal were the most prominent as reported for other mandarin oils (Moshonas and Shaw, 1974; Sawamura, 2000). The terpene aldehydes in the oil included citronellal, geranial, perilla aldehyde, α-sinensal, and β-sinensal, at minor quantities. These aldehydes have been reported in other mandarin oils at varying amounts. Aldehydes are known to be important contributors to the flavor of mandarin oils (Njoroge et al., 2006). Among the alcohols found in the oil, linalool was the most abundant (1.0 and 0.7%). The other relatively prominent alcohols were *iso*-borneol and thymol. The latter is known to be an important contributor to mandarin flavor (Njoroge et al., 2006). *n*-Octanol, l-menthol, decanol, nerol, (*E*)-carveol, and sabinene hydrate occurred at levels less than 0.05 %. The two esters detected in the oil were neryl acetate and geranyl acetate, each at a trace quantity. The oil contained a trace amount of thymol methyl ether, which has not been commonly reported in mandarin oils. (*E*)-Limonene oxide was present at a minor quantity. The mandarin oils from the two regions of Uganda showed close similarities in aroma components. Save for minor variations, the aroma compositions were in agreement with those reported for mandarin oils of other origins. The oils would find valuable applications in the consumer-products industry.

Orange. Uganda produces traditional varieties of common sweet oranges under traditional mixed farming systems, without the use of irrigation, fertilizers, and chemicals. The area under cultivation is about 10,000 ha, and the annual production is 10,000 metric tons (Ministry of Agriculture, Animal Husbandry and Fisheries, Uganda, 2001). A recent study has reported the volatile composition of orange essential oil from Uganda for the first time (Njoroge et al., 2009). The information could be valuable in promoting local production and utilization of the fruit.

The yield of essential oil from the Ugandan orange peel (weight of oil/weight of fruit%) was 0.06%. The oil had a characteristic orange aroma. A total of 51 volatile components were isolated and identified. The components are listed in Table 3.1. Monoterpene hydrocarbons constituted 94.4% of the oil, where the main constituents were limonene (89.7%), myrcene (2.4%), sabinene (1.6%), and α-pinene (0.5%). Sesquiterpene hydrocarbons accounted for 0.3% and β-bisabolene (0.3%) was the most prominent. The total oxygenated compounds accounted for 3.7% of the oil, where aliphatic aldehydes (1.6%), terpene aldehydes (1.4%), and terpene alcohols (1.4%) were the major groups. Linalool (1.2%), octanal (1.3%), α-terpineol (0.2%), and decanal (0.2%) were the most prominent oxygenated compounds in the oil. Some aliphatic aldehydes, including 2-nonenal, 2-isononenal, and (*E*)-2-decenal, rarely reported in orange oils, occurred at trace levels. Terpene aldehydes, including α-sinensal, citronellal, β-sinensal, geranial, and perilla aldehyde, occurred at trace levels. (*E*)-Carvone, a monoterpene ketone, occurred at a trace quantity, while (*Z*)-carvone was not detected. The alcohols present at minor levels were (*Z*)-nerolidol, geraniol, nerol, (*E*)-carveol, terpinen-4-ol, and sabinene hydrate. Esters constituted a minor proportion of the oil, with citronellyl acetate, ethyl acetate, octyl acetate, decyl acetate, and menthyl acetate (*p*-mentha-3-yl acetate) at minor quantities. The oil contained *iso*-amyl acetate, *iso*-safrole, *iso*-amyl isovalerate, (*E*)-sabinene hydrate, and methyl caprate, which are rarely reported in orange oils. The oil contained a trace quantity of methyl methylanthranilate (a nitrogen-containing compound), known to be important for mandarin aroma, and *iso*-safrole (3,4-methylenedioxy-propenyl benzene), an aromatic phenolic ether reported as a prominent compound in the leaf oil of *Piper hispidinervum* (83–93%) (Rocha and Ming, 1999). The Ugandan orange oil could contribute significantly to desirable flavor and fragrances.

3.2.3 Rwanda

Rwanda lies to the western side of Uganda. It has favorable climate, fertile soils, and well-distributed rainfall for *Citrus* fruit production. Sweet oranges are quite popular in the local markets for fresh consumption. They are produced on a small scale mainly in Cyangugu province bordering Burundi and Democratic Republic of Congo. Reports on cultivation and utilization of *Citrus* fruits and the essential oils in the country are scarce. An unprecedented study on the volatile components of essential oil of Rwandan oranges has been reported (Njoroge et al., 2009).

The yield of peel essential oil from the oranges obtained from Cyangugu province (weight of oil/weight of fruit%) was 0.05%. A total of 55 volatile volatile components were isolated and identified. The components are listed in Table 3.1. The main chemical groups were monoterpene hydrocarbons (97.3%), alcohols (1.0%), and aldehhydes (0.8%). Limonene (92.5%) was the most prominent of the monoterpene hydrocarbons, followed by α-pinene (2.4%), myrcene (2.2%), and sabinene (0.2%). Sesquiterpene hydrocarbons constituted a minor quantity (0.1%), with β-bisabolene as the main compound. The total oxygenated compounds constituted 2.3% of the oil. Aldehydes accounted for 0.8%, where octanal (0.6%) and decanal (0.2%) were the main compounds. The other aldehydes occurred at trace levels, including (*E*)-2-undecenal, citronellal, geranial, perilla aldehyde, cinnamic aldehyde, α-sinensal, and β-sinensal. Alcohols accounted for 1.1% of the oil, where linalool (0.9%), α-terpineol (0.1%) and nerol (0.1%) were the most notable. The ester group accounted for 0.2%, represented mainly by ethyl acetate and citronellyl acetate (each at 0.1%).

3.2.4 Burundi

Burundi occupies an area of 25,650 km^2. It is located on the northeastern shoreline of Lake Tanganyika, in east-central Africa, surrounded by Congo, Rwanda, and Tanzania. It lies in the tropical zone between 2° and 4°S, and 29° and 31°E. The altitude ranges between 772 m and 2670 m above sea level. The temperature varies from 17° to 23°C, and the average annual rainfall is about 150 cm. The rainfall pattern is bimodal, with two wet seasons (February to May and September to December). The two dry seasons are from June to August and from December to January. The main fruits produced are bananas, papayas, mangoes, pineapples, and *Citrus*. Mandarins are grown on a small scale for household consumption. The fruits are of good eating quality, with pleasant taste, abundant juice, and rich aroma. The surplus fruit is sold in the local markets and neighboring countries. Few studies have reported on the volatile components of mandarin oil from Burundi (Njoroge et al., 2006).

The fresh fruit was obtained from the capital city, Bujumbura, in May 2004. The average weight of the fruit was 91 g, out of which the flavedo constituted 22% (w/w). The yield of essential oil (weight of oil/weight of fruit) was 0.08%. The oil had a strong characteristic aroma. The volatile constituents are listed in Table 3.1.

Hydrocarbons. The oil contained 12 monoterpene hydrocarbons, amounting to 94.7%. The main constituents were limonene (84.8%), γ-terpinene (5.4%), myrcene (2.2%), and α-pinene (1.1%). The quantities of the major monoterpene hydrocarbons were closely similar to those reported for most mandarin oils

(Shaw, 1979; Sawamura, 2000; Njoroge et al., 2005b). Limonene varies between 57 and 97% among different mandarin varieties (Sawamura, 2000; Mitiku et al., 2002; Njoroge et al., 2005b). The mandarin oil from Burundi exhibited a more complex composition of monoterpene hydrocarbons than reported for most mandarin oils. Sesquiterpene hydrocarbons constituted a low amount (0.2%). Germacrene D and valencene were the main constituents, each at 0.1%. δ- and β-Elemene, (*Z*)-farnesene, β-cubebene, germacrene B, bicyclogermacrene, and β-caryophyllene occurred at <0.05%. The occurrence of these compounds concurred with reports of other mandarin oils (Sawamura, 2000; Njoroge et al., 2005b). One aliphatic hydrocarbon, 1,4,7,10-tetraoxacyclodecane (12-crown-4-ether), was detected. The compound has been reported at a minor quantity in Kenyan oranges and Valencia and Washington navel peel oils (Njoroge et al., 2005a). Methyl-*N*-methyl anthranilate, a compound reported to be a major contributor to tangerine aroma, was not detected in the oil. Thirty-seven oxygenated compounds amounting to 2.4% were identified. Aliphatic aldehydes (0.7%), terpene alcohols (0.7%), and ethers (0.5%) formed the major chemical groups. Among the aliphatic aldehydes, octanal (0.5%) and decanal (0.2%) were the most prominent. Nonanal, dodecanal, (*E*)-2-undecenal, and tridecanal occurred at <0.05%. Perilla aldehyde and α-sinensal were the main terpene aldehydes, each at 0.1%. Citronellal, geranial, and β-sinensal occurred at <0.05%. Aldehydes are known to be important contributors to mandarin flavor, and their constitution in the present oil agreed with previous reports (Shaw, 1979; Sawamura, 2000). Ketones were virtually absent, unlike other similar oils where (*Z*)- and (*E*)-carvone have been indicated. Two aliphatic alcohols, octanol (<0.05%) and decanol (0.1%), were found. Among the 10 terpene alcohols detected (0.7%), linalool was the main constituent (0.7%). l-Menthol, *iso*-borneol, terpinen-4-ol, β-citronellol, nerol, (*Z*)-nerolidol, and thymol each occurred at <0.05%. Three ethers, 1,8-cineole (a monoterpene cyclic ether), thymol methyl ether, and isosafrole (a phenolic ether), were found. The compounds are important in flavor and fragrance industry (Rocha and Ming, 1999; Miyazawa et al., 2001). Esters amounted to 0.2%. The compounds were mostly of the acetate type, including acetyl, octyl, bornyl, terpinyl, geranyl, citronellyl, and neryl acetates. Majority of the esters have been reported in other mandarin oils. (*E*)-Limonene oxide occurred at a trace quantity. The study showed that the qualitative and quantitative characteristics of the Burundian mandarin peel oil were close to those of similar oils from other origins. The variations of some constituents could occur due to environmental influences, origins, varieties, and cultural practices.

3.2.5 Ethiopia

In Ethiopia, *Citrus* fruits are cultivated on a small scale and are mainly utilized for fresh consumption. Temple tangor (mandarin × sweet orange) and Orlando tangelo (Duncan grapefruit × Dancy tangerine) mandarin hybrids are popular for their desirable flavor. The volatile components of the peel oils of Orlando and Temple mandarin hybrids from Ethiopia have been reported and compared to each other, and to other popular mandarins (Mitiku et al., 2002). The fruits were harvested from Nuraera State Farm located in eastern Ethiopia along the Great Rift Valley. The volatile components of the Temple and Orlando are listed in Table 3.1. The volatile composition of cold-pressed oils of mandarin and tangerine are known to be rather different, even though their taxonomy is the same (Boelens, 1991). Sixty-two components representing an average of 99.9% of the total volatile fraction in the essential oils of the two Ethiopian mandarin hybrids were positively identified.

HYDROCARBONS. The volatile compounds were largely constituted by monoterpene hydrocarbons (96.3% in Temple and 99.2% in Orlando). The main compounds of this class in the two samples, respectively, were limonene (93.6 and 96.8%), myrcene (1.8 and 1.7%), α-pinene (0.4 and 0.3%), and sabinene (0.4 and 0.1%). The other monoterpene hydrocarbons present in the oil, including camphene, β-pinene, α-phellandrene, α-terpinene, β-phellandrene, (*Z*)-β-ocimene, (*E*)-β-ocimene, γ-terpinene, and terpinolene, each constituted less than 0.1%. The composition of sesquiterpene hydrocarbons in the mandarin hybrid oils was less than or equal to 0.2%. Those detected included δ-elemene, α-copaene, β-cubebene, β-elemene, β-caryophyllene, α-humulene, germacrene D, and δ-cadinene.

OXYGENATED COMPOUNDS. These constituted the second major class of volatile compounds in the cold-pressed oils of the mandarin hybrids. The peel oil of Temple tangor contained an appreciable quantity of oxygenated compounds (2.8%). Alcohols formed the main class (2.0%), with linalool as the most dominant (1.8%). The other alcohols present in the oil were at levels less than 0.1%. They levels included octanol, α-terpineol, geraniol, and citronellol. In the Orlando oil, total alcohols constituted 0.4%, and linalool, 0.3%. The alcohol composition of the Temple tangor oil appears to be rather characteristic of perfume oils, and it may greatly contribute to differentiating the oil from other citrus oils. Carbonyl compounds constituted 0.8% and 0.3% of the total volatile components of the two cultivars, respectively. Octanal, nonanal, decanal, undecanal, neral, perilla aldehyde, β-sinensal, and α-sinensal occurred in both oils at levels ranging from trace to 0.4%. Nootkatone occurred in the Orlando at a trace quantity, but was absent from the Temple oil. In the two cultivars, esters were the least represented (less than 0.1%). Those detected in the two cultivars included octyl acetate, citronellyl acetate, decyl acetate, and geranyl acetate.

In conclusion, it is clear that the African continent is endowed with good climate and geographical location for increased production of different types of citrus fruits. In addition to fresh consumption and processing of the fruits, the essential oils from citrus peel could be exploited for application in the consumer products industry. There is need for more studies on the flavor chemistry of citrus essential oils from Africa, and to relate the results of the studies to the development of superior citrus cultivars and application of the oils for industrial development.

3.3 THE AMERICAS

Nguyen Thi Thao

Citrus fruits are produced all around the world. According to FAO data, in 2004, among 140 countries that produced citrus fruits, main citrus fruit–producing countries were Brazil (20%) and the United States (14%) (UNCTAD, 2004). Other Latin American countries are also producing a large quantity of citrus fruits. Main producers of orange are Brazil, United States, and Mexico, while major producers of lime are Mexico and Brazil. Mandarins are cultivated mainly in the southern region of Brazil, where they represent an important and strategic economic resource with strong social implications, associated with a small-property culture system. In this section, the data for the composition of citrus essential oils from different countries in the Americas that were reported in the literature will be summarized.

3.3.1 Lemon (*Citrus limon*)

Table 3.2 presents data reported in the literature on the volatile composition of lemon peel oil from Venezuela, Colombia, U.S.–California, and Uruguay.

A total of 51 constituents were identified and quantified by HRGC and GC-MS for fruit peel oil of *C. limon* grown in Venezuela, using an internal standard and response factor (Rodríguez et al., 1998). The major prominent constituent was limonene (65.65%) and the main aldehydes were geranial (1.43%) and neral (0.87%). Among the other monoterpene hydrocarbons, there was a high proportion of β-pinene (11%) and γ-terpinene (9.01%). Oxygenated compounds were found in amounts of 3.97%. Aldehydes were the most abundant constituents of this oxygenated fraction (2.70%), especially the quality indicators: geranial (1.43%) and neral (0.87%), whose levels were very similar to Italian, Californian (Chamblee et al., 1991), and Uruguayan lemon essential oils (Dellacassa, 1997). On the other hand, alcohols were represented in 0.53%, esters in 0.56%, and a small percentage of artifacts was found (0.01%).

In the peel oil of Californian lemon, Chamblee et al. (1991) reported that the monoterpene hydrocarbons was the largest fraction, which accounted for 91.5% of the total volatile components, in which limonene level was 65.65%, followed by β-pinene (11.13%), sabinene (1.85%), α-pinene (1.75%), and myrcene (1.58%). On the other hand, alcohols were represented in 0.51%, aldehydes in 2.32%, sesquiterpene hydrocarbons in 1.24%, ester in 1.18%. Generally, the volatile component of Californian lemon oil was similar to that of Venezuelan lemon oil. An important difference is the content of neral and geranial in Californian lemon oil, whose proportion was lower (1.18%) than those of Venezuelan oil and Uruguayan oil. In addition, the proportion of ketones and oxides in this oil was significantly lower (0.03%) in comparison with this level of Uruguayan and Italian oil (0.11%). Ester compounds were present in minute amounts (0.06%).

TABLE 3.2. Peak-area percent of volatile components in American lemon essential oils

Compounds	Venezuelan[1]	Californian[2]	Uruguayan[3]	Colombian[4]	
				(A)	(B)
Monoterpene Hydrocarbons					
α-thujene	0.42	0.38	0.04–0.4	0.31–0.34	0.33–0.47
α-pinene	1.88	1.75	1.89–1.92	0.8–1.0	1.42–1.53
camphene	0.06	0.06	0.06		
sabinene	1.05	1.85		1.15–3.55	2.25–4.87
β-pinene	11.00	11.13	13.88–14.31	0.65–0.80	0.90–0.99
myrcene	1.01	1.58	1.49–1.58	1.65–1.74	1.55–2.00
α-phellandrene	0.05	0.04	0.07	0.07–0.08	0.06
δ-3-carene	0.01		0.01		
α-terpinene	0.22	0.16	0.18–0.19		
p-cymene	0.10	0.14	0.15	0.65–1.28	0.50–0.59
limonene	65.65	65.65	67.02–67.15	77.27–79.36	77.10–78.90
(*Z*)-β-ocimene			0.05–0.07	tr	tr
(*E*)-β-ocimene	0.09	0.09	0.10–0.12	0.21–0.32	0.18–0.32
γ-terpinene	9.01	8.32	8.81–8.88	7.81–8.85	7.32–7.92
terpinolene	0.39	0.34	0.35–0.36	0.53–0.55	0.42–0.43
cis-epoxylimonene				0.07–0.31	0.12–0.38
trans-sabinene		0.01			
Aldehydes					
octanal	0.07	0.08	0.04	0.20–0.25	0.12–0.17
nonanal	0.12	0.12	0.10–0.12	0.08–0.12	0.09–0.13
citronellal	0.14	0.08	0.08–0.09	0.30–0.40	0.36–0.41
decanal	0.04	0.05	0.04–0.05	0.19–0.34	0.26–0.30
neral	0.87	0.74	0.76–0.81	1.83–2.11	0.98–1.19
geranial	1.44	1.18	1.32–1.38	0.07–0.11	0.03–0.06
undecanal	0.02	0.03	0.02–0.03		
perilladehydes		0.03		0.11–0.18	0.05–0.08
dodecanal/decyl acetate	0.01	0.01	0.01		
thymal				0.02–0.03	0.03–0.05
tetadecanal			0.01		
Alcohols					
octanol	0.05		0.01	0.08–0.12	0.05–0.06
lynalool		0.13	0.12	0.16–0.43	0.18–0.28
1,2-dihydrolinalool				0.04–0.10	0.03–0.10
hydrate/octanol	0.16	0.01			
borneol	0.01	0.11	0.02		
terpinen-4-ol	0.06	0.11	0.04–0.06		
α-terpineol	0.17	0.16	0.16–0.19	0.02–0.05	0.03–0.04

TABLE 3.2. *Continued*

Compounds	Venezuelan[1]	Californian[2]	Uruguayan[3]	Colombian[4]	
				(A)	(B)
citronellol	0.04	0.06	0.02–0.03	0.04–0.08	0.02–0.06
nerol				0.23–0.27	0.05–0.07
geraniol	0.03	0.03	0.03–0.04		
isopulegol				0.27–0.40	0.03
methylthymol				0.05	0.01
decanol				0.03–0.04	0.03
nerolidol		tr			
2,3-dimethyl-3-(4-methyl-3-pentenyl)-2-norbornanol		0.03			
campherenol		0.03			
sesquiterpenol				0.02–0.03	0.01–0.03
α-bisabolol	0.03	0.04	0.02		
β-bisabolol	0.09		0.02		
2,3-dimethyl-3(4-methyl-3-pentenul)-2-norbornanol	0.03		0.02		
Ketones and Oxides					
1,4-cineole				0.33–0.36	0.13–0.20
cis-sabinene hydrate			0.04–0.05	0.05–0.18	0.07–0.21
trans-sabinene hydrate			0.03	0.01–0.06	0.08–0.16
camphor	0.01	0.01	0.01		
piperitone	0.01	0.01	tr		
trans-limonene 1,2-oxides		0.01	0.01		
cis-limonene 1,2-oxides		0.01	0.01		
cis-4,7-dimethylbicyclo [3.2.1]oct-3-en-6-one nootkatone		0.01	0.01		
Esters					
octyl acetate			tr		
bornyl acetate			0.01		
nonyl acetate			0.01		
neryl acetate	0.35		0.33–0.42		
genaryl acetate	0.22		0.31		

TABLE 3.2. *Continued*

Compounds	Venezuelan[1]	Californian[2]	Uruguayan[3]	Colombian[4]	
				(A)	(B)
methyl geranoate		0.01	0.01		
citronellyl acetate		0.03	0.02–0.03		
neryl propionate		0.01			
genaryl propionate		0.01			
undecyl acetate		0.01			
decyl acetate			0.01–0.1		
Sesquiterpene Hydrocarbons					
δ-elemene					
cis-α-bergamotene	0.05	0.03			
β-caryophylene	0.25	0.22		0.04–0.07	0.03–0.06
trans-α-bergamotene	0.41	0.38	0.3–0.34	0.19–0.22	0.18–0.21
trans-β-farnesene	0.04	0.03			
α-humulene	0.02	0.02	0.02		
β-santalene		0.01			
β-farnesene	0.08	0.03			
(*E*)-caryophyllene			0.24–0.26		
sesquiterpene			0.02–0.03		
valencene	0.03		0.02–0.04		
germacrene B	0.11				
β-bisabolene	0.40	0.55	0.44–0.51	0.04–0.09	0.02–0.07
α-muurolene				0.12–0.33	0.24–0.28
(*Z*)-α-bisabolene			0.04		
germacrene D			0.01–0.02		
(*E*)-β-farnesene			0.05		
bicyclogermacrene			0.06–0.07		
γ-elemene	0.03		0.01		

[1]Rodríguez et al., 1998.
[2]Chamblee et al., 1991.
[3]Dellacassa et al., 1997.
[4]Tirado et al., 1995.
(A): Type A oil.
(B): Type B oil.

The data for essential oils of lemon from northern and southern Uruguay are reported by Dellacassa (1997). Generally, the composition of lemon essential oil from the north was not different from that of the oil from the south. Total monoterpene hydrocarbon compounds accounted for 94.64% to 94.81%, which was higher than for the other lemon oils. Limonene content was slightly higher (67%) than the limonene level in Californian (65.65%) and Venezuela lemon oil

(65.65%). The aldehydes were 2.4%, similar to those of Italian oil, but lower than the aldehyde content of Venezuelan oil (2.71%) and higher than Californian oil (2.32%). The total level of alcohol compounds in Uruguayan lemon oil was similar to that of the other lemon oils (0.51%).

The essential oil of Colombian lemon (*C. volkameriana* or *C. limonia* Osbeck: probably the hybrid of *C. lemon* × *C. retiulata*) was determined at different stages of fruit ripeness and by two extraction methods (Tirado et al., 1995). Monoterpene hydrocarbons accounted for 94.3% of total volatile components, followed by aldehydes (2.1%), while the level of alcohol compounds was only 0.47%. The volatile composition of this oil was significantly different from that of the other oils, especially in the higher limonene content (78.9% compared to 65.6–67% of limonene level in the other lemon oils) and lower β-pinene content (0.94%). The total content of sesquiterpene hydrocarbons was also lower than that of the other lemon oils (0.47% in Colombian lemon oil compared to 1.2–1.5% in the other oils). In addition, the linalool content was higher (0.23%). While neral was present in this oil at a level similar to the other lemon oils (0.98%), the geranial content was significantly lower (0.04%). The level of esters was so small that they could not be determined in this study or at trace level.

3.3.2 Sweet Orange (*C. sinensis* (L.) Osbeck)

Table 3.3 summarizes data of the literature on the volatile composition of essential oil from Venezuelan Valencia orange and Colombian orange. Likewise, in different cultivars of sweet orange, the most quantitatively important components in Venezuelan orange oil are monoterpene hydrocarbons, followed by aliphatic aldehydes and linalool (Rodríguez et al., 2003). The composition in the volatile fraction of the oil was 96.83% for total monoterpene hydrocarbons, mainly due to limonene (94.55%), myrcene (1.22%), and α-pinene (0.51%). Volatile aldehydes and alcohols, *n*-octanal, *n*-decanal, geranial, linalool, and α-terpineol, which are important to the flavor and aroma of citrus cold-pressed oils, were found to be the major contributors to the class of oxygenated compounds. Terpene aldehydes were also present in high concentrations. These amounts were higher than those for the same cultivars from Italy, Spain, and Israel.

The volatile composition of Colombian orange essential oils from different extraction methods and the range of individual components are also reported (Tirado, 1995). Orange fruits belonging to different harvesting periods were collected and the peel oils were isolated by both steam distillation (A) and cold pressing (B). Depending on fruit maturity and extraction method, the content of each component varied greatly. For example, the level of geranial was around 0.2% in oil type A, but this compound was present at only 0.02% in oil type B. However, when using the composition of oil type B to compare with the other oil, we can see the following: The Colombian orange oil is somewhat different from the Venezuelan oil. Limonene was present at the highest level (94.55%) followed by octanal (1.55–1.89%), β-pinene (0.63–0.72%), terpinolene (0.58–

TABLE 3.3. Peak-area percent of volatile components in American orange essential oils

Compounds	Venezuelan[1]	Colombian[2]	
		(A)	(B)
Monoterpenes			
α-pinene	0.51	0.28–0.32	0.29–0.53
camphene	0.02	0.27–0.36	0.42–0.52
sabinene	0.42	0.02	0.02–0.03
β-pinene	0.04	0.63–1.05	0.63–0.72
myrcene	1.22	<0.01	
δ-3-carene	0.02	0.04–0.08	0.05–0.07
α-phellandrene		0.02–0.04	0.04–0.05
limonene	94.55	91.03–92.57	93.77–94.55
trans-β-ocimene		0.02–0.03	0.02
γ-terpinene		0.41–1.09	0.02–0.04
terpinolene	0.05	1.83–2.61	0.58–0.78
cis-epoxylimonene		0.02–0.04	0.02–0.37
Aldehydes			
octanal	0.23	1.50–1.64	1.55–1.89
nonanal	0.06		
citronellal	0.06		
decanal	0.45	0.11–0.35	0.26–0.39
neral	0.19	0.12–0.15	0.08
geranial	0.23	0.15–0.23	0.02
undecanal	0.1		
perillaldehyde		0.01–0.03	
dodecanal	0.2		
α-sinensal	0.01		
β-sinensal	0.02		
Alcohols			
octanol	0.04	0.02–0.03	0.02–0.04
linalool	0.48		
terpinen-4-ol		0.11–0.18	0.06–0.23
α-terpineol	0.13		
trans-carveol	0.02		
citronellol	0.11		
nerol	0.01	0.07–0.13	
cis-carveol	0.02		
geraniol	0.02	0.14–0.17	0.10–0.11
isopulegol		0.03–0.05	
nerolidol	0.01		
Ketone			
carvone	0.03		

TABLE 3.3. *Continued*

Compounds	Venezuelan[1]	Colombian[2]	
		(A)	(B)
Esters			
octyl acetate	0.07		
bornyl acetate	0.04		
citronellyl acetate	0.05		
neryl acetate	0.05		
geranyl acetate	0.01		
decyl acetate	0.07		
Sesquiterpenes			
α-copaene	0.07		
β-elemene	0.13		
β-caryophyllene	0.12	0.01–0.02	
δ-elemene		0.07–0.09	0.03–0.08
α-cadinene	0.03		
α-humulene	0.02		
β-farnesene	0.04		
valencene	0.04		
δ-cadinene	0.01	0.03–0.04	0.03
germacrene D		0.02–0.15	0.02

[1]Rodríguez et al., 2003.
[2]Tirado et al., 1995.
(A): Type A oil.
(B): Type B oil.

0.78%), and decanal (0.26–0.39%). The total amount of aldehydes was 1.55%; total aldehydes in orange oil are generally around 1.5% (Shaw, 1979).

3.3.3 Mandarin (*C. reticulata* Blanco, *C. unshiu* Marcovitch, *C. deliciosa*, and *C. clementine* Hort.)

Table 3.4 presents data reported in the literature on the volatile composition of mandarin essential oil from America. These are different cultivars, including Satsuma mandarin (*C. unshiu* Marcovitch), Nova mandarin (*C. reticulata* Blanco cv. *Nova*), and Clementine, which were grown in Uruguay, Brazil, Venezuela, and Colombia. Numerous quantitative values for individual components of mandarin oil are reported (Tirado et al., 1995; Verzera et al., 1998, 2000; Frizzo et al., 2004). These data show the same trend as observed by Shaw (1979): Wider variation in results exists than with any other four major citrus cultivars because of the lager number of mandarin species. The hydrodistilled oil (type A) and cold-pressed oil (type B) of Brazilian and Colombian mandarins are taken as the range of each component depending on the ripening stages of fruit. Aldehydes are important to mandarin flavor, and they are the major class of oxygenated components. The two main aldehydes are octanal and decanal and a wider range of values for both octanal and decanal have been reported.

The oils from Uruguayan Satsuma mandarin were characterized by a high content of limonene (about 91%) and other monoterpenes. Among oxygenated compounds (1%), aliphatic aldehydes constituted about 80% of the carbonyl compound fraction (0.52%); linalool (0.16–0.20%), and α-terpineol (0.09–0.10%) were the main alcohols, and esters were less represented. A large number of sesquiterpenes were present (0.78–0.88%); of these, the main component was (*E*,*E*)-α-farnesene (0.25–0.29%). The oils of Nova mandarin, on the other hand, were rich in monoterpene hydrocarbons (96.7–97.9%). The main component was limonene (91.3–94.2%). Oxygenated compounds were present at higher levels (1.61–2.29%) in which carbonyl compounds were present in 0.8–1%, alcohols in 0.78–1.16%. Aliphatic aldehydes constituted most of the carbonyl fraction; the main component was decanal (0.40–0.32%). Among alcohols, the main component was linalool (0.67–0.88%). Seventeen sesquiterpenes were present in small quantity (0.25–0.31%), among which main components were germacrene D (0.09–0.11%) and δ-cardinene (0.04–0.05%).

The oils of Cai mandarin from Brazil (*C. deliciosa*) were characterized by high content of monoterpene hydrocarbons (91.7–96.12% in type A oil and 92.57–96.71% in type B oil). The main component was limonene; however, this compound was present in lower quantities compared to the other mandarin oils (around 70–75%). Another monoterpene hydrocarbon, γ-terpinene, was also present in significantly high amounts (13.76–19.52%). Among oxygenated compounds, aldehydes were present in 0.96–2.1%, alcohols in 0.81–4.34%, and this fraction was reducing steadily during the development of mandarin fruit. An important compound believed to be characteristic for mandarin flavor, methyl *N*-methlanthranilate, was present at high levels in these oils (0.41–1.45%).

Colombian mandarin (*C. reticulata*) contained high amounts of limonene (83.45–84.29% in type A oil and 89.25–90.05% in type B oil), followed by γ-terpinene (3.35–4.85%), terpinolene (4.45%–5.96% in type A oil and 1.41–1.57% in type B oil), and myrcene (1.45–1.86%). Among alcohols, α-terpinool (0.26–0.35% in type A oil and 0.09–0.10% in type B oil), citronellol (0.14–0.23%), and geraniol (0.12–0.17%) were noteworthy. In addition, the main components of aldehyde group were octanal (0.26–1.05%), decanal (0.14–0.17%), neral (0.08–0.28%), and α-sinensal (0.13–0.23%). Sesquiterpenes were found in small amounts and main components were β-bisabolene (0.05–0.09%) and germacrene D (0.03–0.08%).

Clementine (*C. clementine* Hort.) oils from Uruguay (Nules and Comune varieties) contained high levels of monoterpene hydrocarbons (97%), among which the main components were limonene (more than 93%), followed by myrcene (2%) and sabinene (0.94–1.09%). Specifically, δ-3-carene was present in this fraction (0.03–0.06%). Among oxygenated compounds, which accounted for 1.75–2.37% of the volatile fraction, linalool (0.5–0.7%) and decanal (0.4%)

TABLE 3.4. Peak-area percent of volatile components in American mandarin essential oils

Compounds	Uruguayan Mandarin[1]		Brazilian Mandarin[2]		Uruguayan Clementine[3]		Colombian Mandarin[4]	
	Satsuma	Nova	(A)	(B)	Nules	Comune	(A)	(B)
Monoterpene Hydrocarbons								
α-thujene	0.12	tr	0.38–0.5	0.10–0.53	0.01	0.01	0.11–0.19	0.16–0.19
α-pinene	0.79–0.81	0.48–0.50	1.04–1.44	0.26–1.53	0.55–0.56	0.58	0.39–0.54	0.86–0.93
(A): Type A oil;	tr	tr	0.01	0.01	tr	tr		
(B): Type B oil								
sabinene	0.16–0.17	0.34–0.35	0.17–0.19	0.11–0.17	0.94–0.99	0.98–1.09	0.11–0.17	0.14–0.15
β-pinene	0.23–0.25	0.14	1.01–1.07	0.50–1.17	0.21–0.22	0.21–0.26	0.29–0.46	0.32–0.36
myrcene	1.93–2.01	1.93–1.98	1.53–1.71	1.33–1.78	1.99–2.10	2	1.45–1.49	1.84–1.86
α-phellandrene	0.04	0.03–0.04			0.03	0.03	0.04	0.04
δ-3-carene		0.17–0.19			0.03–0.04	0.03–0.06		
α-terpinene	0.06–0.07	tr	0.32–0.38	0.23–0.32	tr	tr		
1,4-cineole							0.09–0.11	0.08–0.09
p-cymene							0.20–0.36	0.08–0.24
limonene	90.98–91.6	93.13–94.22	70.54–76.41	69.25–72.84	93.5–93.78	92.94–93.29	83.45–84.29	89.25–90.05
(*Z*)-β-ocimene	tr	0.01–0.02			0.01	tr	tr	tr
(*E*)-β-ocimene	0.02–0.03	0.38–0.44	0.01–0.02	0.02–0.03	0.01–0.07	0.04–0.05	0.13–0.14	0.10–0.13
γ-terpinene	3.00–3.34	0.01–0.02	13.76–15.8	15.41–19.52	tr	tr	4.27–4.85	3.35–3.87
terpinolene	0.14–0.15	0.03	0.66–0.83	0.73–1.11	0.01	0.01–0.02	4.55–5.96	1.41–1.57
p-cymenene	tr							
p-mentha-2,4(8)-diene		tr						
cis-epoxylimonene							0.02	
Aldehydes								
octanal	0.19–0.20	0.16–0.17	0.25–0.38	0.06–0.19	0.18–0.31	0.50–0.58	0.39–1.05	0.26–0.49
nonanal	0.05	0.05	0.04–0.06	0.04–0.06	0.01–0.02	0.01		

citronellal	0.04–0.05	0.01	0.04–0.07	0.04–0.1	0.04–0.06	0.06–0.07	0.07–0.13	0.04–0.06
decanal	0.12–0.13	0.3–0.32	0.11–0.15	0.12–0.22	0.36–0.4	0.4	0.10–0.14	0.14–0.17
neral	0.01	0.01–0.03	0.03–0.06	0.01–0.02	0.03–0.04	0.01–0.02	0.13–0.28	0.08–0.10
(*E*)-dec-2-en-1-al	tr	0.01			0.01	0.01		
geranial	0.02	0.04–0.06	0.01–0.04	0.05	0.02–0.03	0.03	0.05–0.12	0.04–0.05
perilla aldehyde	0.05	0.02–0.04	0.16–0.27	0.08–0.14	0.02	0.03–0.04	0.36–0.43	0.08–0.11
(*E*,*Z*)-2,4-decadienal		tr						
undecanal	0.01	0.02	0.01	0.01–0.03	0.01	tr		
(*E*,*E*)-2,4-decadienal		0.03	0.01	0.01	0.01	0.01		
dodecanal	0.02	0.06–0.07	0.02–0.04	0.04–0.27	0.08	0.06–0.08		
(*E*)-dodec-2-en-1-al		0.01–0.02	0.01–0.02	0.02–0.05	0.01	0.01		
tridecanal					tr	tr		
tetradecanal		0.01	0.01	0.01–1.05	tr	0.01		
β-sinensal	tr	0.01–0.02			0.04–0.07	0.05		
α-sinensal	tr	0.02–0.04	0.05–0.28	0.55–0.63	0.21–0.28	0.23–0.24	0.13–0.23	0.18–0.20
Alcohols								
octanol	tr	0.04	0.07–0.21	0.01	0.03	0.01–0.11		
linalool	0.16–0.2	0.67–0.88	0.34–0.69	0.12–0.26	0.46–0.55	0.63–0.67		
p-menth-2-en-1-ol			0.01–0.04					
1-borneol			0.01–0.02	tr				
isopulegol							0.02–0.05	
nonanol							0.09–0.13	
terpinen-4-ol	0.01–0.02	0.01	0.32–0.75	0.06–0.13	0.01	0.01		
α-terpineol	0.09–0.10	0.06–0.08	0.61–1.46	0.29–0.53	0.05–0.07	0.06	0.26–0.35	0.09–0.10
cis-piperitol	0.01	0.01–0.03						
trans-carveol	0.01–0.02	0.01–0.02	0.02–0.03	0.01–0.02				
nerol	tr	0.01			0.02	0.01–0.02	0.08–0.10	
citronellol	0.01	0.01	0.10–0.20	0.03–0.12			0.14–0.23	

TABLE 3.4. *Continued*

Compounds	Uruguayan Mandarin[1]		Brazilian Mandarin[2]		Uruguayan Clementine[3]		Colombian Mandarin[4]	
	Satsuma	Nova	(A)	(B)	Nules	Comune	(A)	(B)
cis-carveol	0.01	tr			0.01	0.01		
geraniol	tr	tr	0.02–0.04	0.16	tr	tr	0.12–0.17	
decanol							0.07–0.10	
perilla alcohol	0.01–0.02	0.02–0.03			0.01	0.01		
p-cymen-7-ol			0.03–0.06	0.02–0.32				
thymol			0.2–0.67	0.05–0.17				
carvacrol				0.02–0.04				
cubebol	tr	tr						
elemol	tr	0.01–0.02						
(*E*)-nerolidol		tr			0.01	tr		
tetradecanol					tr	tr		
germacrene D-4-ol	0.01	0.01						
bulnesol	tr							
Ketones and Oxides								
cis-sabinene hydrate	0.01	0.02	0.03–0.06	0.05–0.09	0.03	0.03		
cis-limonene oxide	tr	0.01–0.05	0.03–0.05	0.01	0.01	0.01		
trans-limonene oxide	0.01	0.01–0.04		nd	0.01–0.03	0.01		
trans-sabinene hydrate	0.02	tr	0.07–0.14	0.12–0.19	tr	tr	0.11–0.33	
(*E*)-myroxide		0.01–0.02						
camphor			0.01–0.03	tr				
cis-pinocamphone		0.01–0.02						

piperitone			0.01–0.02	tr				
carvone	tr	0.02–0.07			tr	tr		
nootkatone	tr	0.01			tr	0.01–0.03		
caryophyllene oxide	tr							
Esters								
heptyl acetate					0.01	0.01		
octyl acetate	tr	tr	0.02–0.04	0.04	tr	0.01		
thymol methyl ether			0.01–0.03	nd				
neodihydro carveol acetate		tr						
α-terpinyl acetate	tr	tr			tr	tr		
citronellyl acetate	0.01	tr	0.01	tr			0.05–0.10	0.07–0.09
neryl acetate	0.02	0.01	0.01	0.05	tr	tr		
geranyl acetate	0.04	tr	0.01	0.01–0.03	tr	tr		
decyl acetate	0.01–0.02	0.01						
methyl *N* -methylanthranilate			0.59–1.45	0.16–0.89	tr	tr		
Sesquiterpene Hydrocarbons								
δ-elemene	0.02–0.03	0.01						
α-cubebene	tr	tr						
α-copaene	0.04	0.02–0.03	0.01–0.02	0.03–0.04	0.04	0.03		
β-cubebene	0.04	0.01	0.01	0.01–1.05	0.04	0.03		
β-elemene	0.02–0.04	0.01			0.01	0.01	0.02–0.10	
β-caryophyllene	0.02	0.01	0.05–0.1	0.06–0.17	0.01	0.01	0.04–0.11	
β-gurjunene					0.02	0.01		
γ-elemene	tr	0.01						

TABLE 3.4. *Continued*

Compounds	Uruguayan Mandarin[1]		Brazilian Mandarin[2]		Uruguayan Clementine[3]		Colombian Mandarin[4]	
	Satsuma	Nova	(A)	(B)	Nules	Comune	(A)	(B)
trans-α-bergamotene	0.01	tr			tr	tr		
α-humulene	0.03	0.02	0.01	0.01–0.12	0.01	0.01		
β-santalene	tr	0.01						
β-bisabolene							0.05–0.09	0.05–0.06
(*Z*)-β-farnesene					0.01	0.01		
(*E*)-β-farnesene					0.01–0.02	0.01–0.02		
γ-muurolene		tr			tr	0.01–0.02		
germacrene D	0.16–0.17	0.09–0.11	0.01	0.02–0.18	0.03–0.04	0.02–0.03	0.03–0.08	0.05–0.08
α-selinene			0.03–0.05	0.01–0.84				
bicyclogermacrene	0.01	tr			0.01	tr		
α-muurolene	tr	tr						
valencene					0.01	0.01		
α-bulnesene	tr	tr						
(*Z*)-α-bisabolene	0.07–0.1				tr	tr		
(*E,E*)-α-farnesene	0.25–0.29	0.02–0.03	0.14–0.22	0.05–0.51	0.04	0.03–0.04		
δ-cadinene	0.07–0.08	0.04–0.05	0.01	0.01–0.03	0.04–0.05	0.03–0.04		
germacrene B	0.03	0.01						

[1]Verzera et al., 2000.
[2]Frizzo et al., 2004.
[3]Verzera et al., 1998.
[4]Tirado et al., 1995.
(A): Type A oil.
(B): Type B oil.

were main components. There were also a large number of sesquiterpenes that were present in small quantities (0.26–0.31%).

3.3.4 Lime (*C. aurantifolia* Swingle)

The volatile fraction of acid lime essential oil has been widely studied for distilled and cold-pressed lime oil, including Key lime oil and Persian lime oil (Guenther and Langenau, 1943; Azzouz et al., 1976; Dugo et al., 1998a; Lota et al., 2002; Chisholm et al., 2003b).

Table 3.5 reports the volatile composition in the literature for Key lime oil and Persian lime oils and lime oil from different geographical origins in the

TABLE 3.5. Peak-area percent of volatile components of American lime essential oils

Compounds	Key Lime		Persian Lime		
	Mexico (A)	Mexico (B)	Mexico (B)	Brazil (B)	Florida (B)
Monoterpene Hydrocarbons					
nonane	0.01–0.02	0.02	tr	0.00	0.00
tricyclene	0.01	0.01	0.01	0.01	0.01
α-thujene	0.36–0.43	0.39	0.39–0.56	0.54	0.55
α-pinene	2.34–2.71	2.44	2.11–2.44	1.96	2.08
camphene	0.11–0.13	0.11	0.07–0.11	0.06	0.06
thuja-2,4(10)-diene	0.01	0.01	tr	tr	tr
sabinene + β-pinene	21.78–25.45	24.33	13.42–13.64	12.41	12.04
6-methyl-5-hepten-2-one	0.01–0.03	0.01	≤0.02	0.06	tr
myrcene	1.26–1.30	1.18	1.47–1.49	1.37	1.43
dehydro-1,8-cineole	tr		tr	tr	tr
decane	tr		tr	tr	tr
α-phellandrene	0.02–0.04	0.03	0.02–0.03	0.02	0.02
δ-3-carene	≤0.01	tr	0.01	0.00	0.01
α-terpinene	0.24–0.35	0.09	0.30	0.31	0.21
p-cymene	0.23–0.39	1.95	0.12–0.20	0.11	0.62
limonene	49.28–49.42	49.38	55.24–56.11	55.17	59.81
(*Z*)-β-ocimene	0.13–0.15	0.13	0.08–0.09	0.04	0.05
(*E*)-β-ocimene	0.38–0.40	0.34	0.17	0.08	0.09
γ-terpinene	7.71–8.04	6.19	13.00	14.51	12.55
terpinolene	0.41–0.49	0.31	0.01	0.66	0.52
Aldehydes					
octanal	0.05–0.07	0.04	0.05	0.04	0.05
nonanal	0.02–0.03	0.02	0.00	0.01	0.01

TABLE 3.5. *Continued*

Compounds	Key Lime		Persian Lime		
	Mexico (A)	Mexico (B)	Mexico (B)	Brazil (B)	Florida (B)
citronellal	0.01	0.03	0.05–0.06	0.04	0.03
decanal	0.20–0.22	0.14	0.06–0.09	0.09	0.07
undecanal	0.02–0.04	0.02	0.01	0.02	0.01
neral	1.06–1.25	1.16	1.16–1.72	1.40	1.11
dodecanal	0.10–0.13	0.08	0.03–0.04	0.05	0.03
tetradecanal	0.05–0.06	0.05	0.03–0.04	0.03	0.05
hexadecanal	0.04–0.07	0.05	0.08–0.09	0.12	0.06
geranial + perilla aldehydes	1.71–2.00	1.97	2.56–2.77	2.33	1.91
Alcohols					
linalool	0.16–0.18	0.17	0.02	0.19	0.16
exo-fenchol	≤0.02	tr	tr	tr	tr
cis-p-menth-2-en-1-ol	0.01–0.02	0.02	≤0.01	0.01	0.01
trans-pinocarveol	0.01–0.02	tr	≤0.01	0.01	0.02
trans-p-menth-2-en-1-ol	≤0.01	0.05	tr	tr	tr
borneol	0.02–0.04	0.02	0.02	0.03	0.01
terpinen-4-ol	0.37–0.71	0.14	0.04–0.11	0.08	0.05
α-terpineol	0.22–0.35	0.21	0.21–0.30	0.36	0.20
nerol	0.02–0.05	0.10	0.06–0.15	0.11	0.07
geraniol	0.03–0.07	0.04	0.03–0.10	0.04	0.02
campherenol	0.05–0.07	0.07	0.05–0.07	0.08	0.06
α-bisabolol	0.07–0.11	0.10	0.07–0.09	0.10	0.08
2,3-dimethyl-3-(4-methyl-3-pentenyl)-2-norbornanol	0.05–0.07	0.07	0.05–0.06	0.07	0.05
Ketones and Oxides					
cis-sabinene hydrate	0.02–0.05	0.01	0.00	0.05	0.03
trans-sabinene hydrate	0.02–0.04	0.02	0.00	0.07	0.04
cis-pinocamphone	0.02	0.02	0.00	0.01	tr
piperitone	tr	tr	tr	tr	tr
Esters					
bornyl acetate	0.01	0.02	≤0.01	0.01	0.01
neryl acetate	0.07–0.09	0.07	0.98–1.15	1.03	0.93
geranyl acetate	0.21–0.29	0.25	0.30–0.31	0.26	0.19

TABLE 3.5. *Continued*

Compounds	Key Lime		Persian Lime		
	Mexico (A)	Mexico (B)	Mexico (B)	Brazil (B)	Florida (B)
Sesquiterpene Hydrocarbons					
dodecane	0.01	0.03	0.01	0.02	0.02
tridecane	0.02–0.03	0.01	tr	0.01	tr
δ-elemene	0.25–0.37	0.07	0.07–0.12	0.04	0.04
β-elemene	0.12–0.22	0.16	0.07–0.09	0.05	0.07
cis-α-bergamotene	0.08–0.10	0.09	0.07–0.08	0.08	0.07
β-caryophyllene	0.96–1.19	0.98	0.67–0.78	0.61	0.48
trans-α-bergamotene	1.13–1.43	1.35	1.08–1.18	1.28	1.06
(*Z*)-β-farnesene	0.01–0.02	0.01	0.01	0.01	0.01
α-humulene	0.10–0.14	0.11	0.06	0.06	0.05
(*E*)-β-farnesene	0.11–0.16	0.12	0.10–0.12	0.12	0.10
β-santalene	0.04–0.06	0.05	0.04–0.05	0.05	0.04
germacrene D	0.26–0.49	0.16	0.10–0.12	0.12	0.07
α-selinene	0.08–0.13	0.08	0.04–0.05	0.04	0.03
(*Z*)-α-bisabolene	0.06–0.21	0.15	0.13–0.14	0.16	0.13
(*E,E*)-α-farnesene + β-bisabolene	2.60–3.79	3.08	1.82–1.99	2.25	1.78
germacrene B	0.45–0.57	0.34	0.15–0.17	0.19	0.11

(A): Type A oil.
(B): Type B oil.

Americas, such as Mexico, Brazil, and U.S.–Florida (Dugo et al., 1997). These data are expressed in relative percentage of peak areas, without taking into account the nonvolatile residue. The authors reported that in the Key lime oil the monoterpene hydrocarbons range from 85% to 88% of the volatile fraction, and the sesquiterpene hydrocarbons go from 6.2% to about 9.0%. The oxygenated compounds represent about 4.7 to 6.0%, among which monoterpene aldehydes were the most abundant, ranging from 2.3 to 3.2%. In Persian lime oil monoterpene hydrocarbons represent 88–90% of the volatile fraction, and sesquiterpene hydrocarbons range from 4 to 5%. Oxygenated compounds represent 5.2 to 7.5%, and monoterpene aldehydes are the most abundant among these components, representing 2.9–4.5%, followed by esters, 1.0–1.5%.

Obviously there was a difference in the composition of the type A and type B oils as seen from the result; this is also in accordance with many analyses for other citrus oils (Shaw, 1979). However, there was no significant difference in volatile composition of lime essential oil from Florida and that from Mexico and Brazil.

3.4 ASIA

3.4.1 China

Masayoshi Sawamura and Xiaolin Yu

China is one of the greatest producers of citrus fruit. The total amount of Chinese production in 2007 was 20,582,000 tons in 1,941,000 hectares. Citrus fruit is commercially produced in 18 provinces of China and its recent production is increased every year, as shown in Table 3.6. Major provinces in which production was more than 2 million tons in 2007 are Hunan, Guangdong, Fujian, Guangxi, Sichuan, and Hubei. The most popular citrus fruit in the world has been sweet orange, with production amounting to 50 million tons in 2006. Brazil produces the greatest volume of this species, followed by the United States, Europe, China, and Mexico. China is the place of origin of sweet orange, whose botanical name *sinensis* refers to China. It is believed that sweet orange was brought into Europe by the Arabs and by Venetian and Portuguese voyagers. Subsequently, many varieties of sweet oranges, such as *Valencia*, navel, blood, and acidless oranges, were bred. Nowadays, China is also one of the countries that mass-produce citrus fruits such as sweet oranges and mandarins. The Chinese generally have a preference for local sweet oranges, which are mostly consumed in the domestic market. Mandarin as a sweet citrus fruit was also born in the center of China. It is said that yuzu (*Citrus junos* Tanaka) as a sour citrus fruit originated in the upper reaches of the Chang Jiang in China. There have been many reports on citrus essential oils and the studies have been reviewed (Shaw, 1979, 1997; Boelens, 1991; Lawrence, 1993; Hugo et al., 1996; Sawamura, 2000; Dugo and Giaccomo, 2002). There are, however, few studies on the essential oil components of citrus fruits in China, although China is a major country of citrus produce (Xiaoyu et al., 1998). The author will here introduce the volatile constituents of several typical varieties of Chinese sweet oranges and mandarins.

Sweet Orange. Four kinds of fresh sweet oranges were obtained in the harvest season, November, in Guagzhou. *Citrus sinensis* Osbeck var. *Hongjian*, called *hong jang chen* in Chinese, and *C. sinensis* Osbeck var. *Anliu*, called *luo gang chen*, were obtained at an orchard in Luo gang in Guangzhou (25 km from the center of Guagzhou). *C. sinensis* Osbeck var. *Sihui*, called *sihui chen*, was harvested at the Shigou Experimental Farm in Sihui City in Guangdong Province (75 km far away from Guangzhou). *C. sinensis* Osbeck var. *Washington navel*, called *qi chen*, which was produced in Jiangxi Province (200 km from Guangzhou; bordering Guangdong Province), was purchased at the wholesale market in Guanzhou. The peel oils were extracted by the cold-pressing method (Sawamura, 2000). A Shimadzu gas chromatograph GC-14A equipped with a flame ionization detector was used. Two capillary columns were used; the first was a DB-Wax column, 60 m × 0.25 mm with a film thickness of 0.25 μm (J&W Scientific, Folsom, CA), and the second was a DB-1 column, 60 m × 0.25 mm

TABLE 3.6. Cultivation area and product of citrus fruits in China

(Unit: (×1000))

Year	2003		2004		2005		2006		2007	
Province	ha	tons	ha	tons	ha	tons	ha	tons	ha	tons
Hunan	260	1,728	276	1,879	296	2,120	314	2,508	326	2,779
Guangdong	150	1,351	176	1,591	196	1,827	225	2,244	244	2,568
Fujian	164	1,944	166	2,068	170	2,153	170	2,267	170	2,386
Guangxi	122	1,521	134	1,719	141	1,877	152	2,055	165	2,347
Sichuan	192	1,862	202	1,988	207	2,137	216	2,058	223	2,325
Hubei	110	1,241	125	1,308	143	1,463	159	1,811	189	2,166
Zhejiang	125	1,767	124	2,010	123	1,481	120	1,805	123	1,987
Jiangxi	186	620	217	844	215	1,098	229	1,394	263	1,957
Chongqing	96	752	98	799	109	909	110	847	114	1,044
Yunnan	25	133	26	166	28	211	29	244	32	281
Shanghai	10	174	11	185	9	180	11	197	11	240
Shanxi	17	99	18	117	20	168	22	163	23	224
Guizhou	34	150	36	158	39	172	37	177	38	191
Jiangsu	3	54	4	48	4	52	5	48	4	47
Henan	8	30	10	35	10	36	10	37	10	38
Hainan	3	15	3	23	4	20	4	27	4	30
Anhui	2	11	2	13	4	12	3	13	3	19
Gansu	0	3	0	3	0	3	0	3	0	3
Total	1,506	13,454	1,627	14,958	1,717	15,919	1,815	17,898	1,941	20,582

with a film thickness of 0.25 μm (J&W Scientific, Folsom, CA). The column temperature was programmed from 70°C (2 min) to 230°C (20 min) at a programmed rate of 2°C/min. The injector and detector temperatures were 250°C. Nitrogen was the carrier gas at a flow rate of 2 mL/min. The compounds were identified by our mass library of GC-MS and retention indices, which were determined for all constituents by using a homologous series of *n*-alkanes (C_7–C_{27}).

The yields of cold-pressed oils from *Hongjian*, *Anliu*, *Sihui*, and *Washington navel* oranges were 0.01%, 0.06%, 0.04%, and 0.04% (weight of oil/weight of fruit), respectively. The oil constituents are presented in Table 3.7. The components are listed in order of their elution on the DB-Wax column. A classification based on functional groups is also summarized there. The methodology for sample preparation and the subsequent analytical conditions have been carefully consistent. The majority of the oil components was limonene, the proportion of which was commonly more than 93%. Thus the quantitative data based on peak relative area percent could be comparable to each other, although an internal standard was not employed in this experiment. Furthermore, each sample was supplied from one of the most popular production areas at the same harvest season. These analytical values are worth characterizing and comparing to each other.

HONGJIAN. This variety has a delicious taste with a good balance of sweet and sour and its flesh is red. The Chinese use it, in general, as a gift in the lunar New Year season because of its superlative quality and high cost. The peel oil composition, consisting of 53 compounds, was nearly the same as in other Chinese orange peel oils as reported in most studies of orange peel oils (Lawrence, 1992; Sawamura, 2000). The most abundant compound was limonene (93.6%) followed by myrcene (2.0%), sabinene (0.7%), α-pinene (0.4%), and β-phellandrene (0.3%). These monoterpene hydrocarbons were found to be present at almost the same level in the four samples analyzed here, and were also nearly equivalent, except for sabinene, to earlier estimates of Valencia orange from Florida (Shaw, 1979; Owusu-Yaw et al., 1986; Boelens, 1991; Lawrence, 1992), Spain (Boelens, 1991), Italy (Boelens, 1991; Verzera et al., 1996), Israel (Boelens, 1991), Japan (Boelens, 1991), Ethiopia (Mitiku et al., 2000), and Vietnam (Minh Tu et al., 2002a), as reported. The sabinene content of *Valencia* oranges has been reported to be 0.2–0.5%. Chinese sweet oranges, however, were found to contain a comparatively high percent of sabinene. The rather higher content of δ-3-carene might be used as an indicator to distinguish sweet orange (*C. sinensis* Osbeck) from bitter orange (*C. aurantium* L.) (Giacomo and Mincione, 1994). This compound was found to be present at more than 0.04% in 164 oil samples of the oils of eight cultivars of Italian sweet orange (Verzera et al., 1996). δ-3-Carene was identified and quantified at a level of 0.1% in all the cold-pressed orange oils from China analyzed here, where the level was in accord with that of Vietnam orange oil, which we reported previously (Minh Tu, 2002a). Valencene, a sesquiterpene, was detected in the range of 0.02–0.41% in Italian *Valencia* orange (Giacomo and Mincione, 1994). According to our previous reports, it was not

TABLE 3.7. Volatile components of Chinese sweet orange and mandarin

Compound	Sweet Orange				Mandarin		
	Hongjian	*Anliu*	*Sihui*	*Washington Navel*	*Ponkan*	*Unhsiu*	*Shatang*
α-pinene	0.4	0.5	0.5	0.5	1.0	0.9	0.5
camphene	*	*	*	*	*	*	*
β-pinene	**	**	**	**	0.4	0.3	**
sabinene	0.7	0.8	0.8	0.7	0.2	0.1	0.8
δ-3-carene	0.1	0.1	0.1	0.1	—	—	—
myrcene	2.0	2.0	2.1	2.0	1.9	1.8	2.1
α-phellandrene	**	**	**	**	**	**	**
α-terpinene	—	—	—	—	0.1	0.1	—
limonene	93.6	94.2	93.6	94.4	88.6	90.0	93.6
β-phellandrene	0.3	0.3	0.3	0.3	0.3	0.3	0.3
(*Z*)-β-ocimene	*	*	*	*	*	*	*
1,8-cineole	nd	*	nd	nd	—	—	—
(*E*)-β-ocimene	**	**	**	0.1	—	—	**
γ-terpinene	—	—	—	—	5.0	3.5	—
p-cymene	*	*	*	nd	0.1	0.1	*
terpinolene	*	0.3	*	*	0.3	0.2	*
octanal	0.4	*	0.2	0.4	0.2	0.1	0.2
tetradecane	nd	nd	*	nd	—	—	—
nonanal	0.1	**	**	**	**	**	**
cis-limonene oxide	*	nd	**	**	**	—	**
trans-limonene oxide	**	**	nd	nd	—	—	nd
citronellal	0.1	0.1	0.1	**	0.1	0.1	0.1
decanal	0.3	0.2	0.1	0.2	0.2	0.2	0.1
linalool	0.7	0.4	0.4	0.4	0.5	0.2	0.4
β-cubebene	*	*	nd	nd	—	—	—
octanol	**	*	**	**	*	*	**
α-cedrene	nd	nd	nd	**	**	*	—
β-elemene	*	nd	*	nd	—	*	—

TABLE 3.7. *Continued*

Compound	Sweet Orange				Mandarin		
	Hongjian	*Anliu*	*Sihui*	*Washington Navel*	*Ponkan*	*Unhsiu*	*Shatang*
terpinen-4-ol	nd	**	nd	nd	—	—	—
β-caryophyllene	**	**	nd	**	—	**	nd
undecanal	**	nd	**	*	—	—	**
(*E*)-β-farnesene	0.1	0.1	**	**	**	—	**
α-humulene	*	nd	nd	*	—	**	nd
neral	0.2	0.2	0.2	0.1	**	**	0.2
terpinyl acetate[a]	**	nd	*	nd	—	—	—
α-terpineol	0.1	0.1	0.1	0.1	0.1	0.1	0.1
dodecanal	0.1	**	**	**	**	**	**
germacrene D	**	**	**	**	0.1	0.2	**
valencene	**	nd	*	nd	—	—	—
neryl acetate	nd	**	nd	**	—	0.1	—
geranial	0.3	0.2	0.2	0.2	**	**	0.2
carvone	nd	nd	nd	**	—	—	—
bicyclogermacrene	nd	nd	nd	*	—	—	—
α-farnesene[b]	0.1	0.1	0.1	**	—	*	—
geranyl acetate	*	*	*	*	—	—	—
β-citronellol	**	**	**	*	0.1	0.1	—
bisabolene	**	*	nd	nd	*	—	—
sesquiphellandrene	**	*	*	nd	—	**	—
cumin aldehyde	*	nd	*	nd	*	—	—
perillaldehyde	**	**	**	*	**	**	—
octadecane	**	nd	nd	nd	—	—	—
cis-carveol	*	nd	nd	*	—	**	—
geraniol	**	**	**	**	—	—	—
isopiperitone	nd	*	nd	*	*	—	nd
nerol	*	*	*	*	—	*	—
perilla alcohol	*	nd	nd	*	—	—	—
dehydrocarveol	nd	**	**	**	—	—	—
(*E*)-2-dodecenal	*	nd	nd	nd	—	—	—

(*Z*)-nerolidol	nd	*	nd	**	—	—	—
(*E*)-nerolidol	*	**	*	nd	*	—	*
limonene diepoxide	**	nd	nd	nd	—	—	—
β-elemol	*	nd	nd	nd	—	—	—
cedrol	*	nd	nd	nd	—	—	—
(*Z,E*)-farnelsol	nd	*	nd	nd	*	—	nd
β-sinensal	**	nd	*	nd	*	—	*
α-sinensal	**	**	nd	**	*	—	nd
Hydrocarbons							
Aliphatics	**	nd	*	nd	—	nd	*
Monoterpenes	97.1	98.2	97.4	98.0	97.9	97.3	97.3
Sesquiterpenes	0.2	0.2	0.1	**	0.1	0.2	0.1
Aldehydes							
Aliphatics	0.9	0.2	0.3	0.6	0.4	0.3	0.3
Terpenes	0.6	0.5	0.5	0.3	0.1	0.1	0.5
Alcohols	0.8	0.5	0.5	0.5	0.7	0.4	0.5
Ketones	nd	nd	nd	**	nd	nd	**
Esters	**	**	*	**	**	0.1	*
Oxides	**	**	**	**	**	**	**
Miscellaneous	nd	*	nd	nd	*	nd	nd
Total	99.6	99.6	98.8	99.4	99.2	98.4	98.6

[a]Correct isomer not identified.
[b]Correct geometrical isomer not identified.
Nd: Not detected.
*: Peak area detected less than 0.005%.
**: Peak area detected not less than 0.005% and less than 0.05%.

appreciably present in the cold-pressed oils from Japan (Dugo et al., 1994), but was detected in Ethiopian (Mitiku et al., 2000) (<0.005%) and Vietnamese (Minh Tu, 2002a) (<0.05%) oils. It was detected in *Hongjian* at a level of <0.05%. Octadecane was detected only in the *Hongjian* oil. The aldehydes were the major composition after the hydrocarbons. As reported in earlier reviews on sweet orange oils (Shaw, 1979; Lawrence, 1992; Mitiku et al., 2000; Sawamura, 2000; Minh Tu, 2002a), octanal and decanal were detected in amounts of 0.4% and 0.3%, respectively. Either α- or β-sinensal was detected at <0.05% as well as in the cold-pressed oils from California, Florida, and Israel (Boelens, 1991). Alcohols have been identified as being the most important contributor to orange flavor (Shaw, 1979; Wolford et al., 1971). In this study, the contents of linalool and α-terpineol were 0.7% and 0.1%, respectively. α-Terpineol is known to be a contributor to off-flavor in stored orange juice (Tatum et al., 1967). This compound was found to be present at the same percent in the four oranges. Citronellol, *cis*-carveol, geraniol, nerol, perilla alcohol, (*E*)-nerolidol, elemol, and cedrol were detected in trace amounts. *cis*- and *trans*-Carveol were the newly identified compounds in sweet orange oils from Ethiopia (Mitiku et al., 2000), but only *cis*-carveol was detected in the cold-pressed oil of *Hongjian* and *Washington* navel oranges. Trace amounts of esters such as terpinyl acetate and geranyl acetate, and oxides such as *cis*- and *trans*-limonene oxides and limonene diepoxide, were detected in *Hongjian*.

Anliu. This variety is one of the most popular sweet oranges in China, having white flesh and a taste that is not so much sour as sweet. For this reason, it may be cheaper than *Hongjian*. Commercially it can be either sold soon after harvest or stored for nearly half a year. As shown in Table 3.6, 45 compounds were identified in *Anliu* cold-pressed oil. The hydrocarbon group accounted for most of the oil (98.4%), while limonene (94.2%) of the 13 monoterpene hydrocarbons (98.2%) accounted for the predominant part, as was also the case in the other oranges. The content of terpinolene (0.3%) was noted, because it was present to a small extent in the other three types of oranges. There were comparatively few sesquiterpenes, and α-cedrene, β-elemene, α-humulene, and valencene were not detected. The total content of aldehydes and alcohols was 1.2%, which was the lowest among the four samples. Octanal is an important flavor substance giving a sweet and citrusy aroma (Minh Tu et al., 2002a), but its content was <0.005% in *Anliu* in comparison to more than 0.2% in the other three oranges. Undecanal, (*E*)-2-dodecenal, and β-sinensal were not detected, either. Linalool was the major compound of the alcohols, whose content of 0.4% was the same as that of *Sihui* and *Washington navel*. According to previous reports (Shaw, 1979; Boelens, 1991; Mitiku et al., 2000; Sawamura, 2000; Minh Tu et al., 2002a), terpinen-4-ol is usually minimally detected in sweet orange oils. It was present at <0.05% in *Anliu* oil, but could not be detected in the other three varieties. Among the miscellaneous substances, 1,8-cineole was found in a trace amount, but it was absent in the other three samples.

SIHUI. Sihui city is one of the famous citrus fruit production districts in China, known for its high quality. The *Sihui* variety has a sweet taste and is usually stored until the following January or February, that is, the lunar New Year season. At least 42 compounds were detected in *Sihui* sweet orange oil. The major hydrocarbon was limonene (93.6%), followed by myrcene (2.1%), sabinene (0.8%), α-pinene (0.5%), and β-phellandrene (0.3%). Tetradecane, an aliphatic hydrocarbon, was detected only in *Sihui* oil. α-Farnesene was predominant in *Sihui* (0.1%) as well as in *Hongjian* and *Anliu*. There were fewer sesquiterpenes in the *Sihui* oil than in the other varieties, except for β-elemene, (*E*)-β-farnesene, germacrene D, valencene, and sesquiphellandrene in a trace amount. The composition of aldehydes and alcohols in *Sihui* was similar to that in *Anliu*.

WASHINGTON NAVEL. The navel orange is very popular, not only in China, but also around the world. This fruit is usually brought to markets soon after the harvest in China. It is said that the navel orange also originated in South China and was subsequently brought to Portugal and then to California, where the *Washington navel* was bred (Hodgson, 1967). The chemical composition of the *Washington navel* orange oil comprised 44 compounds. The proportion of monoterpene hydrocarbons in this variety was almost the same as that in *Hongjian*, *Anliu*, and *Sihui* oranges. The total hydrocarbons including monoterpenes and sesequiterpenes accounted for 98.0% in the absence of aliphatic hydrocarbons. The content of limonene was 94.4%, close to that in our previous data for Japanese *Washington navel* (*C. sinensis* Osbeck forma *Ogawa navel*) cold-pressed oil, 94.0% (Sawamura, 2000). Aliphatic aldehydes such as octanal and decanal were present in greater proportions than terpene aldehydes such as citronellal, neral, and geranial in *Washington navel* (Sawamura, 2000). The contents of octanal and decanal were 0.4% and 0.2%, respectively, just the same as our previous data on the *Washington navel* orange from Japan (Sawamura, 2000). The composition of Japanese *Washington navel* oil prepared by SDE was also similar to that of cold-pressed oil (Sugisawa et al., 1989). α- and β-Sinensal are believed to be characteristic aroma compounds of sweet orange essence. Both sinensals were detected in navel oranges at a level of <0.05% (Sugisawa, 1989; Sawamura, 2000). In the present samples from China, α-sinensal was detected at a level of <0.05% in *Hongjian*, *Anliu*, and *Washington navel*, but β-sinensal was not detected in *Anliu* or *Washington navel*. Neral and geranial were dominant among the terpene aldehydes, which is in agreement with previous reports (Sugisawa, 1989; Sawamura, 2000). Regarding alcohols, the proportions of linalool and α-terpineol were 0.4% and 0.1%, respectively. These data agree with the author's previous data (Sawamura, 2000). Among the ketones, carvone was detected in a trace amount, although it was not detected in the other three types of sweet oranges. The author's group has found either *cis*- or *trans*-limonene oxide in the sweet oranges from China as well as in the *Valencia* oranges from Ethiopia (Mitiku et al., 2000) and from Vietnam (Minh Tu, 2002a). This compound has not been reported in other sweet oranges (Sugisawa, 1989; Usai et al., 1992).

The authors did not detect nootkatone in the present four sweet oranges from China under examination here, as was the case for Japanese (Sawamura, 2000), Ethiopian (Mitiku et al., 2000), and Vietnamese oranges (Minh Tu et al., 2002a), although these results were obtained for other sweet oranges by many researchers (Boelens, 1991; Dugo et al., 1996; Giacomo and Mincione, 1994; Lawrence, 1993; Moshonas and Shaw, 1979; Shaw, 1977; Sugisawa et al., 1989; Verzera et al., 1996; Wolford et al., 1971). The detection of nootkatone may depend on the method of preparation of the essential oil. Preparation of essential oil samples has been always carried out here under the same conditions, without heating, solvents, or evaporation in the process of extraction (Dugo et al., 1994; Sawamura, 2001), in order to obtain consistent oil samples that are as natural as possible.

In conclusion, the peel oil compositions of four kinds of sweet oranges in China, *Citrus sinensis* Osbeck var. *Hongjian*, *C. sinensis* Osbeck var. *Anliu*, *C. sinensis* Osbeck var. *Sihui*, and *C. sinensis* Osbeck var. *Wahington navel*, were investigated by GC and GC-MS. The essential oils were extracted by the cold-pressing method. Between 42 and 53 compounds were quantitatively determined for each variety. Their percentages, respectively, were >97.3%, >98.4%, >97.5%, and >98.0% in hydrocarbons; >1.5%, >0.7%, >0.8%, and >0.9% in total aldehydes; 0.8%, 0.5%, 0.5%, and 0.5% in alcohols. Either *cis*- or *trans*-limonene oxide was detected in a small amount, with *Hongjian* containing both limonene oxides. δ-3-Carene was commonly quantified at a level of 0.1% in all the samples. The content of aliphatic aldehydes, including octanal, nonanal, decanal, and dodecanal, exceeded that of terpene aldehydes such as neral and geranial in *Hongjian* (0.9%) and *Washington navel* (0.6%), whereas the aliphatic aldehydes in *Anliu* and *Sihui* were present to a lesser degree than the terpene aldehydes. Either α- or β-sinensal was detected in trace amounts in each of the four samples. Linalool was the major alcohol in all of the samples. Nootkatone was not detected.

Mandarin. The place of origin of mandarins is said to be around Assam, the northwest region of India. They say *Citrus indica*, the most primitive species, and its various mutants are still found there. After some of them were brought into China, the species of mandarin or tangerine developed enormously. *C. reticulata* covers all the varieties of mandarins or tangerines as a scientific name classified by Swingle. *C. unshiu* or Satsuma mandarin, which was brought to Japan and improved, is now one of the biggest commercial citrus fruits in the world, along with orange and grapefruit. On the other hand, the mandarins or tangerines introduced to the Mediterranean countries bore other popular mandarins such as Mediterranean mandarins and *Clementine* in Europe, and *Dancy* tangerine in the United States. *Ponkan* is said to have originated from the district Suntala, India, and moved to China around the tenth century. It was introduced into Japan in the nineteenth century. The common property of *C. reticulata* is that the fruit can be easily peeled and its taste is a good balance of sweetness and sourness. Today *C. reticulata* is widely cultivated all over the world. Sawamura (2000) has studied the compositions of essential oils of several mandarin types from Japan, Vietnam, and Kenya. There has been little compositional information on Chinese mandarins as well as oranges. This section will deal with volatile components of some Chinese mandarins. Three kinds of fresh mandarins were obtained in the harvest season in Guagzhou. *Citrus unshiu* Marcovitch was purchased at the wholesale market, Tian ping ja, in Guanzhou, and was produced in Jiangxi Province (200 km from Guangzhou; bordering Guangdong Province). *C. reticulata* Blanco var. *Ponkan* was obtained at an orchard in Luo gang in Guangzhou (25 km from the center of Guagzhou). *C. reticulata* Blanco var. *Shatang* was harvested at the Shigou Experimental Farm in Sihui City in Guangdong Province (75 km from Guangzhou).

The yields of cold-pressed oils from *Unshiu*, *Ponkan*, and *Shatang* mandarins were 0.02%, 0.05%, 0.04%, and 0.04% (weight of oil/weight of fruit), respectively. The mean weight of the fruit was 117 g, 194 g, and 31 g, respectively. The oil constituents are presented in Table 3.6. The major oil component was limonene, of which the proportion was commonly more than 88.6%. The quantitative data based on peak relative area percent could be comparable to the previous data by Sawamura (2000), because the oil extraction method and the GC conditions are almost the same. Furthermore, each sample was supplied from one of the most popular production areas and at the same harvest season. These analytical values are worth characterizing and comparing to each other.

UNSHIU. This variety is very popular and it does not cost so much in China. As shown in Table 3.6, the major component was limonene (90.0%), followed by γ-terpinene (3.5%). According to the previous report on *C. unshiu* var. *Okitsu-wase*, which is the most popular Satsuma mandarin in Japan, the proportions of limonene and γ-terpinene were 89.3% and 4.0%. The composition of other monoterpene hydrocarbons was also similar to that of *Okitsu-wase*, except β-phellandrene (Sawamura, 2000). The level of β-phellandrene was higher (0.3%) than that of *Okitsu-wase* (trace amount). Among sesquiterpene hydrocarbons, α-farnesene and germacrene D were noticeable (0.3%). However, β-elemene was not detected, although it was detected at a level of 0.7%. Decanal is one of the characteristic compounds of mandarins. The level of Chinese *unshiu* was as much as 0.2%. Other aldehydes such as octanal, nonanal, and citronellal in *unshiu* were comparable to *Okitsu-wase*. Linalool is a commonly important component of essential oils presenting a floral odor. Its proportion was 0.2%. In the previous paper, nonanal and decanal were not detected in Korean and Japanese Satsuma mandarin (*Miyagawa-wase*). According to GC-O of the Satsuma mandarin it is suggested that the sweet and fruity flavor of Korean mandarin resulted from terpinolene and linalool, and the herbaceous note of Japanese mandarin resulted from α-humullene, neral, *l*-carvone, and perillaldehyde. These organoleptic analyses did not seem to be important in the aldehydes, such as octanal, nonanal, and decanal.

PONKAN. This variety is one of the most popular mandarins in Southeast Asian countries, particularly in tropical zones like Taiwan, having a good aroma and a taste that is more sweet than sour. The Chinese and Japanese store it, in general, for a few months after harvest in November to reduce the acidity. It is intended to be sold in the lunar New Year season in China. The proportion of *Ponkan* essential oil components shown in Table 3.6 was similar to the result reported previously (Sawamura, 2000). The peel oil composition consisted of 54 compounds. The hydrocarbon group accounted for most of the oil (98.0%), while limonene (88.6%) of the 13 monoterpene hydrocarbons (97.9%) accounted for the predominant part, as was also the case in the other mandarins (*Unshiu* and *Shatang*). The levels of limonene (88.6%) and sabinene (0.2%) of Chinese *Ponkan* (88.6%) was less than those of Japanese Ponkan (89.9% and 0.6%, respectively). The total content of aliphatic aldehydes (0.9%) such as octanal, nonanal, and decanal, was noted, because it was present to a small extent in the other types of mandarins.

SHATANG. The taste of *Shatang* is very sweet and it is a favorite mandarin for the Chinese. As shown in Table 3.6, the major component was limonene (93.6%), followed by myrcene (2.1%), sabinene (0.8%), and α-pinene (0.5%). Although γ-terpinene is one of the common compounds in citrus essential oils, it was not detected in *Shatang* or in *Clementine*. These varieties would be rare in the sense of γ-terpinene content. The proportion of neral and geranial (0.2%), on the other hand, was predominant compared to that of *Ponkan* and *Unshiu*. These two aldehydes seem to be characteristic in *Shatang*, because their content is trace or nothing in mandarin oils (Sawamura, 2000). The level of sesquiterpenes was commonly low in these three varieties.

3.4.2 Indonesia

C. Hanny Wijaya

Citrus species are commonly known by Indonesians especially as table fruits and juices. Citrus plants are also widely used as spices/herbs as well as medical treatments (Rukmana, 2000; Sunarjono, 2008). As in many other countries, there are various citrus species available in Indonesia, including oranges, mandarins, pummelos, citrons, lemons, limes, and kumquats. Some citrus species have been recognized and cultivated by Indonesian people, that is, citruses locally named as "Jeruk keprok" and its family (*Citrus nobilis* Lour.); "Jeruk manis" and its family (*Citrus aurantium* Linn.); "Jeruk sitrun" and is family (*Citrus medica* Linn.); "Jeruk besar" (*Citrus maxima* Merr.); "Jeruk grapefruit" (*Citrus paradisi* Macf.); "Jeruk kasturi" (*Citrus mitis* Blanco); "Jeruk sambal" (*Citrus amblycarpa* Hassk.); "Jeruk purut" (*Citrus hystrix* D. C.); and "Kamquat" (*Fortunella japonica Thunb*) (Sarwono, 1994; Sunarjono, 2008).

There are also several different varieties or cultivars in each species; for example, "Jeruk keprok" (*Citrus nobilis* Lour.) includes "Jeruk mandarin" (*Citrus nobilis* var. *chrysocarpa*), "Jeruk siam" (*Citrus nobilis* var. *microcarpa*), " Jeruk jepun" (*Citrus nobilis* var. *typica*), and "Jeruk keprok Satsuma" (*Citrus nobilis* var. *reticulata*) (Sarwono, 1994). Moreover, "Jeruk siam" itself is known by several names pertaining to the region where it was cultivated, such as "Jeruk pontianak" or "Jeruk tebas," "Jeruk garut," "Jeruk madang," "Jeruk medan," "Jeruk jatibarang," "Jeruk kroya," "Jeruk palembang," and so on (Sarwono 1994; Tim Penulis, 2007). At least 160 cultivars of citrus are cultivated throughout Indonesia (Maryoto, 2004). The citrus diversity in Indonesia might be related to the report of Webber et al. (1967), which stated that the various species of the genus *Citrus* are believed to have originated from the tropical and subtropical regions of Asia and the Malay archipelago (Fellers, 1985).

Some local *Citrus* (Jeruk) have been newly developed in Indonesia. Some outstanding varieties are "Jeruk keprok garut," "tejakula," "soe," "siompu," "keprok kacang," "Jeruk besar sikoning," "bali," "Jeruk manis punten," "batu," "betawi," and "Madura," but these varieties have not been released yet; several further steps are needed. Qualified varieties can be released by the assessment team and National Cultivar Center—Ministry of Agriculure if then pass judgment as CVPD free and virus free. Some other important citrus species (although the economic value is low) are "Jeruk RI," "Jeruk JC," "Jeruk tonsil" (*Poncirus trifoliate*), "Jeruk uwik" (*C. cleopatra*), and "Jeruk tanum" (*C. aurantium*) (Sunarjono, 2008).

Indonesian citruses are not only fulfilling national consumption needs but are also exporting commodities. The fruit production increased significantly in 2002. The total production of all citruses during 2001–2002 reached 691.4 tons and 968.1 tons. In the same timeframe, citrus export also increased sharply. The total export quantity in 2001 reached 1919.7 tons, while in 1998 it was only 408.3 tons (Biro Pusat Statistik, 2002; Sunarjono, 2008). The local citrus trading in Indonesia, however, is currently highly displaced by imported citrus.

To strengthen local citrus development, a three-year (2008–2011) ACIAR-funded project regarding market development for citrus from eastern Indonesia, with the specific objective of using "Jeruk keprok" as a model for developing awareness of quality parameters, product differentiation, and the importance of careful post-harvest handling, and of introducing and fostering market-driven business practices in the "Jeruk keprok" supply chain, thereby forging a stronger link between farmers and the marketplace, has been conducted by Taverner and team (ACIAR, 2008). Among important citrus-producing regions in Indonesia are Garut, Batu, Pujon, Tebas, Samarinda, Soe, Molo, Punten, Tawangmagu, Brastagi, Selayar, Jambi, and Solok (Sunarjono, 2008).

Utilization of citrus flavors in food products is also popular. Usage as flavorings can be in its original form—juice (extract), or essential oil. The utilized parts of the plant are not only the fruit but also the leaves, such as in "Jeruk purut." Due to hybridization, there are many varieties of citrus in Indonesian regions that have distinct flavors and are known only by locals (Dharmawan et al., 2008).

Reports on locally known citrus volatile components, more prominently the active-flavor components, are still very limited. Based on this writer's knowledge and on literature studies, there are two kinds of citrus that have intensively been investigated regarding their volatiles, that is, the fruit of "Jeruk pontianak" and the leaf of "Jeruk purut."

Jeruk pontianak (*Citrus nobilis* Lour. var. *microcarpa* Hassk.). "Jeruk pontianak," known also as "Jeruk tebas," is actually included in the "Jeruk siam" family (*Citrus nobilis* var. *microcarpa* Hassk.). According to Sarwono (1994), this species originated in Thailand (Siam), and it entered West Kalimantan in 1936, being cultivated first in the Tebas region. The pioneers were Yung Kung, Bung Kim, and Bong Kim In from Segaran village. In 1944, it was expanded by H. A. Rani and Lim Kim Sin in Bekut village and its surroundings. In 1955, this citrus species was expanded into thousands of hectares of cultivation land in the Tebas region.

The characteristics of this fruit are its thin and a bit sticky skin (difficult to be detached from its fruit pulp), round shape, and smaller size than "Jeruk keprok," which has a thick skin. The fruit pulp is soft in texture, containing a lot of water and having a sweet taste with a nice aroma. The skin is fairly thin, shiny, and yellowish-green-colored (Tim Penulis, 2007) (Figure 3.6). According to Sunarjono (2008), as one of the "Jeruk siam," this citrus is better if cultivated in lowland. The change in skin color depends on the intensity of sunlight exposure. When cultivated in humid lowland with less sunlight exposure, it will maintain its green color even if the fruit has matured already.

This "siam" cultivar is well known by Indonesians due to its distinct sweetness. It is assumed that the market demand for "Jeruk siam" is approximately 60% of all Indonesian citrus. The export potential of this cultivar has not been optimally developed. The main export destinations are Singapore, Taiwan, and

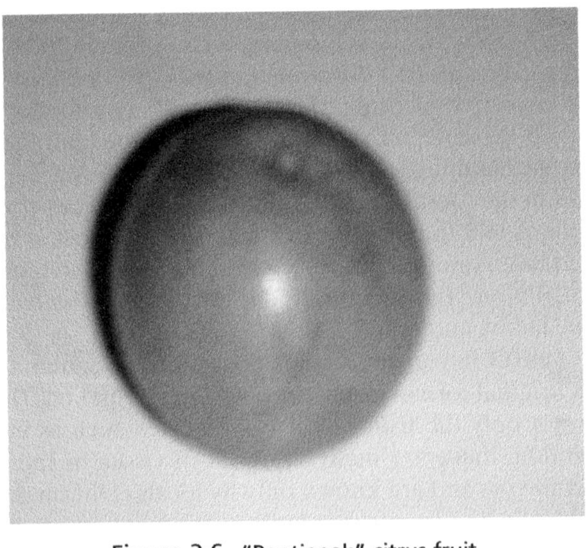

Figure 3.6. "Pontianak" citrus fruit.

Hong Kong. Besides Asian countries, this species is also exported to Holland, France, Belgium, and Luxemburg, although not in significant quantities (Tim Penulis, 2007).

Characterization studies of the volatile compounds in Pontianak juice and peel oil have been undertaken by several groups of researchers. In 1995, Nugroho extracted and characterized the peel oil of Pontianak by the cold-pressed method and reported that limonene and myrcene comprised around 95% and 2.4% of the volatile compounds, respectively. This finding is reconfirmed by Dharmawan et al. (2008), which reported that the major compound of Pontianak peel oil was limonene (96.3%), followed by myrcene (2.0%). Moreover, Dharmawan et al. (2008) also reported several other compounds that were not previously reported, that is, α-thunjene, camphene, α-camphene, α-phellandrene, γ-terpinene, terpinolene, limonene oxide, carvone, perrillaldehyde, and α-copaene. Thirty-two compounds were detected in Pontianak peel oil and they are mainly terpenes, esters, alcohols, and carbonyl compounds (Dharmawan et al., 2008). The absence of some important contributor compounds to the mandarin family such as thymol and methyl-*N*-methyl anthranilate (MNMA) (Shaw, 1991) in "Jeruk pontianak" shows that this citrus is a mandarin with a unique characteristic flavor.

The characterization of volatiles in freshly squeezed Pontianak citrus juice has been conducted by Dharwawan et al. (2007). The volatiles from the headspace of the Pontianak juice were isolated by solid-phase microextraction (SPME) prior to separation with a gas chromatograph (GC) and identification by mass spectrometry (MS). There were 51 volatiles that could be characterized in freshly squeezed Pontianak citrus juice. Similar to other citrus cultivars, limonene was the major compound (almost 90% of the total volatiles) present in the Pontianak juice. The other major contributors to citrus-like flavor (Ahmed et al., 1978) were octanal, decanal, linalool, ethyl butyrate, acetaldehyde, citral, citronellal, dodecanal, limonene, myrcene, nonanal, α-pinene, and (*E*)-2-hexenal. Similar to the peel oil, even though Pontianak is a mandarin, except for β–pinene and γ-terpinene the rest of the important flavor contributors of mandarin (thymol, MNMA, and α-sinensal) were not found in Pontianak citrus juice.

The identification of aroma-active compounds in Pontianak citrus peel oil has been initiated by Fischer et al. (2008). Further studies have been conducted by Dharmawan et al. (2009). Forty-one aroma-active volatiles were characterized by using gas chromatography–olfactometry (GC-O) and aroma extract dilution analysis (AEDA) techniques. The aroma-active compounds of Pontianak citrus peel oil are shown in Table 3.8. The main identified compounds are dominated by saturated and unsaturated aldehydes with FD factors from 16 to 512, such as nonanal, decanal, undecanal, (*Z*)-5-dodecanal, and (*E*,*Z*)-2,6,dodecadienal. (*Z*)-5-Dodecanal has rarely been reported in citrus fruits.

The compounds having the highest FD factor (2048) were α-pinene, β-pinene, linalool, 2-methoxy-3-(2-methylpropyl) pyrazine, and a few unknown compounds; those exhibited woody, metallic, green, earthy, sulfuric, and citrus-like odor quality. Limonene, which is the most abundant compound exhibited an FD factor of 1024.

TABLE 3.8. Aroma-active compounds (FD ≥ 2) in "Pontianak" citrus peel oil

Peak No.	RI[a]	Compound[b]	Odor Quality[c]	FD[d]
1	963	α-pinene	woody, piney, citrusy	2048
2	1003	β-myrcene	sulfury, mango-like, metallic	128
3	1014	β-pinene	metallic, citrusy, woody	2048
4	1059	limonene	orange-like, fruity	1024
5	1114	linalool	floral, green	2048
6	1120	nonanal	soapy, aldehydic	128
7	1160	1-phenylethyl mercaptan[e]	tarry, sulfury	256
8	1166	citronellal	lemongrass-like	128
9	1170	(*E,Z*)-2-6-nonadien-1-ol	cucumber-like	64
10	1174	(*E*)-2-nonenal	melon-like, fatty	256
11	1181	1-nonanol	fresh, green	4
12	1187	camphor	fruity, green, grassy	128
13	1193	2-metoxy-3-(2-methylpropyl) pyrazine[e]	chili-like-peppery	2048
14	1203	unknown	earthy, tarry, sulfury	2048
15	1208	unknown	citrusy, soapy	512
16	1211	4-terpineol	floral, fresh	8
17	1218	decanal	soapy, aldehydic	512
18	1228	unknown	sweet, floral	128
19	1229	unknown	earthy	2048
20	1236	citronellol	citrusy, fruity	64
21	1240	nerol	citrusy, roselike	8
22	1246	*trans*-carveol	sulfury, fruity	2
23	1255	neral	floral, green	2
24	1260	geraniol	fruity, citrusy	128
25	1271	L-carvone	minty	256
26	1276	(*E*)-2-decenal	fatty, aldehydic	16
27	1279	1-decanol	fresh, floral	2
28	1284	geranial	lemon-like	8
29	1309	perilla aldehyde	almond-like, floral	64
30	1319	undecanal	soapy, aldehydic	128
31	1335	(*E,E*)-2,4-decadienal	fatty, oily	256
32	1344	unknown	earthy	64
33	1353	unknown	floral, green	2048
34	1365	neryl acetate	green, citrusy	4
35	1379	unknown	floral	256
36	1393	geranyl-acetate	citrusy	2
37	1405	(*Z*)-5-dodecenal	soapy, citrusy	128
38	1421	dodecanal	soapy, aldehydic	128
39	1465	(*E,Z*)-2,6-dodecadienal	fruity, soapy	256
40	1482	(*E*)-2-dodecenal	fatty, citrusy	512
41	1490	unknown	oily, creamy	128

[a]Experimental linear retention index on a DB5-MS column.
[b]The compound was identified by comparing its retention time and mass spectrum with the reference standard.
[c]Odor quality perceived through the sniffing port.
[d]FD factor of the odor-active compound.
[e]The MS signal was too weak for interpretation. The compound was identified based on similar odor quality perceived at the sniffing port and the retention time of its odor detection with the standard compound.

Source: Dharmawan et al. (2009).

In addition, the previously reported compound (Fischer et al., 2008), 1-penylethyl mercaptan, with an FD factor of 246, has also been found. The odor of this compound was described as sulfurous and resinous, resembling that of the whole fruits, and was reported to be part of the composition of the Pontianak citrus oil (Ficher et al., 2008; Dharmawan et al., 2009). Both 1-penylethyl mercaptan and (*Z*)-5-dodecanal were documented to have unique characteristics contributing to the flavor of Pontianak citrus oil.

Based on the GC-O results, an odor-activity value (OAV) and relative flavor activity (RFA) can be determined for an aroma model reconstitution (Buettner and Schieberle, 2001; Choi et al., 2001; Sawamura et al., 2004; Dharmawan et al., 2009). A model solution derived from AOV resembling the original aroma of the peel oil for the green, fatty, fresh, peely, floral, and tarry attributes has been developed by Dharmawan et al. (2009). The synthetic blend has been judged by the panelists as being closest to Pontianak oil. The result of the omission test verified the significance of (*Z*)-5-dodecenal and 1-phenyl mercaptan as key compounds in the aroma of Pontianak citrus peel oil (Dharmawan et al., 2009).

***Jeruk purut (Citrus hystrix* D. C.).** "Jeruk purut" (Indonesian) or "Kaffir limoen" (Dutch) is also included in the Rutaceae family (Katzer, 1998). The fruit is smaller than a human fist, pear-like in shape, having thick skin and a lot of wrinkles, and it contains essential oils that give a nice aroma (Figure 3.7). The fruit pulp is green-yellowish in color, sour in taste, and sometimes gives a bitter taste (Sarwono, 1994). The leaves are broadly oval to oval-oblong shaped, blunt edged, and have one petiole. The leaves have wide foliage that is greenish-yellow, and have a nice, fresh aroma (Sarwono, 1994) (Figure 3.7).

Known as Indonesian lime, "Jeruk purut" (*Citrus hystrix* D. C.) is one of the citrus plants that is widely used as natural flavoring in various foods and beverages in Indonesia and other Asian countries (Sato et al., 1990; Mohammad, 1992; Anonim, 2009). The leaves of "Jeruk purut," called "Som makrut" in Thailand, "Suwangi limau" or "Purut limau" in Malaysia, and "Daun jeruk purut" in Indonesia, are utilized to give the unique oriental flavor to "tom yam" soup,

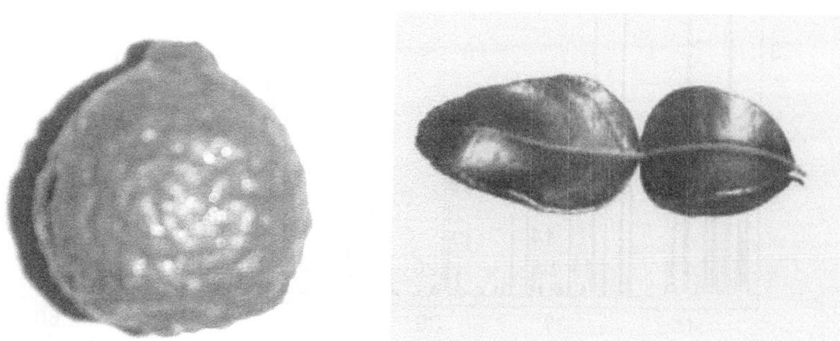

Figure 3.7. Fruit and leaf of kaffir lime.

curries, "laksa," and many other cuisines, cookies, and cakes. Besides as flavoring agents, the purut leaves are also utilized as a main ingredient in traditional medicines and are even used in some Malaysian traditional ceremonies (Mohammad, 1992).

The common names in English are Indonesian lime, Indonesian lime leaves, Kaffir lime, Makrut lime, Mauritius papeda, and Porcupine orange, Thai Mai makrut, Thai lime, or Wild lime (Anonim, 2009). According to Pudil et al. (1998), the flavor of "Jeruk purut" leaves extract is similar to that typical of citrus flavors, but it is harsher, reminding the panelists of citrus leaves, and almost unknown in the European countries.

In Indonesia, the fruit of "Jeruk purut" is utilized as cooking flavoring to diminish the stinking odor in fish. However, the fruit of "Jeruk purut" is mainly used for cleaning mixtures and body treatments instead of being food material (Sarwono, 1994).

Investigation of "Jeruk purut" oil composition already has been reported by several authors (Lawrence et al., 1971; Sato et al., 1990; Wijaya, 1995; Jantan et al., 1996; Pudil et al., 1996). It was reported that the oil mainly contains citronellal, citronellol, and nerol. Sato et al. (1990) have confirmed citronellal in the L-form as a principal component of the oil. The compilation of composition of "Jeruk purut" oil published by Pudil et al. (1996) can be seen in Table 3.7. More than 30 constituents were characterized in the oil. Besides the main compounds, pinene, sabinene, terpinen-4-ol, linalool, *p*-menthen-3-ol, and citronellyl acetate were among the compounds found in the essential oil. A review of the oil constituents has been written by Lawrence (1993).

It is commonly known that essential oil of citrus is sensitive to oxidation. Pudil et al. (1998) have studied the changes of "Jeruk purut" essential oil during

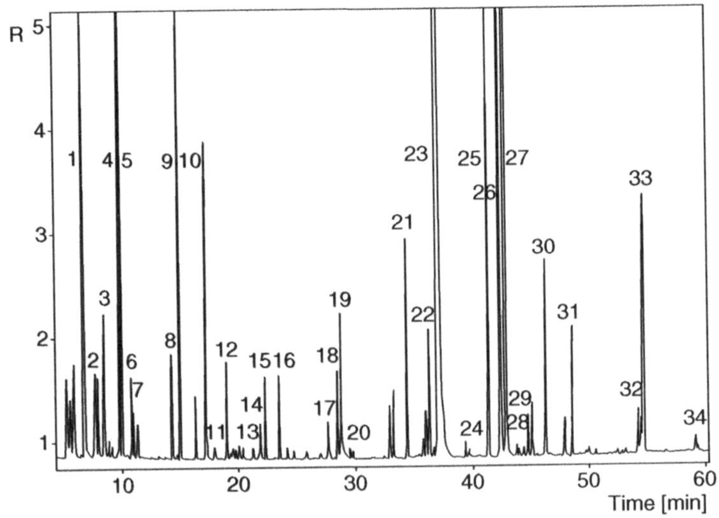

Figure 3.8. GLC headspace analysis of slightly oxidized kaffir lime oil (Pudil et al. 1998).

auto-oxidation. A gas chromatogram of slightly oxidized oil and the main identified components of the slightly oxidized oil are shown in Figure 3.8 and Table 3.9, respectively. During auto-oxidation under simulated storage conditions, the content of citronellal decreased rapidly, and followed the first-order reaction kinetics. Typical oxidation products of monoterpenes represented the main oxidation products. Based on sensory evaluation, however, the odor characteristic is affected marginally. Sensory profiles of "Jeruk purut" oil stored during different periods is shown in Figure 3.9.

The study has also reported that an added antioxidant, such as rosemary extract or 1,4-dihydropyridines, not only inhibits the oxidation but also influences the composition of oxidation products (Pudil et al., 1998). The formation of acetone and linalool oxides was efficiently inhibited by the rosemary extract, but both 1,4-dihydropyridines (Diludine and OSI 7284) were ineffective. In the formation of *p*-mentha-1,4(8)-diene and *p*-ment-8-en-ol, however, the 1,4-dihydropyridines showed moderate antioxidant activity.

Furthermore, the study reported the utilization possibilities of the oxidized oils. Based on the sensory panel's opinion, the application of oxidized "Jeruk purut" oil (24 months stored) will be best in cosmetic or daily-care products, although some foods still could be successfully flavored as well. The reverse ranking was found for the shorter-stored oil (3 months), which showed it will be more suitable in foods. The area of application seems to depend on the actual chemical composition and thus the aroma profile of the oil.

A series of studies regarding the possibility of producing a flavoring agent that is more practical in its utilization and has longer shelf-life have been conducted by Wijaya and team (Wijaya, 1995; Wijaya et al., 2000; Wijaya and Apriyantono, 2003). Five methods of extraction have been applied in the liquid flavor preparation: (1) simultaneous distillation-extraction (Likens-Nickerson); (2) steam distillation; (3) water distillation; (4) maceration; and (5) percolation. The simultaneous distillation-extraction (Likens-Nickerson) method provided the best aroma. However, except in the extract of percolation, in terms of sensory quality, there was no significant difference among the obtained extracts. The water distillation extract gave the highest yield.

Pilot plant research has been further conducted in order to study the distillation parameters in producing "Jeruk purut" essential oil in maximum extract yield and preferable sensory quality (Wijaya et al., 2000). The research results showed that the essential oils obtained from sliced "Jeruk purut" leaves were fresher. Chopping treatment increased the acid number and reduced the percentage of citronellal. The height of the material in the distillation kettle has positive correlation to the yield, but shows no relationship to the density, the refractive index, or the solubility index of the oil. Recommended distillation parameters that give an optimum physicochemical quality, sensory acceptability, and the lowest cost prediction have been reported.

According to Wijaya (1995), the best "Jeruk purut" flavor powder can be produced by encapsulating the water-distilled oil in the mixture of gum Arabic–maltodextrin as carrier and spray-drying. Addition of proper anti-caking and

TABLE 3.9. Main identified components of slightly oxidized kaffir lime oil

Peak No.	RT (min)	RI	Indentification	Note
1	6.63	825	acetone	
2	7.61	891	methanol	
3	8.37	934	ethanol	
4	9.79	989	chloroform	air contamination
5	10.01	1000	n-decane	internal standard
6	10.83	1023	α-pinene	
7	11.00	1028	α-phellandrene	
8	14.27	1107	β-pinene	
9	14.94	1123	β-phellandrene	
10	17.16	1166	β-myrcene	
11	17.99	1182	α-terpinene	
12	19.05	1198	limonene	
13	21.25	1240	*cis*-ocimene	
14	21.85	1255	γ-terpinene	
15	22.29	1257	*trans*-ocimene	
16	23.46	1274	*p*-mentha-1.4(8)-diene	
17	27.69	1342	3-hydroxycyclopentanone	
18	28.53	1356	4-methyl-(2-methyl-1-propenyl)-tetrahydropyrane	
19	28.84	1361	2,2,6 -trimethylcyclohexanone	
20	29.61	1371	octahydro-3A -methyl-*cis*-2*H*-inden-2-one	
21	34.51	1446	*cis*-linalool oxide	
22	36.39	1475	*trans*-linalool oxide	
23	37.15	1485	citronellal	
24	39.79	1528	sesquiterpene	2-cubebene (tentative)
25	41,40	1552	linalool	
26	42.42	1568	*p*-menth-8-en-3-ol	unidentified
27	42.89	1575	*p*-menth-8-en-3-ol	unidentified
28	43.86	1590	sesquiterpene	caryophyllene (tentative)
29	44.43	1599	terpinen-4-ol	
30	46.33	1617	citronellyl formate	
31	48.61	1636	citronellyl acetate	
32	54.33	1681	geranyl acetate	
33	54.76	1684	citronellol	
34	59.23	1840	sesquiterpene	nerolidol (tentative)

Source: Pudil et al. (1998).

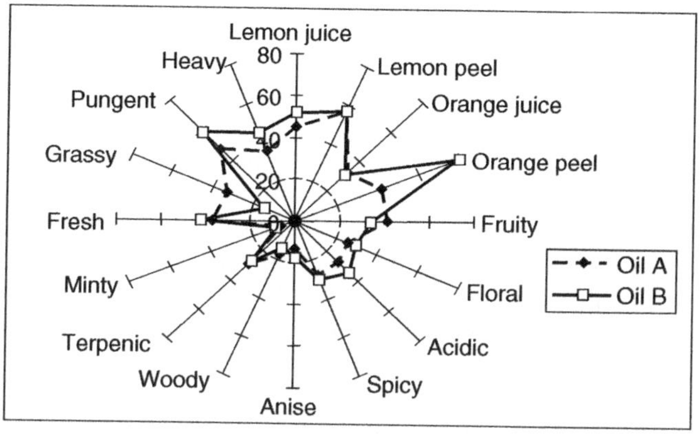

Figure 3.9. Odor profiles of important components of *Citrus hystrix* oil. A: stored 24 months at −15°C. B: stored 3 months at −15°C (Pudil et al. 1998).

packaging will extend the shelf-life of the flavor powder up to three years (prediction test). The sensory evaluation results showed that until six weeks' storage no deviation in flavor couled be detected and the flavor was still acceptable to the panelists.

Closing Remarks. There are still many locally developed cultivars, species, or subspecies such as Cinakonde, Batu, and Pulung from *C. reticulata* Blanco; Nambangan, Sambas, and Sri Nyonya from *C. maxima* Merr.; and Pacitan, Kupang, and Punten from *C. sinensis* Osbeck (Hardiyanto et al., 2007) that have not yet been investigated on their flavor profiles. There is still a challenge to obtain more information regarding the odor-active compounds of citrus families in Indonesia. Even though it has not played its role optimally yet, information on citrus in Indonesia can be accessed through the web address for "Masyarakat Jeruk Indonesia (Indonesian Citrus Society)," http://www.citrus-indonesia.com, or via e-mail at mji@citrus-indonesia.com.

3.4.3 Japan

Nguyen Thi Lan-Phi and Masayoshi Sawamura

Citrus fruits are the most popular fruits in the world; they have a pleasant aroma and taste, and are a source of vitamin C. There are a great number of *Citrus* varieties widely distributed around the world, of which *Citrus unshiu* or Satsuma mandarin is the major fruit among those produced in Japan. Other fruit varieties grown in Japan are tachibana (*C. tachibana* Tanaka), kumquat (*Fortunella*), ichang-papeda (*C. ichangensis*), lime (*C. aurantifolia*), lemon (*C. limon*), sweet oranges (*C. sinensis*), bitter/sour oranges (*C. aurantium*), mandarins (*C. reticulata* Blanco), pummelos (*C. grandis* Osbeck), and grapefruits (*C. paradisi*). Many of these fruits are of Chinese origin, but have been modified or specially bred for cultivation in Japan. Citrus fruits are used not only as a Vitamin C daily supplement, but also for extraction of essential oil, the most popular source of many perfumes and fragrance essences. The essential oil is extracted from the outer part of the peel containing volatile aroma compounds that contribute to the unique aroma of each citrus fruit. A great number of studies on the volatile compounds of Japanese citrus essential oil have been carried out (Sawamura, 2000). The results indicate that the different citrus varieties have different volatile compound profiles. Therefore, the aim of this section is to summarize and clarify the volatile composition of Japanese citrus essential oils that have been studied so far.

Tachibana (C. tachibana). Tachibana is said to be native to south-western Japan and is believed to be one of the oldest citrus species in Japan. The peel oil has a sweet, green, juicy and mandarin-like odor (Ubukata et al., 2002). The main components of Tachibana oil (see Table 3.10) are limonene (80.12%), γ-terpinene (8.07%), myrcene (2.66%) and linalool (2.03%) (Sawamura, 2000). A similar composition was also reported by Ubukata et al. (2002), though linalool content (9.13%) exceeded its level in common citrus peel oils. The lower level of limonene (63.2–76.8%), a higher amount of γ-terpinene (8.5–13.1%), and a wide range of linalool content (0.8–5.1%) were quantified in tachibana oil from Shizuoka, Tokushima, and Kochi prefectures (Fujita et al., 2005).

Ichang-Papeda (C. ichangensis). Although they belong to the same species as classified by Swingle, the volatile components of hanayu, kabosu, yuko, mochiyu, sudachi, naoshichi, yuzu, and seedless yuzu peel oils exhibit different characteristics. The characteristic of this group is having a low level (less than 0.5%) of aldehydes and esters, where sesquiterpene hydrocarbons, made up mostly of *trans*-β-farnesene, and alcohol (by linalool) were predominant in the remaining group besides monoterpene hydrocarbons (91.6–98.7%).

Yuzu (*Citrus junos* Sieb. ex Tanaka) is the most well-known among almost 70 sour citrus cultivars in Japan. Due to its distinctive flavor and wide uses, yuzu has attracted many researchers (Tajima et al., 1990; Njoroge et al., 1994a, 1996b; Song et al., 1999; Song et al., 2000; Sawamura, 2000, 2005; Sawamura et al., 2006; Lan Phi and Sawamura, 2008; Miyazato et al., 2008; Lan Phi et al., 2009; Miyazawa et al., 2009) to study its chemical composition and aroma. As in the other citrus fruits, the main component of yuzu is limonene (60–70%). The results published for more than 70% of limonene were the relative percentage of peak areas. Other major compounds in yuzu oil are γ-terpinene, β-phellandrene, and myrcene. Besides monoterpene hydrocarbons, alcohols and sesquiterpene hydrocarbons predominate in the volatile fraction of yuzu peel oil. A recent study has concluded that yuzu peel oil contains (*E*)-non-6-enal and (6*Z*,8*E*)-undeca-6,8,10-trien-3-one (Yuzunone), which were not identified in the peel of other citrus species, and (6*Z*,8*E*)-undeca-6,8,10-trien-4-ol (Yuzuol) was identified for the first time in nature (Miyazawa et al., 2009).

Naoshichi (*C. taguma-sudachi* Hort. ex Y. Tanaka) is a large, sour citrus fruit with an average weight of 18–25 g/fruit (6–8 cm in diameter). Hydrocarbons made up for more than 99% of the total oil, particularly limonene (>90%), and *trans*-β-farnesene content was reported much higher than in other sour citrus fruits. Most of the oxygenated components are present in trace amounts (less than 0.1%), where the two straight-chain aliphatic aldehydes, decanal (0.3%) and octanal (0.1%), were prominent (Njoroge et al., 1996a). The oil contains up to 98% of monoterpene hydrocarbons made up mostly of limonene, γ-terpinene, myrcene, and α-pinene.

The chemical compositions of kabosu (*C. sphaerocarpa* Hort. ex Tanaka), yuko (*C. yuko* Hort. ex Tanaka) (Njoroge et al., 1994b; Minh Tu et al., 2002b), mochiyu (*C. inflata* Hort. ex Tanaka), and sudachi (*C. sudachi* Hort. ex Shirai) (Njoroge et al., 1995) were in agreement with the data in Table 3.10. Myrcene occurred at a remarkable concentration in mochiyu (19.52%) and kabosu (16.96%) peel oils. Hanayu (*C. hanaju* Hort. ex Shirai) and yuko were rather similar in the oil composition. Besides limonene, both oils have a high level of α-pinene and α-terpinene and unusual richness in γ-terpinene (10.34 and 21.15%).

Lime (C. aurantifolia). Lime is one of the smallest fruits in the citrus family. In Japan, Tahiti lime (*C. latifolia*) and Mexican lime (*C. aurantifolia*) have been investigated (Njoroge et al., 1996a; Sawamura, 2000), although lime is scarcely produced. Limonene content is the lowest among all citrus fruits ranging between 50 and 60%. The proportion of γ-terpinene (17%), β-pinene (13%), α-pinene (3.2%), sabinene (2%), and myrcene (1%) together with neryl acetate (1.4%), geranial (2.3%), and neral (1.2%) made up most of the oil (Njoroge et al., 1996a), and is responsible for the distinctive aroma of Tahiti lime oil. Citral includes neral (β-citral) and geranial (α-citral), and these two isomers have been known as quality-controlling values of lemon and lime oils. Geranial was present at 5.14% in a Tahiti lime oil sample reported by Sawamura (2000). The sesquiterpene hydrocarbons were dominated by α-bergamotene. Camphene, β-pinene, sabinene, *trans*-sabinene hydrate, and *cis*- and *trans*-geraniols were reported as the characteristic components of lime oil (Sawamura, 2000).

Lemon (C. limon). Japan imports about 70,000 tons every year, while more than 4300 tons per year are produced in western Japan. *Lisbon* is one of the most suitable varieties to be cultivated in Japan, since it has comparatively stronger resistance against the cold climate. The cold-pressed oil of lemon (*C. limon* Burmann forma *Lisbon*) grown in Japan includes more than a hundred volatile components. Aldehydes (2.10%) and esters (0.63%) are predominant, and bicyclogermacrene and α-bergamotene are significant sesquiterpene hydrocarbons of the investigated lemon oil (Njoroge et al., 1994a). β-Bisabolene and α-bergamotene are likely the characteristic compounds of lemon flavor (Sawamura, 2000).

TABLE 3.10. Volatile components of Japanese citrus essential oils

Compounds	*C. ichangensis*							*C. tachibana*		*C. indica*	*C. latifolia*	*C. limon*
	HAN	KAB	MOC	NAO	SUD	YUK	YUZ	TAC	TAU*	SHI	TAL	LEM
Monoterpenes												
α-pinene	2.64	0.75	0.37	0.99	1.70	3.55	1.74	1.17	0.94	2.91	3.20	2.55
camphene	0.01	tr	tr	tr	0.01	0.01	0.01	0.01	—	0.01	0.10	0.08
β-pinene	0.80	0.19	0.10	0.25	0.39	1.43	0.58	1.87	1.63	2.08	13.00	13.96
sabinene	0.59	0.12	0.14	0.17	0.52	0.68	0.40	0.68	0.33	0.16	2.00	2.32
myrcene	0.66	16.96	19.52	1.83	0.61	0.70	1.09	2.66	1.56	1.19	1.30	1.43
α-phellandrene	tr	0.01	tr	tr	tr	tr	0.51	tr	0.13	0.35	tr	—
α-terpinene	1.70	tr	—	tr	1.41	2.18	tr	tr	0.19	0.22	0.30	0.03
limonene	72.24	77.11	78.40	90.69	76.46	64.90	77.48	80.12	71.40	51.84	52.20	64.62
β-phellandrene	2.91	tr	tr	tr	3.92	2.95	1.63	tr	0.25	0.40	nq	nq
cis-β-ocimene	0.02	tr	0.01	0.01	0.01	0.01	0.01	0.02	0.03	0.01	tr	0.04
γ-terpinene	10.34	2.80	tr	4.17	2.70	21.15	7.64	8.07	7.78	28.30	17.00	10.25
p-cymene	3.19	0.10	—	0.03	5.15	0.21	0.17	0.09	0.14	2.28	0.10	0.03
terpinolene	0.46	0.13	0.01	0.16	0.13	0.90	0.35	0.66	0.56	1.45	0.70	0.41
Sesquiterpenes												
α-cubebene	—	tr	—	—	—	—	0.04	—	—	—	tr	tr
δ-elemene	0.03	—	0.03	0.01	0.04	—	0.17	0.15	0.12	0.01	0.10	—
α-copaene	0.02	0.07	—	—	0.06	0.01	0.05	0.04	0.04	0.05	—	—
β-cubebene	0.03	0.06	—	—	0.05	0.01	0.06	0.03	—	tr	tr	nq
α-bergamotene	—	—	—	—	—	—	tr	0.02	—	—	0.80	0.21
β-elemene	0.08	0.06	0.01	tr	1.29	0.40	0.06	0.08	0.06	tr	0.10	—
β-caryophyllene	0.01	0.20	0.01	tr	0.14	0.04	0.30	0.18	0.19	2.02	—	0.25
cis-β-farnesene	0.02	—	0.01	0.03	0.47	—	—	—	—	—	—	—
α-humulene	tr	0.02	tr	—	tr	0.03	0.03	0.04	0.06	0.03	tr	nq
trans-β-farnesene	0.92	0.49	0.26	0.86	0.39	0.10	0.96	—	—	—	0.10	0.02

δ-muurolene	—	—	—	—	—	—	tr	—	—	—	—	nq
germacrene-D	0.26	0.10	0.06	0.03	0.26	0.03	0.29	0.25	0.24	0.19	0.10	—
bicyclogermacrene	0.27	0.04	0.06	0.09	—	0.01	1.48	0.44	0.32	0.22	—	—
β-bisabolene	—	—	—	—	0.70	—	—	—	—	—	—	0.31
valencene	0.09	0.11	—	—	—	—	0.04	0.09	—	—	—	—
α-farnesene	—	—	—	—	—	—	—	—	0.01	1.80	—	—
δ-cadinene	—	—	0.01	—	0.19	0.12	tr	—	0.11	—	—	—
germacrene-B	0.18	—	0.02	—	0.41	tr	tr	0.17	0.15	0.04	0.10	—
Aldehydes												
octanal	0.02	0.09	—	0.08	0.03	0.01	tr	0.02	0.09	tr	tr	0.04
nonanal	0.01	0.05	—	0.01	0.01	tr	0.01	—	0.01	0.02	tr	0.14
citronellal	—	—	0.01	tr	0.06	—	tr	0.02	0.01	0.05	0.10	0.03
decanal	0.05	0.20	tr	0.30	0.04	0.01	0.09	0.03	0.05	0.17	0.10	0.01
undecanal	—	0.02	—	0.01	0.01	—	tr	—	—	0.01	tr	nq
neral	tr	tr	0.01	—	0.04	—	tr	0.01	0.03		1.20	0.61
dodecanal	—	0.01	—	0.05	—	—	—	—	—	tr	—	0.02
geranial	—	—	—	—	—	—	tr	—	0.05	—	2.30	1.13
perillaldehyde	0.01	—	0.03	0.02	—	0.03	0.03	—	0.02	tr	—	0.04
β-sinensal	tr	—	—	tr	tr	—	—	—	—	—	—	—
α-sinensal	—	—	—	—	—	—	—	—	—	tr	—	—
Alcohols												
linalool	1.31	0.06	0.09	0.10	0.45	0.17	2.65	2.03	9.13	2.18	0.20	0.15
n-octanol	—	—	—	—	0.03	—	—	—	—	0.05	—	—
terpinen-4-ol	0.03	tr	—	tr	0.01	0.04	0.01	0.01	0.19	0.01	—	tr
α-terpineol	0.30	0.03	0.02	0.03	0.12	0.18	0.11	0.09	0.49	0.35	0.40	0.30
citronellol	0.06	0.02	0.01	—	0.08	0.01	—	—	tr	0.08	—	0.01
cis-geraniol	—	—	0.03	—	—	0.01	0.02	0.01	—	tr	—	—
perillyl alcohol	0.03	—	—	0.01	—	—	0.01	—	—	—	—	—
thymol	—	—	—	—	—	—	0.1	—	0.01	0.10	tr	0.01

TABLE 3.10. *Continued*

Compounds	*C. ichangensis*							*C. tachibana*		*C. indica*	*C. latifolia*	*C. limon*
	HAN	KAB	MOC	NAO	SUD	YUK	YUZ	TAC	TAU*	SHI	TAL	LEM
Esters												
heptyl acetate	0.01	—	—	—	—	—	—	—	—	—	—	tr
octyl acetate	0.04	tr	—	0.01	—	—	—	—	—	—	—	—
linalyl acetate	—	—	—	—	—	—	0.02	—	—	—	tr	0.01
neryl acetate	0.01	—	—	—	—	—	—	—	0.01	—	1.40	0.31
geranyl acetate	0.01	tr	0.02	0.01	—	—	—	0.02	—	tr	1.00	0.23
Oxides												
(*Z*)-linalol oxide	tr	—	—	—	—	—	—	—	0.03	—	—	—
(*Z*)-limonene oxide	0.01	—	—	—	0.20	—	tr	—	—	0.01	—	0.07
(*E*)-limonene oxide	tr	tr	tr	—	—	—	tr	—	—	tr	—	0.04
Ketones												
piperitone	0.01	—	—	—	tr	0.01	0.04	—	—	0.98	—	—
(+)-carvone	—	—	—	—	0.23	—	—	—	—	—	—	—

tr: Trace, weight percent quantified less than 0.005%.
nq: Detected but not quantified.
C. ichangensis: HAN (Hanayu), KAB (Kabosu), MOC (Mochiyu), NAO (Naoshichi), SUD (Sudachi), YUK (Yuko), YUZ (Yuzu).
C. tachibana: TAC (Tachibana), TAU (Ukon-no-tachibana); *, Ubukata et al. (2002).
C. indica: SHI (Shiikuwasha).
C. latifolia: TAL (Tahiti lime).
C. limon: LEM (Lemon).

Sweet Orange (C. sinensis). Representatives of this group are omishima navel (*C. sinensis* Osbeck forma *Omishima navel*), funadoko (*C. funadoko* Hort. ex Y. Tanaka), hyuganatsu (*C. tamurana* Hort. ex Tanaka), iyokan (*C. iyo* Hort. ex Tanaka), and ujukitsu (*C. ujukitsu* Hort. ex Shirai). The composition of the sweet orange group is shown in Table 3.11.

Hyuganatsu (*C. tamurana* Hort. ex Tanaka) is one of the predominant citrus crops in Japan. The volatile components of hyuganatsu peel oil isolated by cold-pressing were mainly composed of limonene (84.0%), the most abundant compound in citrus oil. Beside limonene, the abundant monoterpene hydrocarbons were γ-terpinene (6.9%), myrcene (2.2%), α-pinene (1.2%). Among sesquiterpene hydrocarbons identified, *trans*-β-farneserne was present at the highest amount. Linalool (1.0%) was predominant in the oxygenated group that contributed to the characteristics of hyuganatsu flavor (Choi and Sawamura, 2000).

It is reported that α- and β-sinensal are characteristic components of sweet orange. α-Sinensal has orange-like flavor, but β-sinensal has a metallic or fish odor, becoming more unpleasant at higher concentration. Ujukitsu oil has been proved to inhibit the formation of *N*-nitrosodimethylamine (NDMA) more effectively than other citrus oils (Sawamura et al., 1999). Although belonging to the *C. sinensis* species, the volatile profile of ujukitsu is quite different from sweet orange oils with a rather low level of limonene (59.2%) and an abnormal amount of myrcene (25.3%). The two isomers of α- and β-sinensals were also absent from ujukitsu oil volatiles. Other aldehydes such as octanal, decanal, neral, and geranial also dominated in the oxygenated fraction and γ-terpinene occurs in trace amounts (Sawamura, 2000).

Bitter/Sour Orange (C. aurantium). Representatives of this group are daidai (*C. aurantium* Linn. var. *Cyathifera* Y. Tanaka), kabusu (*C. aurantium* Linn. forma *Kabusu*), konejime (*C. neo-aurantium* Tanaka), and tokosu (*C. aurantium* Linn.). Daidai, a sour Japanese citrus fruit, is rich in hydrocarbons (~97%). Geranial, octanal, linalyl acetate, and *cis*-limonene oxide were found as the characteristic components of daidai (Sawamura, 2000).

Mandarin (C. reticulata Blanco). Representatives of this group are imamura unshu (*C. unshiu* Marcov. forma *Imamura*), miyagawa-wase unshu (*C. unshiu* Marcov. forma *Miyagawa-wase*), okitsu-wase unshu (*C. unshiu* Marcov. var. praecox Tanaka cv. *Okitsu-wase*), sanpo-wase unshu (*C. unshiu* Marcov. forma *Sanpo-wase*), mukakukishu (*C. kinokuni* Hort. ex. Tanaka), and ponkan (*C. reticulata* Blanco). The volatile composition is also listed in Table 3.10.

Satsuma mandarin (*C. unshiu*) is one of the most produced and famous Japanese citrus fruits in the world, though it is also cultivated in Spain, the United States and the other countries. The recent annual production of Satsuma mandarin in Japan accounts for approximately 1 million tons. In Japanese mandarins, monoterpene hydrocarbons amounted to 96.0–98.6%, of which the limonene level ranges from 85 to 91%, followed by γ-terpinene (3.5–6.0%) and myrcene (1.6–1.8%), of the total oil. The level of oxygenated compounds is rather low,

TABLE 3.11. Volatile components of Japanese citrus essential oils

Compounds	*C. aurantium*				*C. sinensis*					*C. reticulate*					
	DAI	KBU	KON	TOK	OMI	FUN	HYU	IYO	UJU	UN1	UN2	UN3	UN4	MKI	PON
Monoterpenes															
α-pinene	0.51	0.54	0.90	0.47	0.57	1.60	1.42	1.21	1.35	1.14	1.01	0.99	1.05	0.40	1.21
camphene	tr	0.01	tr	0.01	tr	0.01	0.01	tr	0.01	tr	0.09	tr	tr	0.01	0.01
β-pinene	0.18	0.91	1.31	0.69	0.05	1.63	0.79	0.33	0.43	0.31	0.24	0.28	0.26	2.57	0.28
sabinene	0.19	0.26	0.28	0.30	1.61	0.16	0.20	0.23	0.26	0.18	0.15	0.19	0.2	tr	0.57
myrcene	1.73	1.65	1.73	1.64	1.87	1.61	1.81	1.75	25.33	1.75	1.79	1.68	1.8	1.63	1.83
α-phellandrene	tr	tr	0.03	tr	tr	tr	tr	tr	0.01	tr	tr	tr	tr	tr	tr
α-terpinene	—	—	0.06	—	—	0.02	0.02	tr	0.04	tr	tr	tr	tr	0.01	tr
limonene	95.85	92.03	88.91	94.36	93.91	83.07	84.52	88.17	59.23	89.74	90.57	89.3	90.23	84.86	89.88
β-phellandrene	tr	tr	—	tr	tr	tr	tr	tr	tr	tr	tr	tr	tr	tr	tr
cis-β-ocimene	0.01	0.01	—	0.01	tr	0.02	0.02	0.01	0.01	tr	tr	tr	tr	tr	tr
γ-terpinene	tr	—	3.55	—	tr	8.15	7.46	5.36	7.60	4.61	3.50	3.97	3.67	5.99	4.54
p-cymene	—	—	0.01	—	—	0.11	0.03	0.11	0.04	0.14	0.19	0.24	0.16	0.2	0.05
terpinolene	tr	tr	0.14	tr	tr	0.37	0.32	0.21	0.33	0.19	0.14	0.17	0.15	0.28	0.19
Sesquiterpenes															
δ-elemene	—	tr	0.11	0.02	—	0.13	—	0.21	0.08	0.07	0.09	0.11	0.10	0.05	0.02
α-copaene	—	—	0.07	tr	0.01	0.02	0.02	0.01	0.03	0.05	0.04	0.05	0.04	0.01	tr
β-cubebene	—	—	0.06	—	tr	tr	tr	0.01	0.02	0.05	0.04	0.04	0.03	tr	—
α-bergamotene	—	—	—	—	—	—	0.11	—	0.03	—	—	—	—	—	—
β-elemene	—	—	0.09	0.03	tr	0.04	0.01	0.04	0.04	0.29	0.45	0.66	0.47	0.02	0.01
β-caryophyllene	0.02	0.01	0.11	0.18	0.02	0.06	0.06	0.03	0.09	0.03	0.05	0.07	0.05	0.01	—
cis-β-farnesene	—	—	—	—	0.01	—	0.03	—	—	—	—	—	—	—	—
α-humulene	—	—	0.01	0.05	—	0.01	tr	0.01	0.02	0.05	0.07	0.10	0.07	0.01	—
trans-β-farnesene	0.01	0.02	0.27	—	0.03	—	0.5	—	—	—	—	tr	tr	tr	0.01
δ-muurolene	—	—	—	—	—	—	0.01	—	—	—	—	—	—	—	—

germacrene-D	0.04	0.04	0.08	0.47	0.02	0.25	0.06	0.25	0.16	0.13	0.15	0.18	0.15	0.1	0.02
bicyclogermacrene	—	—	—	0.28	—	tr	0.11	—	0.29	0.04	0.06	0.06	0.05	0.04	—
β-bisabolene	—	—	—	—	—	—	—	0.04	—	—	—	—	—	—	—
valencene	—	—	—	0.02	—	—	0.03	0.02	—	—	—	—	—	—	—
α-farnesene	—	—	0.13	—	0.03	0.08	—	0.01	—	0.06	0.44	0.71	0.48	1.08	0.02
δ-cadinene	—	—	—	—	—	—	—	—	0.05	—	—	—	—	—	—
germacrene-B	—	—	—	0.01	—	0.05	—	0.06	0.09	0.02	—	0.03	0.02	0.02	0.02
Aldehydes															
octanal	0.09	0.14	0.06	tr	0.38	0.41	0.03	0.07	tr	0.01	0.07	0.1	0.1	0.13	0.21
nonanal	0.01	0.02	0.01	0.01	0.03	0.02	0.01	0.02	—	0.01	0.01	0.02	0.02	0.04	0.22
citronellal	—	—	0.02	—	0.01	0.02	0.15	tr	0.01	0.02	0.03	0.03	0.03	0.01	0.06
decanal	0.07	0.07	0.05	0.01	0.15	0.24	0.02	0.07	tr	0.05	0.06	0.07	0.07	0.18	0.12
undecanal	tr	0.01	0.02	0.01	tr	tr	—	tr	—	tr	tr	0.01	tr	0.01	0.01
neral	0.02	0.03	0.06	0.01	0.09	0.01	0.03	0.01	0.07	—	tr	tr	tr	—	0.01
dodecanal	0.01	0.01	0.08	tr	0.02	0.04	tr	tr	—	—	—	0.01	0.01	0.01	0.02
geranial	—	0.08	—	—	0.15	—	—	—	—	tr	—	tr	—	—	0.01
perillaldehyde	0.01	0.01	0.02	0.02	0.01	0.01	0.01	0.03	0.01	—	0.02	0.02	0.02	0.01	0.02
β-sinensal	—	—	—	—	0.05	—	—	0.01	—	—	—	—	—	—	0.02
α-sinensal	—	—	—	—	0.03	0.11	—	0.03	—	—	—	—	—	—	0.05
Alcohols															
linalool	0.18	1.04	0.72	0.15	0.57	1.43	1.32	1.33	0.64	0.32	0.35	0.51	0.41	0.78	0.58
n-octanol	—	—	tr	—	0.01	0.01	0.01	tr	—	—	—	—	—	0.07	0.01
terpinen-4-ol	—	—	0.05	—	tr	tr	0.01	0.01	0.01	0.01	0.01	0.01	0.01	0.02	tr
α-terpineol	0.04	0.04	0.14	0.04	0.07	0.13	0.11	0.08	0.05	0.08	0.06	0.08	0.07	0.1	0.08
citronellol	—	—	—	—	0.01	0.01	0.03	0.01	—	0.01	0.01	0.01	0.01	0.03	0.02
cis-geraniol	—	—	0.03	0.01	0.01	tr	—	—	0.05	—	—	—	—	tr	0.01
trans-geraniol	—	—	tr	—	tr	—	—	—	tr	—	—	—	—	—	—
perillyl alcohol	0.01	0.02	tr	—	—	—	—	—	—	—	—	—	—	—	—
thymol	—	—	—	—	—	—	—	—	—	—	—	—	—	0.07	0.02

TABLE 3.11. *Continued*

Compounds	*C. aurantium*				*C. sinensis*					*C. reticulate*					
	DAI	KBU	KON	TOK	OMI	FUN	HYU	IYO	UJU	UN1	UN2	UN3	UN4	MKI	PON
Esters															
heptyl acetate	tr	tr	—	—	—	—	—	—	—	—	—	—	—	—	—
octyl acetate	0.04	0.07	—	—	—	0.02	—	0.01	—	—	—	—	—	—	—
linalyl acetate	—	—	—	—	—	—	—	—	—	—	—	—	—	—	—
neryl acetate	tr	—	—	—	—	—	—	—	—	—	—	—	—	—	—
geranyl acetate	0.06	0.09	0.03	0.01	0.01	0.10	0.02	0.05	0.01	0.04	0.03	0.18	0.04	0.05	tr
Oxides															
(*Z*)-linalol oxide	—	—	tr	—	—	—	—	—	—	—	—	—	—	—	—
(*Z*)-limonene oxide	—	—	tr	0.04	tr	tr	0.01	—	—	—	—	—	—	tr	—
(*E*)-limonene oxide	—	—	0.01	0.03	tr	—	—	—	—	—	—	—	—	tr	—
Ketones															
piperitone	—	—	—	—	—	—	—	—	tr	—	—	—	—	—	—
(+)-carvone	tr	tr	—	—	—	—	—	—	—	—	—	—	—	—	—
nootkatone	—	—	—	—	0.01	—	—	—	—	—	—	—	—	—	—

tr: Trace, weight percent quantified less than 0.005%.
nq: Detected but not quantified.
C. aurantium: DAI (Daidai), KBU (Kabusu), KON (Konejime), TOK (Tokosu).
C. sinensis: OMI (Omishima navel), FUN (Funadoko), HYU (Hyuganatsu), IYO (Iyokan), UJU (Ujukitsu).
C. reticulata: UN1 (Imamura unshu), UN2 (Miyagawa-wase unshu), UN3 (Okitsu-wase unshu), UN4 (Sanpo-wase unshu); MKI (Mukakukishu), PON (Ponkan).

while the components are represented by the sesquiterpenes such as β-elemene, α-farnesene, germacrene D, and α-humulene (Sawamura, 2000). The sesquiterpene hydrocarbons usually appear in lime oil, α-bergamotene, *cis*-β-farnesene, β-bisabolene, valencene, and δ-cardinene. Decanal is an important oil component of mandarin, such as Satsuma mandarin.

Pummelo (C. grandis). Swingle classified grapefruit and pummelo into different species. Grapefruit is considered, however, to be a hybrid of pummelo according to Tanaka. Thus, both of them are categorized into the zabon or buntan group. The high level of nootkatone is commonly used to differentiate grapefruit and pummelos from others (less than 0.01%) in the *Citrus* family.

PUMMELO OR SHADDOCK (*C. grandis*). This cultivar is also called *zabon* or *buntan* in Japanese, and was introduced to Japan in the 1770s. The representatives of pummelos cultivated in Japan are anseikan (*C. grandis* Osbeck var. *anseikan* Hort. ex Tanaka), banhakuyu (*C. grandis* Osbeck forma *Banhakuyu*), banokan (*C. grandis* Osbeck forma *Banokan* Hort. ex Tanaka), egami-buntan (*C. grandis* Osbeck forma *Egami*), hirado-buntan (*C. grandis* Osbeck *Hirado*), suisyo-buntan (*C. grandis* Osbeck forma *Suisyo*), tanigawa-buntan (*C. grandis* Osbeck *Mato* × *C. sulcata* Hort. ex *Takahashi*), Tosa-buntan (*C. grandis* Osbeck forma *Tosa*), uchimurasaki (*C. grandis* Osbeck forma *Benikawa*), uwa-pummelo (*C. grandis* Osbeck forma *Uwa-pummelo*), and hayasaki (*C. grandis* Osbeck forma *Hirado* × *C. grandis* Osbeck forma *Buntan* Hayata), a new artificial hybrid of Mato- and Hirado-buntan. The composition of Japanese pummelo excludes α- and β-sinensal, though the two components usually appear in sweet orange oils. More careful studies on Japanese pummelo oils have been carried out by Sawamura et al. (1989; 1990).

Banhakuyu or banpeiyu (*C. grandis* Osbeck forma *Banhakuyu*) is the largest of the citrus fruits, with average weight of more than 2 kg. The peel oil possesses a metallic, green, and citrusy aroma (Katayama et al., 2002). Its composition shows a low concentration of limonene compared to other citrus (48.7–55.4%), while that of myrcene exceeded 35.1% (Sawamura, 2000; Katayama et al., 2002).

Tosa-buntan (*C. grandis* Osbeck forma *Tosa*), grown mainly in southwestern Japan, is the most popular among the pummelos. Twenty-eight compounds were identified and quantified in the cold-pressed and steam-distilled oils under reduced pressure with subsequent solvent extraction using glass capillary GC and GC-MS (Sawamura and Kuriyama, 1988). The major components in the cold-pressed oil were monoterpenes, including limonene (86.19%), γ-terpinene (5.78%), myrcene (3.53%), and α-pinene (1.22%). Among minor oxygenated components, decanal (0.29%), linalool (0.24%), citronellal (0.18%), and nootkatone (0.21%) made up most of the remainder (Sawamura and Kuriyama, 1988; Sawamura et al., 2001).

Eight different pummelo varieties have been investigated (Sawamura et al., 1991). The most predominant components were limonene, γ-terpinene, α-terpinene, and myrcene. The quantities of γ-terpinene in these varieties varied from 5 to 7% in Tosa-buntan, banokan, akano-buntan, and Vietnam-buntan to less than 0.2% in the others. β-Cubebene is relatively abudant among the sesquiterpene hydrocarbons. Oxygenated compounds such as octanal, decanal, citronellal, and nootkatone significantly contributed to the pleasant aroma of pummelo oils. The main data are collected in Table 3.12.

Grapefruits (*C. paradisi*). Representatives of grapefruit are hassaku (*C. Hassaku* Hort. ex Tanaka), hyoukan (*C. ampullaceal* Hort. ex Tanaka), kawachibankan (*C. kawachinensis* Hort. ex Y. Tanaka), kawano-natsudaidai (*C. natsudaidai* Hayata), kinkoji (*C. obovoidea* Hort. ex Tanaka), kinukawa (*C. glaberrima* Hort. ex Tanaka), narutokan (*C. medioglobosa* Hort. ex Tanaka), natsudaidai (*C. natsudaidai* Hayata), otachibana (*C. otachibana* Hort. ex Tanaka), sanbokan (*C. sulcata* Hort. ex Tanaka), tengu (*C. tengu* Hort. ex Tanaka), and yamabuki (*C. yamabuki* Hort. ex Y. Tanaka). Their composition is shown in Table 3.13. It is reported that nootkatone and 1-*p*-menthen-8-thiol contribute to grapefruit flavor. The threshold value of nootkatone is about 1 ppm, and that of 1-*p*-menthen-8-thiol is really 10^{-4} ppb (Sawamura, 2000).

Sanbokan is a Japanese citrus with the aroma character of grapefruit type. The essential oil of sanbokan peel contains mainly limonene (89.0%), γ-terpinene (5.15%), myrcene (1.7%), α-pinene (1.12%), and linalool (0.87%) (Table 3.13).

Hybrids and Unidentified Citrus Species. Along with the famous citrus fruits listed above, there have been various hybrids and unidentified citrus species that have been used to analyze their volatile composition (Table 3.13). Tangors such as ariake (*C. sinensis* Osbeck forma *Seike navel* × *C. clementina* Hort. ex Tanaka) and kiyomi (*C. unshiu* Marcov. × *C. sinensis* Osbeck) and tangors-tangerines such as tsunoka (*C. reticulata* Blanco × *C. sinensis* Osbeck × *C. unshiu* Marcov. var. praecox Tanaka cv. *Okitsu-wase*) seem to have inherited the character of *C. sinensis*, because those fruits contained both α-sinensal and β-sinensal. However, tangelos such as minneola (Duncan × Dancy tangerine), Sampson (Grapefruit × Dancy tangerine), and orland (Duncan × Dancy tangerine) and tangerine-tangelos such as nova (Clementine × Orland) and fairchild (Clementine × Orland) also contain either α-sinensal or β-sinensal, although Duncan, grapefruit, dancy tangerine, and clementine, which are parents of their hybrids, own no sinensal.

Shiranui (*C. unshiu* Marcov. × *C. sinensis* Osbeck × *C. reticulata* Blanco), also called *Dekopon* in Japanese, is a hybrid of kiyomi and ponkan. Limonene, a characteristic component of ponkan oil, presented at high levels (91.8%) in Shiranui oil (Song et al., 2006).

In addition, some unidentified species such as kiyookadaidai (*C. sp.*) and ozu (*C. ozu* Hort. ex Y. Tanaka) have been investigated. Kiyookadaidai is one of a great number of sour citrus varieties, which has a unique and pleasant aroma. Sawamura (2000) reported that myrcene was the most abundant (about 50%) among 36 compounds detected in kiyookadaidai cold-pressed oil, whereas limonene content was only around 20%. It was found that myrcene, (*Z*)-ocimene,

TABLE 3.12. Volatile components of Japanese citrus essential oils

Compounds	C. grandis														
	ANS	BAH	BAN	EGA	HAY	HIR	SU1	TNI	TOB	UCH	UWA	HON	ANS	BAO	AKA
Monoterpenes															
α-pinene	0.45	0.26	1.19	0.55	0.68	0.49	1.4	1.63	1.24	0.43	0.49	0.57	0.39	1.33	1.13
camphene	tr	tr	0.01	0.01	0.02	tr	0.01	0.01	0.01	tr	tr	—	—	—	—
β-pinene	0.10	0.15	0.87	2.44	3.73	0.57	0.51	0.56	0.85	0.79	0.02	1.76	0.12	0.98	0.46
sabinene	0.12	0.09	0.24	0.24	tr	0.36	0.28	0.3	0.32	0.29	0.1	0.48	0.13	0.26	0.15
myrcene	1.74	39.30	1.73	1.69	1.75	1.77	1.79	1.78	1.78	3.18	1.71	1.30	1.29	1.15	1.17
α-phellandrene	tr	tr	tr	tr	tr	—	tr	tr	tr	tr	—	—	—	—	—
α-terpinene	—	—	0.02	—	—	—	tr	tr	tr	tr	—	—	—	0.16	0.13
limonene	96.15	55.41	85.81	94.41	91.82	95.69	87.36	84.22	88.76	92.33	96.96	77.95	77.73	66.52	74.63
β-phellandrene	tr	tr	tr	tr	tr	tr	tr	tr	tr	tr	—	—	—	—	—
cis-β-ocimene	0.01	tr	0.01	tr	0.01	0.01	tr	0.01	0.01	tr	tr	—	—	—	—
γ-terpinene	tr	0.22	8.09	tr	—	—	6.71	8.49	5.41	0.11	—	0.10	0.20	6.93	5.54
p-cymene	—	—	0.09	—	—	—	0.04	0.07	0.05	tr	—	0.01	—	0.17	0.10
terpinolene	0.01	0.02	0.34	tr	0.01	tr	0.27	0.34	0.2	tr	tr	—	0.01	0.67	0.51
Sesquiterpenes															
α-cubebene	tr	—	—	—	—	—	tr	—	—	—	—	—	—	—	—
δ-elemene	0.03	—	0.06	0.05	0.04	0.05	0.03	0.03	0.05	—	0.02	—	—	—	—
α-copaene	0.05	0.04	tr	—	—	—	0.01	0.06	0.07	—	0.02	—	0.10	0.06	—
β-cubebene	0.04	0.01	0.01	—	—	—	0.04	0.05	0.06	tr	0.02	0.61	0.14	1.14	0.79
β-elemene	0.02	—	0.02	tr	0.02	0.02	0.02	0.02	0.02	0.12	0.01	0.05	0.04	0.05	0.14
β-caryophyllene	0.03	0.12	tr	0.05	0.02	0.01	0.03	0.05	0.03	0.05	0.01	—	—	0.02	0.02
α-humulene	—	—	tr	0.01	0.02	—	0.01	0.02	0.01	tr	tr	—	—	—	—

TABLE 3.12. *Continued*

Compounds	*C. grandis*														
	ANS	BAH	BAN	EGA	HAY	HIR	SU1	TNI	TOB	UCH	UWA	HON	ANS	BAO	AKA
trans-β-farnesene	—	—	0.03	—	—	—	—	—	—	—	—	—	—	—	—
germacrene-D	0.06	—	0.44	0.11	0.42	0.34	0.06	0.07	0.09	—	0.04	—	—	—	—
bicyclogermacrene	—	—	—	—	—	0.03	—	0.02	—	—	tr	—	—	—	—
β-bisabolene	—	—	—	—	—	—	0.02	—	—	—	—	—	—	—	—
valencene	—	—	—	—	—	—	—	—	—	0.03	—	—	0.02	0.04	0.04
α-farnesene	—	—	—	tr	tr	tr	—	—	—	—	—	—	—	—	—
δ-cadinene	0.07	0.08	0.04	—	—	—	0.06	0.07	0.08	tr	0.03	—	0.16	0.10	0.02
germacrene-B	tr	—	0.02	0.02	0.02	0.01	0.01	—	0.01	—	0.01	—	—	—	—
Aldehydes															
octanal	0.03	—	0.24	tr	tr	—	0.35	0.23	0.19	0.02	tr	—	0.05	0.20	0.07
nonanal	0.01	—	0.05	—	—	—	0.02	0.03	0.03	0.02	—	—	0.01	0.10	0.02
citronellal	—	—	—	—	—	—	0.07	0.06	0.06	tr	0.12	—	0.12	0.08	0.01
decanal	0.02	0.04	0.19	—	—	—	0.22	0.19	0.15	0.06	—	—	0.04	0.59	0.31
undecanal	—	—	0.01	—	—	—	tr	tr	0.01	—	—	—	—	0.02	—
neral	0.08	0.22	0.02	0.06	0.04	0.09	0.04	0.02	0.05	tr	0.02	0.19	0.18	0.02	0.04
dodecanal	—	—	0.01	—	—	—	0.03	0.02	0.02	—	—	—	—	—	—
geranial	0.36	0.33	0.03	0.08	0.07	0.15	0.06	0.05	0.08	0.23	0.07	0.31	0.79	0.28	0.13
perillaldehyde	tr	—	0.01	—	tr	0.01	0.01	0.01	0.01	—	tr	—	0.01	0.01	0.01
Alcohols															
linalool	0.10	0.39	0.12	0.07	0.08	0.07	0.09	1.27	0.1	0.21	0.07	0.19	0.26	0.12	0.16
n-octanol	—	—	tr	—	—	—	tr	tr	tr	—	—	—	0.05	0.20	0.07

terpinen-4-ol	—	—	0.03	—	tr	—	0.01	0.01	0.01	tr	—	0.02	0.06	0.02	0.07
α-terpineol	0.05	0.06	0.10	0.05	0.07	0.04	0.09	0.11	0.07	0.07	0.04	0.14	0.12	0.10	0.16
citronellol	—	—	tr	—	—	—	0.01	0.01	tr	tr	0.01	0.02	0.01	0.01	0.03
cis-geraniol	0.02	—	0.08	—	—	—	—	—	—	tr	tr	0.02	0.07	0.01	0.07
trans-geraniol	—	—	tr	—	tr	—	—	—	—	0.04	—	—	—	—	—
Esters															
heptyl acetate	—	—	—	—	—	—	tr	—	—	—	—	—	—	—	—
octyl acetate	—	—	0.01	—	—	—	0.06	—	—	—	—	0.01	tr	0.01	0.14
neryl acetate	—	—	—	—	—	—	—	—	—	—	—	—	—	—	—
geranyl acetate	tr	—	tr	0.05	0.05	0.02	0.04	0.02	0.01	—	0.01	0.03	0.02	0.02	0.04
Oxides															
(*Z*)-limonene oxide	—	—	—	—	tr	—	—	—	—	0.04	—	0.01	0.03	0.19	0.07
(*E*)-limonene oxide	tr	—	tr	0.01	—	tr	—	—	tr	0.01	—	—	—	—	—
Ketones															
(+)-carvone	—	—	—	—	—	—	—	—	—	—	—	—	—	—	—
nootkatone	0.01	0.06	0.01	0.03	0.07	0.04	0.01	0.03	0.05	0.14	0.02	0.28	0.03	0.16	0.46

tr: Trace, weight percent quantified less than 0.005%.
nq: Detected but not quantified.
C. grandis: ANS (Anseikan), BAH (Banhakuyu), BAN (Banokan), EGA (Egami-buntan), HAY (Hayasaki), HIR (Hirado-buntan), SU1 (Suisyo-buntan), TNI (Tanigawa-buntan), TOB (Tosa-buntan), UCH (Uchimurasaki), UWA (Uwa-pummelo), HON (Honda-buntan), ANS (Anseikan), BAO (Banokan), AKA (Akano-buntan).

TABLE 3.13. Volatile components of Japanese citrus essential oils

Compounds	*C. paradisi*								
	HAS	HYO	KAW	KAN	KIN	KIK	NTK	NAT	OTA
Monoterpenes									
α-pinene	0.24	0.51	1.06	1.19	1.17	0.95	1.34	1.14	1.52
camphene	0.01	tr	0.01	0.01	0.01	0.01	0.01	tr	0.01
β-pinene	0.36	0.08	0.63	0.37	0.41	0.72	0.58	0.33	0.54
sabinene	0.27	0.12	0.3	0.18	0.14	0.17	0.18	0.16	0.28
myrcene	1.8	1.75	1.76	1.78	1.71	1.41	1.65	1.71	1.83
α-phellandrene	tr	tr	tr	tr	tr	tr	tr	tr	tr
α-terpinene	tr	—	tr	tr	0.01	0.02	0.01	tr	tr
limonene	89.77	96.18	89.83	89.79	88.95	78.84	86.7	90.24	86.03
β-phellandrene	tr	tr	tr	tr	tr	tr	tr	tr	tr
cis-β-ocimene	0.01	0.01	0.01	0.01	0.01	0.02	7.15	tr	0.01
γ-terpinene	5.56	tr	5.16	5.01	5.56	6.87	0.3	4.86	7.68
p-cymene	0.03	—	0.03	0.08	0.17	1.34	0.31	0.04	0.12
terpinolene	0.22	tr	0.2	0.22	0.23	0.33	0.33	0.19	0.31
Sesquiterpenes									
α-cubebene	—	—	—	—	—	—	—	—	—
δ-elemene	0.02	0.05	0.01	—	0.05	0.16	0.06	—	0.01
α-copaene	0.02	0.04	0.01	0.02	0.06	0.02	0.01	0.02	0.06
β-cubebene	0.01	0.04	—	0.04	0.08	tr	tr	0.01	0.05
α-bergamotene	—	—	—	—	—	—	—	—	—
β-elemene	tr	0.04	—	0.01	0.03	0.15	0.06	0.01	0.02
β-caryophyllene	0.01	0.06	0.01	0.03	0.07	0.06	tr	0.02	0.04
cis-β-farnesene	—	—	tr	—	—	—	—	—	—
α-humulene	tr	tr	—	tr	0.01	0.01	0.02	0.01	tr
trans-β-farnesene	—	0.07	0.08	—	0.05	—	—	—	—
germacrene-D	0.03	0.07	0.01	0.13	0.13	0.43	0.11	0.16	0.06
bicyclogermacrene	—	0.01	—	0.01	—	—	—	tr	tr
valencene	—	—	—	—	—	—	0.02	—	—
α-farnesene	—	0.12	tr	0.06	0.08	0.24	—	0.03	—
δ-cadinene	0.02	—	—	—	—	—	—	0.02	0.07
germacrene-B	0.01	0.01	tr	—	0.03	0.12	0.02	—	0.01
Aldehydes									
octanal	0.09	—	0.28	0.28	0.24	0.42	tr	0.33	0.05
nonanal	0.01	—	0.02	0.04	0.02	0.7	0.06	0.04	0.01
citronellal	0.01	0.01	—	—	0.06	0.05	0.04	—	0.06
decanal	0.1	—	0.17	0.19	0.19	0.45	0.47	0.19	0.10
undecanal	0.01	—	0.01	0.01	tr	0.02	0.01	tr	tr
neral	0.02	tr	0.07	0.01	0.02	0.04	0.03	tr	0.01
dodecanal	0.01	—	0.01	0.03	0.01	0.05	0.01	0.02	0.01
geranial	0.05	0.12	0.12	0.07	0.04	0.32	0.12	0.05	0.05

			Hybrid					Unidentified		*Fortunella*
SAN	TEN	YAM	ARI	KIY	TSU	ISU	SNU	KID	OZU	KUM
1.12	0.52	1.07	0.54	0.46	0.88	1.17	0.70	0.82	0.69	0.39
0.01	tr	0.01	tr	tr	tr	tr		0.01	tr	tr
0.4	0.03	0.48	0.01	0.02	0.27	0.31	0.08	1.13	0.02	0.03
0.16	0.11	0.16	0.10	0.42	1.02	0.17	1.65	1.86	0.01	0.07
1.7	1.59	1.68	1.61	1.74	1.72	1.69	2.55	50.03	0.25	1.74
tr	tr	—	tr	tr	tr	—	0.04	—	1.90	tr
tr	—	0.01	—	—	tr	tr		6.46	—	—
89.0	95.99	90.08	95.06	95.62	87.4	90.55	91.82	21.67	93.93	96.65
tr	tr	tr	tr	tr	tr	tr	0.56	—	1.43	tr
0.01	0.01	tr	0.01	tr	0.01	—		—	0.01	0.01
5.15	tr	4.46	0.03	tr	3.92	5.00		8.43	0.01	0.04
0.1	tr	0.08	0.02	tr	0.85	0.06		0.61	tr	tr
0.22	tr	0.19	0.01	0.01	0.18	0.20	0.01	0.05	0.01	0.01
—	—	—	—	—	tr	—	—	—	—	—
0.17	—	0.17	—	—	—	0.01	0.03	0.03	0.01	0.06
0.01	0.01	—	0.06	0.03	0.09	0.03	—	—	—	0.01
tr	0.01	—	0.06	—	0.09	0.03	tr	0.03	—	0.01
—	—	—	—	—	—	—	—	—	—	tr
0.03	—	0.04	0.12	0.02	0.14	0.01	0.01	—	0.01	—
tr	0.02	tr	0.07	0.02	tr	0.05	—	—	0.05	0.01
—	—	—	tr	0.01	—	—	—	—	—	—
0.01	—	tr	tr	—	0.01	tr	0.01	—	tr	0.01
0.04	0.01	0.05	0.09	0.10	0.27	—	—	—	0.06	—
0.25	0.03	0.41	0.07	0.02	0.08	0.03	0.05	0.3	0.42	0.29
—	—	0.07	0.46	—	—	—	0.03	—	tr	—
0.03	—	—	—	—	—	—	0.12	—	—	—
—	0.01	0.03	0.11	0.06	0.13	—	0.74	—	—	0.01
—	—	—	—	—	—	—	0.06	—	—	—
0.06	—	0.04	—	—	—	—		0.03	—	0.05
0.1	0.14	0.02	tr	0.12	0.26	0.05	0.08	—	—	tr
0.02	0.03	0.01	—	0.06	0.1	0.02	0.02	—	—	tr
—	—	—	0.01	0.02	0.02	0.03	0.10	0.07	0.01	—
0.06	0.14	0.04	0.01	0.1	0.3	0.08	0.33	0.03	—	0.01
0.01	0.01	0.01	—	0.01	0.02	0.01	0.02	—	—	—
0.01	0.03	0.01	0.01	0.04	0.06	—	—	1.45	tr	—
0.01	0.06	tr	0.03	—	0.08	0.01	0.09	—	—	—
0.17	0.04	0.02	—	—	—	—	—	2.70	—	—

TABLE 3.13. *Continued*

Compounds	*C. paradisi*								
	HAS	HYO	KAW	KAN	KIN	KIK	NTK	NAT	OTA
perillaldehyde	0.02	—	0.01	0.02	0.01	0.24	0.01	0.03	0.01
β-sinensal	—	—	—	—	—	—	—	—	—
α-sinensal	—	—	—	—	—	—	—	—	—
Alcohols									
linalool	0.12	0.04	0.12	0.08	0.08	5.05	0.16	0.09	0.74
n-octanol	—	—	tr	0.02	—	0.04	0.11	0.03	—
terpinen-4-ol	0.01	—	0.02	tr	tr	tr	0.04	0.01	0.01
α-terpineol	0.09	0.01	0.08	0.08	0.11	0.01	0.12	0.08	0.05
citronellol	tr	0.01	0.01	tr	tr	tr	0.03	—	0.01
cis-geraniol	—	—	tr	—	—	0.01	0.01	tr	—
trans-geraniol	—	—	—	—	—	tr	tr	tr	—
perillyl alcohol	—	—	—	0.01	—	0.02	—	—	—
thymol	—	—	—	—	—	—	—	—	—
Esters									
heptyl acetate	—	—	—	tr	—	tr	—	—	—
octyl acetate	tr	—	0.01	0.05	0.01	0.05	—	0.03	—
linalyl acetate	—	—	—	—	—	—	—	—	—
neryl acetate	—	0.01	—	—	—	—	—	—	tr
geranyl acetate	0.02	0.22	—	0.04	0.12	0.08	tr	0.04	0.03
Oxides									
(*Z*)-linalol oxide	—	—	—	—	—	—	—	tr	—
(*Z*)-limonene oxide	—	—	tr	—	tr	0.03	0.01	—	—
(*E*)-limonene oxide	0.01	tr	—	tr	—	0.04	0.06	—	—
Ketones									
piperitone	—	—	—	—	—	—	—	—	—
(+)-carvone	—	—	—	—	—	tr	—	—	—
nootkatone	0.02	0.03	0.02	0.01	tr	tr	0.01	0.01	0.04

tr: Trace, weight percent quantified less than 0.005%.
nq: Detected but not quantified.
C. paradisi: HAS (Hassaku), HYO (Hyoukan), KAW (Kawachi-bankan), KAN (Kawano-natsudaidai), KIN (Kinkoji), KIK (Kinukawa), NTK (Narutokan), NAT (Natsudaidai), OTA (Otachibana), SAN (Sanbokan), TEN (Tengu), YAM (Yamabuki).
Tangor: ARI (Ariake), KIY (Kiyomi).
Tangor-tangerine: TSU (Tsunoka).
Tangelo: ISU (Imamura unshu × Suisyo-buntan).
Tangor-mandarin: SNU (Shiranui).
Unidentified: KID (Kiyookadaidai), OZU (Ozu).
Fortunella: KUM (Kumquat/Marukinkan).

			Hybrid					Unidentified		*Fortunella*
SAN	TEN	YAM	ARI	KIY	TSU	ISU	SNU	KID	OZU	KUM
0.01	0.01	tr	0.15	0.02	0.02	0.01	0.02	—	0.03	0.02
—	—	—	0.04	0.09	0.25	—	—	—	—	—
—	tr	—	0.03	0.05	0.06	—	—	—	—	—
0.87	0.06	0.04	0.02	0.12	0.3	0.05	0.14	0.34	0.1	0.08
tr	0.02	tr	—	0.01	0.12	tr	—	0.02	—	—
0.02	tr	0.02	—	—	0.05	0.01	—	0.01	tr	—
0.04	0.02	0.11	tr	0.05	0.14	0.05	0.02	0.3	0.08	0.01
tr	0.03	0.01	0.01	0.01	—	0.03	0.07	0.16	tr	—
tr	0.01	—	0.01	0.01	0.03	—	—	1.42	0.03	—
—	—	—	—	—	tr	—	—	0.15	—	—
—	0.01	0.01	0.04	—	—	—	—	—	—	0.02
—	—	0.05	—	—	—	—	—	—	—	—
—	tr	0.02	—	—	tr	—		0.03	—	tr
0.01	0.03	0.31	—	—	0.01	0.03	tr	—	—	0.02
—	—	—	0.01	—	0.01	—		0.01	—	—
—	—	—	—	—	—	—	0.01	—	—	—
tr	—	0.05	0.1	0.05	0.03	0.04	0.03	0.4	—	0.11
—	—	—	—	—	—	—	tr	0.05	—	—
—	0.08	0.01	0.01	tr	0.03	tr	0.04	—	tr	—
tr	0.03	tr	0.06	tr	tr	tr	—	0.02	—	—
—	—	—	—	—	—	—	—	0.04	—	—
tr	0.14	—	—	—	—	—	—	—	—	0.02
tr	tr	0.04	0.02	0.01	—	—	0.08	—	—	—

and α-bergamotene were the odor-characteristic compounds, reproducing a kiyoodaidai-like odor (Minh Tu et al., 2003).

Kumquat (Fortunella). Kumquat, called *kinkan* in Japanese, is a group of small oval fruits with typical citrus aroma that actually belong to the genus *Fortunella* of the Rutaceae family, including the genus *Citrus*. Sawamura (2000) reported 40 chemical components in the marukinkan or round-type of kumquat (*Fortunella japonica* Swingle). The peel oil composition is composed principally of limonene, which makes up about 97% of the total oil (Table 3.13). Monoterpene hydrocarbon (>98.9%) and sesquiterpene hydrocarbon (>0.4%) composed most of the oil volatile. Oxygenated compounds including alcohols, aldehydes, esters, and ketones occupy only less than 0.3% of the total oil. Similar results were also published for round kumquat as studied by Umano et al. (1994).

Closing Remarks. Citrus fruits have been cultivated in Japan anciently and developed day by day using up-to-date crossing techniques. The major citrus species have attracted much research to find out the characteristics of each cultivar for utilization and for creating new products and also improving brands. It is, therefore, very important to investigate and discriminate the aroma composition of a certain citrus oil. The volatile compositions are different among different species and even different varieties of the same species. The most common component occurring at high concentrations in citrus essential oils is limonene. In Japanese citrus, limonene content ranges from 50% to 97% of the total oil volatiles. The lowest limonene levels were reported for *C. indica* and lime oil and the highest content for bitter orange, pummelo, and their hybrids. Due to the highest level of limonene, Japanese citrus oils are dominated by monoterpene hydrocarbons (>90%). The second most abundant components are myrcene and/or γ-terpinene. In some varieties, such as kabosu, mochiyu, banhakuyu, kiyookadaidai, and ujukitsu, myrcene compounds occur at unusual levels (17–50%). The normal level of myrcene was in the range of 1–2%. Regarding γ-terpinene, its content varies widely among species and cultivars. The richest γ-terpinene level was reported for shiikuwasha (*C. depressa* Hayata) and yuko (*C. yuko* Hort. ex Tanaka) of Indica and Ichang-papeda species, respectively. Nootkatone, a characteristic compound of grapefruit and pummelo oils, was not found in Ichang-papeda, tachibana, kumquat, Indica, Tahiti lime, or lemon essential oils. α-Bergamotene is likely a factor to distinguish lime oil from others due to its high concentration and its absence from Ichang-papeda, pummelo, grapefruit, bitter orange, and even the mandarin oils investigated.

3.4.4 Korea

Hee-Sun Song

There are not many kinds of citrus cultivated in Korea. However, the cultivation history of citrus is 1000 years old. Among citrus, commercial crops are yuza

(*Citrus junos*; Yuzu), onjugaml (*Citrus unshiu*; Satsuma mandarin), hallabong (*C. unshiu* × *C. sinensis* × *C. reticulata*; Shiranui), setoka ([*Kiyomi* × *Encore* No. 2] × *Murcott*; Setoka), cheunggyeun (*Citrus unshiu* × *C. sinensis*; Kiyomi), and kumquat (*Fortunella japonica*; Geumgyul).

The essential oils of Korean citrus fruits have been focused on very little; therefore, the research reports have not been often presented (Kang et al., 2006; Baik et al., 2008). The first report on the flavors of Korean citrus was about yuzu in 1975 (Jung, 1975); since then, some research about the flavors and essential oils of Korean citrus has been constantly reported (Lee et al., 1997; 2005). However, the method of identification of flavor components has not been highly developed. After 1998, various reports of Korean citrus flavors were presented, which were systemically studied by using retention index (RI), co-injection of standard compounds, and sensory evaluation, including GC-O (gas chromatography–olfactometry). The volatile composition of Korean citrus fruits and the flavor characteristic compounds so far reported are summarized and listed in Tables 3.14 and 3.15, respectively.

Yuzu (Yuza). The volatile flavors of Korean yuzu were first reported in 1975 (Jung, 1975). In this study, yuzu extract was prepared by hydrodistillation, and three flavor compounds—α-pinene, limonene, and *p*-cymene—were identified (Jung, 1975). The goal of this research was to study organic acids, nonvolatile organic acids, and aromatic compounds and to find the proper method for the processing of yuzu tea. Yuza tea is a favorite of Koreans because of its unique flavor. Yuzu with sugar or honey is fermented for three days or one week; after that, it is diluted with hot water as tea.

Yuzu essential oil was prepared by the solvent extraction method using methylene chloride. Limonene was suggested as the major compound, followed by α-pinene, sabinene, myrcene, terpinene, terpinolene, α-copaene, isocaryopyllene, β-selinene, and elemene, of 28 flavor components identified (Lee et al., 1987b).

Yuzu juice-extraction methods were importantly regarded in the research of yuzu flavor. Jeong et al. (1994) used three extraction methods for getting yuzu juice from whole fruit, including flesh and peel: rotary-crushing and screening, pressing, and belt-pressing. However, they used the solvent extraction method for preparing a flavor extract sample from yuzu juice. They reported 12 volatile compounds as major flavor components of yuzu juice among 74 peak components detected. The ratio of limonene was highest, at a level of 76%, and the second was γ-terpinene (11%). The other 10 components were α-pinene, β-pinene, myrcene, α-terpinene, *p*-cymene, terpinolene, linalool, β-farnesene, γ-elemene, and α-terpineol. Using the belt-press method was more effective than the other two extraction methods for obtaining yuzu flavor components.

The studies on yuzu flavor or yuzu essential oil have focused on the development of new food products or material and development of industrial techniques in Korea until 1995. Kim et al. (1996) also reported volatile compounds of yuzu peel. They used freeze-dried yuzu peel at −70°C. Its volatile compounds were extracted using supercritical CO_2 under 4000 psi at 40°C (Lee and Chun, 2002).

TABLE 3.14. Volatile flavor components of Korean citrus essential oils

Compounds	Yuzu					Mandarin		Shiranui				Kumquat		Setoka	Kiyomi
	CPO-Jeju	CPO-Jindo	SD-Peel	SD-Fruit	SPME-Tea	CPO-Peel	SD-Flesh	Open Field	Green-house	SPME-Peel	SPME-Flesh	CPO-Peel	SD-Fruit	CPO-Peel	CPO-Peel
ethyl acetate	0	0	0	0	0	0	0	0	0	tr	tr	1.1	0	0	0
α-thujene	0	0	0.4	0	0.2	0	0	0	0	0	0	0	0	0	0
α-pinene	2.0	1.9	1.5	1.4	0.9	0.9	0.4	0.6	0.7	0.7	0.3	0.4	0	0.7	0.8
β-pinene	0.7	0.8	0.8	0	0.6	0.4	0	0.2	0.1	0.1	0.1	tr	1.9	tr	tr
sabinene	0.4	0.4	0.2	0.6	0	0	0	3.6	1.8	3.0	1.4	tr	0	0.7	0.9
myrcene	1.1	1.1	2.0	1.9	1.5	2.1	tr	2.4	2.6	1.9	1.4	1.8	0	1.9	2.4
α-phellandrene	1.3	1.3	0.5	0	0.6	tr	0	tr	tr	0.1	tr	0	0	tr	tr
α-terpinene	0.2	0.2	0	0	0.4	0.1	0.4	0	0	tr	0.1	0	0	tr	tr
limonene	75.0	72	80	72.4	63.6	86.7	62.6	86.4	89.4	89.1	64.7	93.7	97.0	77.3	87.5
β-phellandrene	2.1	2.2	0	0	0	0.3	0	0.5	0.5	1.4	0.7	0	0	0.3	0.4
cis-β-ocimene	0	0	0	0	0	0	0	tr	tr	0.4	0.3	0	0	0	0
(*E*)-β-ocimene	0	0	0	0	0.3	0	0	1	0.6	0	0	0	0	0	0.2
γ-terpinene	9.5	9.4	9.3	3.4	14.3	4.8	0	0	0	1.3	1.5	0.3	0.2	0.1	tr
p-cymene	0.4	0.4	0.2	0	0.1	0.3	0	0	0	0.1	0.1	tr	0	tr	0
terpinolene	0.4	0.4	0.5	0.8	0.9	0.2	0.5	tr	tr	tr	0.1	0.1	0	tr	tr
octanal	tr	0.1	0	9.6	0	0.1	2.7	0.5	0.6	tr	0.1	0	0	0.2	0.3
citronellal	0	0	0	0	0	tr	0.6	0.2	0.2	tr	0.1	tr	0	0.1	tr
pentadecane	0	0	0	0	0	0.2	0	0.5	0.6	0	0	tr	0	0	0
decanal	0.1	0.1	0	0	0.1	0	0.1	0.5	0.6	0	0	0	0	0.5	0.3
linalool	3.3	4.7	1.2	1.7	1.6	0.7	0.1	1.2	0.5	0.2	0.9	0.1	0.1	0.7	0.2
β-caryophyllene	0.1	0.2	0.2	0.2	0.9	0.2	0	0	0	tr	0.1	tr	0	0	0.1
thujyl alcohol	0	0	0	0	0	0	0	0	0	0	0	0	0	0.7	tr
cis-β-farnesene	0	0	0	0	0	tr	0	0	0	tr	0.1	0	0	0.2	0.7
trans-β-farnesene	0.6	1.0	0.6	0.7	2.7	tr	0	0	0	0	0	tr	0	0	0.1
α-humulene	tr	tr	0	0	0	0.1	0	tr	tr	0	0	tr	0	0.6	tr
(*E*)-verbenol	0	0	0	0	0	0	0	0	0	0	0	0	0	0.3	0
neral	0	0	0	0	0	0.1	0	tr	tr	0	0	tr	0	0.3	tr
terpinyl acetate	0	0	0	0	0	tr	0	0	0	tr	tr	tr	0	0.5	0
α-terpineol	0.2	0.2	0.1	0.7	0.2	0.2	3.7	0.2	0.1	tr	0.1	tr	0.4	0.4	0.3

dodecanal	0	0	0	0	tr	tr	0	tr	0	tr	tr	tr	0	0.5	0
germacrene D	0.2	0.2	0	0	1.1	tr	0	tr	tr	0	0	0	0	0	0.2
valencene	0	0	0	0	0	tr	0.1	tr	tr	0.1	0.6	tr	0	tr	0.5
geranial	0	0	0	0	0	0	0	0	0	tr	tr	0	0	tr	0.3
bicyclogermacrene	1.0	1.3	0	0	4.6	0.6	0	0.1	tr	tr	0.1	tr	0	0	0
l-carvone	0	0	0	0	0	0.1	0	0	0	0	0	0.4	0	0.7	0.1
cis-linalool pyran oxide	0	0	0	0	0	0	0	0	0	0.1	0.5	0	0	0	0
α-farnesene	0	0	0	0	0.2	0	0	1.3	1.1	0	0	0	0	0.4	0.5
geranyl acetate	0	0	0	0	0	tr	0	0	0	0	0	tr	0.1	0.5	0.2
citronellol	0	0	0	0	0	tr	0.7	0.2	0.2	0.1	0.1	tr	0	0.2	0
perillyl aldehyde	tr	tr	0	0	0	tr	0	0.1	0.1	0	0	0	0	0.3	0.1
carvone oxide	0	0	0	0	0	0	0	0	0	0	0	tr	0	0.4	0
germacrene B	tr	tr	0	0	0.9	tr	0	0	0	0	0	0	0	0	0
cis-carveol	0.1	0.2	0	0	0	tr	0.4	0	0	0	0	tr	0	1	tr
(*E*)-2-dodecenal	0	0	0	0	0	0	0	0	0	0	0	0	0	1.8	0.2
trans-carveol	0	0	0	0	0	0	0	tr	tr	0	0	0	0	0.7	0
cis-nerolidol	0	0	0	0	0	tr	0	0	0	0	0	0.1	0	4.2	0
trans-nerolidol	0.2	0.3	0	0	tr	0	0	0.1	tr	0	0	tr	0	0	tr
thymol	0.1	0.2	0.1	0	0.1	0	0	0	0	0	0	0	0	0	0
β-sinensal	0	0	0	0	0	0	0	0	0	0	0	tr	0	0.4	0.8
α-sinensal	0	0	0	0	0	0	0	0	0	0	0	0	0	0.4	0.5
farnesol	0	0	0	0	0	0	0.5	0	0	0	0	0	0	0	0
nootkatone	0	0	0	0	0	0	0	tr	tr	0	0	0	0	0.1	0.2
Total identified components	62.0	62.0	26.0	28.0	41.0	85.0	25.0	44.0	45.0	43.0	43.0	82.0	10.0	74.0	65
Hydrocarbons	95.4	93.4	97.6	82.8	95.5	97.1	65	96.1	96.8	98.2	72.2	96.7	99	82.6	94.5
Oxygenated compounds	4.1	6.0	1.7	12.0	3.2	1.9	9.7	3.4	2.6	0.6	2.5	2.4	1.1	16.8	4.9
Alcohols	3.9	5.6	1.7	2.4	3.1	1.0	5.2	1.7	0.8	0.3	1.3	0.6	0.6	8.8	0.7
Aldehydes	0.1	0.2	0	9.6	0.1	0.3	4.3	1.5	1.7	0.1	0.5	0.2	0	4.9	2.7
Esters	0	0	0	0	0	0.2	0.2	0.2	0.1	0.1	0.1	1.3	0.5	1.7	1.2
Ketones and oxides	0.2	0.4	0	0	0	0.2	0	tr	tr	0.1	0.6	0.3	0	1.4	0.3

TABLE 3.15. Characteristics of volatile profile of Korean citrus essential oils

Common Name	Scientific Name	Oil Type	Major Compound	Characteristic of Volatile Profile
Yuza (Yuzu)	*Citrus junos* Sieb. ex Tanaka	CPO-peel	limonene, linalool, γ -terpinene, β-phellandrene, α-pinene	• Relatively low proportion of limonene among hydrocarbon compounds
		SD-peel	limonene, linalool, γ -terpinene, α-pinene	• High proportion of alcohol group
		SD-fruit	limonene, octanal, terpinene, myrcene, linalool, α-terpinene	• Abundance of octanal
Onjugam (Mandarin)	*Citrus unshiu* Marcov. forma *Miyagawa-wase*	CPO-peel	limonene, γ-terpinene, myrcene, α-pinene	• Relatively high proportions of γ-terpinene and bicyclogemacrene • Ordor-active impact component by GC-O: terpinolene and linalool
		SD-flesh	limonene, α-terpineol, octanal	• Low proportion of hydrocarbon group • Abundance of octanal and α-terpineol
Hallabong (Shiranui)	*C. unshiu* × *C. sinensis* × *C. reticulata*	CPO-peel	limonene, sabinene, myrcene	• Abundance of sabinene and myrcene • Ordor-active impact component by GC-O: citronellal and citronellyl acetate • Ordor-active impact component by GC-O: citronellal and citronellyl acetate
		SPME-flesh	limonene, sabinene, myrcene, γ-terpinene	• Abundance of valencene and linalool pyran oxide
Geumgyul (Kumquat)	*Fortunella japonica* Swingle	CPO-peel	limonene, myrcene, ethyl acetate	• Abundance of ethyl acetate • Ordor-active impact component by GC-O: citronellyl formate and citronellyl acetate

Setoka	[*Kiyomi* × *Encore* No. 2] × *Murcott*	CPO-peel	limonene, (*Z*)-nerolidol, myrcene, (*E*)-2-dodecenal, *cis*-carveol	• Abundance of (*Z*)-nerolidol, (*E*)-2-dodecenal, carvone, and α-terpinyl acetate
Cheunggyeun (Kiyomi)	*Citrus unshiu* × *C. sinensis*	CPO-peel	limonene, myrcene, sabinene, α-pinene, β-sinensal	• Abundance of valencene and α- and β-sinensal • High proportion of aldehyde group
Jigak	*Citrus aurantium* L.	SD-peel	limonene, myrcene, linalool, α-terpineol	• Abundance of α-terpineol and linalool
Joadeung	*Citrus aurantium* L.	SD-peel		
Dangyuja	*Citrus grandis*	SD-peel	limonene, myrcene, linalool, γ-terpinene	• Abundance of myrcene
Sadungam	*Citrus pseudogulgul*	SD-peel	limonene, γ-terpinene, myrcene	• Abundance of γ-terpinene
Hagyul	*C. natudaidai* Hayata	SD-peel	limonene, γ-terpinene, myrcene	• Abundance of decanal and γ-terpinene
Gamwhagyul	*Citrus natsudaidai* Hayata	SD-peel	limonene, myrcene, linalool, γ-terpinene	• High proportion of alcohol group
Ihyangha	*C. tamurana* Hort. ex Tanaka	SD-peel	limonene, myrcene, linalool, γ-terpinene, sabinene	• High proportion of alcohol group
Chunggyul	*Citrus sinensis*	SD-peel	limonene, myrcene	• Abundance of limonene
Dongjunggyul	*Citrus erythrosa*	SD-peel	limonene, myrcene, β-pinene	• Abundance of myrcene
Gamja	*Citrus benikoji*	SD-peel	limonene, myrcene, β-pinene	• Abundance of limonene
Byunggyul	*Citrus platymamma*	SD-peel	limonene, myrcene, linalool	• Abundance of myrcene
Pyungyul	*Citrus tangerine* Hort. ex Tanaka	SD-peel	limonene, myrcene, linalool, β-pinene, geranyl acetate	• Low limonene level • Abundance of geranyl acetate
Seminole	*Citrus paradisi* Mac. × *C. tangerina* Hort. ex Tanaka	SD-peel	limonene, myrcene, linalool, γ-terpinene, α-terpineol	• Abundance of linalool and γ-terpinene

The yield of volatile compounds was 0.11 g/CO_2 (L) and maximum yield was 8.8 g/yuzu peel (kg). Twenty-two aroma compounds were identified and nine compounds (*dl*-limonene, γ-terpinene, linalool, sabinene, β-myrcene, α-pinene, β-farnesene, α-terpineol, and terpinolene) were suggested as major flavor components of yuzu peel extract by supercritical CO_2. α-Pinene, β-myrcene, and *dl*-limonene decreased gradually, while α-terpineol and β-farnesene increased as the consumption of CO_2 increased.

Song et al. (1999) compared volatile composition of yuzu peel oil from Japan and Korea. Yuzu peel oil was prepared by the cold-pressing method using no chemical solvent. Sixty-two flavor components were identified. Korean yuzu peel oils usually had lower levels of monoterpene hydrocarbons but were relatively more abundant in oxygenated compounds than those from Japan.

Kim et al. (2003) reported the aroma compounds of yuzu tea in the research of the aroma dilution method using GC injector split ratio for volatile compounds extracted by headspace solid-phase microextraction. They suggested linalool and decanal as the most intense aroma-active compounds of yuzu tea.

Satsuma Mandarin (Onjugaml). Satsuma mandarin has been a representative commercial citrus fruit in Korea, although recently Shiranui together with Kiyomi and Setoka has begun to replace these fruits. The essential oil of Korean mandarin juice from the edible portion was extracted by steam distillation using methylene chloride (Lee et al., 1987a). The 31 components were identified and limonene (62.6%), terpineol (3.7%) and octanal (2.7%) were the major components from its essential oil.

The 85 aroma components were identified from Korean mandarin cold-pressed peel oil (Choi and Sawamura, 2002). Its abundant compounds were limonene, γ-terpinene, myrcne, and α-pinene, and terpinolene and linalool were suggested as the character impact odorants related to the sweet and fruity flavor of Korean mandarin by GC-O.

Shiranui (Hallabong). Shiranui, a hybrid variety, was bred by crossing Kiyomi (*Citrus unshiu* Marcov. × *C. sinensis* Osbeck) and Nakano No. 3′ Ponkan (*Citrus reticulata* Blanco) at the Kunchinotsu Branch of the Fruit Tree Research Station in Nagasaki Prefecture (Japan) in 1972 (Matsumoto, 2001). It was recently brought from Japan to Korea and then named Hallabong in 1998, as its round shape with a folded neck looks like Mt. Halla with its crater in Korea (Ko and Kim, 2001). This fruit tastes sweet like orange and has seedless flesh. Shiranui has a large diameter of 8 to 10 cm and an average weight of 350 g.

There are several research reports about Korean Shiranui oil and flavor: character impact odorants of citrus Hallabong (Choi, 2003), headspace-SPME analysis of Hallabong (Choi and Min, 2004), volatile flavor properties of Hallabong grown in open field and greenhouse by GC/GC-MS and sensory evaluation (Song et al., 2005), and the comparison of volatile profiles between Korean and Japanese Shiranui (Song et al., 2006).

One hundred and nine aroma components have been identified from Korean Shiranui (Choi, 2003; Choi and Min, 2004; Song et al., 2005). Limonene (86–91%), sabinene (1.8–3.6%), myrcene (1.9–2.6%), and linalool (0.5–1.2%) were major compounds in Shiranui CPO (Choi, 2003; Song et al., 2005). Citronellal and citronellyl acetate have been regarded as the character impact odorants of Shiranui CPO and citronellal was suggested as giving the most odor-active character by GC-O (Choi, 2003).

The difference in volatile profile between open-field and greenhouse oils was significantly characterized by identification and quantity of alcohol group (Song et al., 2005). The total alcohols in the open-field and greenhouse oils accounted for 1.8% and 0.8%, respectively. Among alcohols, the level of linalool was relatively high in open-field oil (1.2%); however, it accounted for 0.5% in greenhouse oil. Flavor properties of fresh Shiranui peel and flesh were also examined by sensory evaluation. Flavor properties of fresh Hallabong grown in open field were relatively stronger on both peel and flesh by sensory analysis. Sweetness was strong in Hallabong flesh from open field, and sourness in that from greenhouse. The sensory evaluation of the preference in consideration of taste and aroma was significantly high in Hallabong grown in open field ($P < 0.01$). From the present study, the stronger flavor properties and the preference of Hallabong from open field by sensory evaluation seem to be associated with the high level of linalool in its peel oil, and the composition of monoterpene hydrocarbons such as sabinene and (*E*)-β-ocimene (Song et al., 2005).

For the research of Korean Shiranui aroma, an analysis method of headspace-SPME was employed (Choi and Min, 2004). In the headspace of its flavedo, 43 compounds, representing 98.8% of total volatile flavors, were characterized, with limonene (89.1%) being the most abundant compound, followed by sabinene (3.0%), myrcene (1.9%), β-phellandrene (1.4%), and γ-terpinene (1.3%). Monoterpene hydrocarbons were predominant in Hallabong aroma. Major hydrocarbons detected in the edible portion were limonene (64.7%), γ-terpinene (1.5%), myrcene (1.4%), and sabinene (1.4%) (Choi and Min, 2004).

Kumquat (Geumgyul). There are two reports related to the flavor profile of Korean kumquat oil. One is solvent-extracted oil (SEO) and the other is cold-pressed peel oil (Kwang et al., 1992; Choi, 2005). From kumquat SEO, 46 aroma components were identified and limonene (96.5%), β-pinene (1.9%), α-terpineoil (0.4%) were the major components. Specifically, α-terpineol (32.0%) was the most abundant in its diethyl ether fraction (Kwang et al., 1992). The major compounds of Kumquat CPO were limonene (93.7%), myrcene (1.8%), and ethyl acetate (1.1%) (Choi, 2005). Citonellyl formate and citronellyl acetate were regarded as the characteristic odor components of the kumquat peel oil from the results of GC-O, including FD-factor, relative flavor activities, and GC-sniffing. Especially, citronellyl acetate has been suggested as a powerful key component of kumquat (Choi, 2005).

Kiyomi (Cheunggyeun). Among the 65 components quantified in Korean Kiyomi oil, 25 terpene hydrocarbons and 40 oxygenated compounds were identified, with peak weight percentages measuring 94.5% and 4.9%, respectively (Song, 2008). Its major compounds were limonene (87.5%), myrcene (2.4%), sabinene (0.9%), α-pinene (0.8%), β-sinensal (0.8%), (*Z*)-β-farnesene (0.7%), neryl acetate (0.6%), valencene (0.5%), α-farnesene (0.5%), and α-sinensal (0.5%). Valencene and α- and β-sinensal were regarded as the most abundant components of Korean Kiyomi peel oil (Song, 2008).

Setoka (Setoka). Korean Setoka fruit is 200–280g in weight, orange to deep-orange in color, and the shape is flat like mandarin. The rind is thin; therefore the fruit peels easily. The flesh is smooth and juicy. Its aroma is similar to that of orange or mandarin. For this season Shiranui, Setoka, and Kiyomi are harvested from February to April in Korea. They are more popular in spring than the other sweet citrus such as mandarins or oranges because of their freshness and pleasant aroma. The major components of Setoka CPO, among 74 components identified, were limonene (77.3%), (*Z*)-nerolidol (4.2%), myrcene (1.9%), (*E*)-2-dodecenal (1.8%), and *cis*-carveol (1.0%). And a significant feature of Setoka CPO has been suggested to be its relative abundance of (*Z*)-nerolidol, (*E*)-2-dodecenal, carvone, and α-terpinyl acetate (Song and Sawamura, 2007).

3.4.5 Vietnam

Nguyen Thi Lan-Phi

Citrus is one of the most important fruit crops in the world today. In Vietnam, citrus fruits are grown in seven ecological regions, including three major subregions in the north of Vietnam (the mountainous midland region, the Red River Delta, and the northern central coast), in total accounting for 35–40% of citrus production in Vietnam, the Mekong River Delta in the south of Vietnam accounting for 55–60% of citrus production, and the rest concentrated in the central provinces. The citrus-growing areas have increased year by year and citrus fruit production reached 800,000 tons in 2005 (Agro, 2006). The harvesting season that gives the highest production is normally September to December. The citrus fruits grown in Vietnam are diversified and each citrus crop varies with the agro-ecological region; orange (*Citrus sinensis* L. Osbeck), mandarin (*Citrus reticulata* Blanco), pummelo (*C. grandis* (L.) Osbeck), and lime (*C. aurantifolia* Swingle and *C. limonia* Osbeck) are found to be the most popular species harvested all over the country.

Despite the fact that there have been numerous studies on citrus oils of various citrus varieties in the world, there have been very few studies on citrus oils in Vietnam, especially the less common species. This section will focus on the volatile composition of the essential oils of different Vietnamese citrus fruits such as orange (*Citrus sinensis* L. Osbeck), mandarin (*Citrus reticulata* Blanco), pummelo (*C. grandis* (L.) Osbeck), and lime (*C. aurantifolia* Swingle and *C.*

limonia Osbeck), especially those citrus fruits that are of major economic importance.

***Orange (Citrus sinensis* (L). Osbeck).** The Vietnamese sweet orange cultivated in Xa Doai is of medium size with average weight of 192 g. The yield of cold-pressed oil accounts for 0.04% (w/w) of the whole fruit. The volatile compounds presenting in this citrus oil are listed in Table 3.16 in the order of their elution in GC-MS with DB-wax column. The volatile compounds are categorized into groups of monoterpene hydrocarbons, sesquiterpene hydrocarbons, oxygenated compounds including aldehydes, alcohols, esters, ketones, and oxides, and others. A total of 81 volatile compounds have been identified in Xa Doai orange. The composition of monoterpene hydrocarbons consisted of 17 compounds. The most abundant compound was limonene (90.42%), followed by myrcene (2.81%) and α-pinene (0.81%). Myrcene is the second most abundant component of almost citrus oils. The OXD oil can be distinguished from the other hybrids by its high content of δ-3-carene (0.30%). This compound was identified at the lower level of 0.1% or less in sweet orange oil previously studied (Tirado et al., 1995; Minh Tu et al., 2002a). Valencene, a sesquiterpene compound, is believed to play an important role in orange aroma and its concentration has been traditionally used to determine the commercial value of orange oil. Valencene is present in the small amount of 0.02% (Minh Tu et al., 2002a). The two isomers, (*Z*,*E*)- and (*E*,*E*)-α-farnesene, were present at the small amounts of from trace to 0.04%.

Hydrocarbons and aldehydes are the two groups of compounds most extensively quantified in orange oil (Shaw, 1979). In this study, the quantitative values of straight-chain aldehydes from C_8 to C_{11} ranged from trace to 0.15%. Of this, octanal (0.11%) and decanal (0.15%) were predominant compounds. Although neral and geranial are characterstic components of lemon and lime oils, they were present at levels of 0.24% and 0.33%, respectively, and contain of 45% of total aldehydes identified in this sweet orange oil. The two isomeric aldehydes, α- and β-sinensal, which are characteristic components of sweet orange oils (Sawamura, 2000), were quantitated at the same amount (0.09%) in Xa Doai orange oil. Shaw (1979) reviewed a similar amount of these components in orange oil (less than 0.1%); however, the β-isomer predominated over the α-isomer.

Alcohols have been reported to be most important to orange flavor and some of them are the main constituents, including linalool, α-terpineol, and terpinen-4-ol (Shaw, 1979). The amount of linalool in Xa Doai orange was 0.73% and α-terpineol was detected at the considerably high level of 0.26%. This compound, however, is a product of acidic and microbial degradation of limonene and also a contributor to off-flavor in stored orange juice (Shaw, 1979). (*Z*)- and (*E*)-Carveol were identified in sweet orange oils from Ethiopia (Mitiku et al., 2000), but neither was detected in the oil from Vietnam (Minh Tu et al., 2002a). (*E*)-Carveol was quantified at an amount from trace to 0.02%, while (*Z*)-carveol was absent in Xa Doai orange oil. 7-Methyl-3-methylene-6-octen-1-ol and (*R*,*S*)-(+)-*p*-menth-1-en-9-ol were identified for the first time in these orange peel oils.

TABLE 3.16. Volatile components (%w/w) of several Vietnamese citrus essential oils

Compound	Orange	Mandarin		Pummelo			Lime		
	OXD	MHG	MVL	PVG	PPT	PNR	PEL	DLL	BTL
				Hydrocarbons					
Aliphatics									
undecane	—	tr	tr	—	—	—	—	0.01	0.01
tridecane	—	tr	tr	—	—	—	—	0.01	0.01
tetradecane	—	tr	tr	—	—	—	—	—	—
pentadecane	—	—	tr	—	—	—	—	—	—
Monoterpenes									
α-pinene	0.81	2.14	0.93	0.58	0.70	1.69	0.26	0.70	2.87
camphene	tr	0.01	0.01	0.01	tr	0.01	tr	0.20	0.13
β-pinene	0.05	0.89	0.60	0.53	0.23	0.76	0.05	5.81	18.54
sabinene	0.99	0.27	0.33	0.29	0.23	0.22	0.11	1.49	4.52
δ-3-carene	0.30	tr	—	—	—	tr	0.01	—	—
myrcene	2.81	2.30	2.79	18.00	2.63	1.97	2.11	1.69	1.21
α-phellandrene	0.09	0.09	0.06	0.05	0.05	0.07	0.02	0.07	0.05
α-terpinene	0.01	0.32	—	—	—	0.26	—	0.39	0.16
limonene	90.42	74.46	91.58	66.35	85.83	70.46	73.50	59.60	41.40
β-phellandrene	0.58	0.43	0.53	0.46	0.46	0.37	0.23	0.45	0.73
(*Z*)-β-ocimene	0.01	0.01	0.01	0.01	0.02	0.01	0.59	0.16	0.22
thujene	0.01	tr	tr	tr	tr	tr	—	0.01	0.01
γ-terpinene	0.01	12.65	tr	0.40	0.01	11.09	0.87	15.59	7.13
(*E*)-β-ocimene	0.06	tr	0.04	0.01	0.65	0.00	0.59	—	0.22
p-cymene	tr	0.48	tr	—	tr	0.26	—	0.29	0.09
terpinolene	0.07	0.70	0.01	0.02	0.01	0.53	0.02	0.93	0.36
(+)-4-carene	0.01	tr	—	—	—	—	—	—	—
α-pyronene[t]	—	—	—	—	—	—	0.01	—	—
α-*p*-dimethylstyrene	—	tr	—	—	—	—	—	—	—
Sesquiterpenes									
fenchene	—	—	—	—	—	tr	—	—	—
α-cubebene	tr	tr	—	—	tr	tr	—	—	—
guaiene	tr	—	—	—	—	—	—	—	—
α-copaene	0.09	0.11	0.01	tr	tr	0.04	—	0.03	—
β-cubebene	0.07	0.08	—	—	—	0.03	—	0.13	—
α-cedrene	—	—	—	—	—	—	tr	—	0.02
longifolene	—	—	—	—	tr	—	—	—	—
(*Z*)-α-bergamotene	—	—	—	—	—	—	0.04	0.07	0.15
(*E*)-α-bergamotene	—	—	—	—	—	—	0.63	1.14	2.29
β-elemene	0.01	0.04	0.03	0.03	0.03	0.07	0.02	0.02	0.20
epi-bicyclosesqui-phellandrene[t]	0.05	—	—	—	—	—	—	—	—
β-caryophyllene	0.06	0.05	nd	0.44	0.53	0.21	0.38	0.97	2.11
(+)-aromadendrene	—	—	—	—	—	—	—	0.03	0.07
γ-elemene	—	—	—	—	—	—	0.01	—	0.05
β-santalene	—	—	—	—	—	—	0.03	0.04	0.09

TABLE 3.16. *Continued*

Compound	Orange	Mandarin		Pummelo			Lime		
	OXD	MHG	MVL	PVG	PPT	PNR	PEL	DLL	BTL
(*Z*)-β-farnesene	—	—	—	—	0.01	—	nq	0.08	0.17
α-humulene	0.03	0.08	0.03	0.04	0.05	0.20	0.03	0.10	0.26
(*E*)-β-farnesene	0.01	—	—	—	—	0.02	nq	0.05	0.11
farnesene	—	—	—	—	—	—	0.49	—	—
β-himachalene[t]	—	—	—	—	—	—	tr	—	—
α-selinene	—	—	—	—	—	—	—	—	0.03
δ-elemene	0.01	0.01	0.01	0.02	—	0.04	0.14	0.03	0.40
germacrene D	0.24	0.65	0.30	3.56	6.37	1.81	0.07	1.28	0.77
(*Z*,*E*)-α-farnesene	tr	—	—	0.03	—	0.02	—	—	0.06
valencene	0.02	0.02	tr	0.06	—	0.11	—	—	0.13
α-muurolene	0.02	0.02	—	0.03	—	0.10	—	—	—
γ-selinene	—	—	—	2.04	—	—	—	—	—
β-bisabolene	—	—	—	—	—	—	1.62	1.85	3.71
bicyclogermacrene	0.09	0.14	—	0.30	0.58	—	—	—	—
(*E*,*E*)-α-farnesene	0.04	0.17	—	0.06	0.02	0.07	—	1.52	2.34
δ-cadinene	0.21	0.01	0.19	0.04	0.05	0.21	—	—	0.26
β-selinene[t]	—	—	—	0.03	—	—	0.03	—	—
β-sesquiphellandrene	tr	—	tr	—	—	—	—	—	—
(*Z*)-α-bisabolene	—	—	—	—	—	0.08	—	0.06	0.23
germacrene B	—	0.05	—	—	—	—	0.03	0.03	1.28
β-guaiene	—	—	0.07	—	0.01	0.31	—	—	—
			Aldehydes						
heptanal	—	—	—	—	—	—	tr	—	—
octanal	0.11	0.04	0.15	tr	tr	0.35	0.32	0.14	0.03
nonanal	0.02	0.01	0.06	—	—	0.10	0.39	0.03	0.02
2-methyl octanal[t]	—	—	—	—	—	—	0.02	—	—
citronellal	0.08	0.06	0.02	0.02	0.01	0.09	0.14	0.77	0.06
decanal	0.15	0.06	0.17	tr	tr	0.39	0.63	0.17	0.27
undecanal	0.01	0.02	0.06	—	—	0.07	0.38	—	—
p-menth-1-en-9-al	0.01	0.01	0.01	—	—	—	—	—	—
(*E*)-2-decenal	—	—	—	—	—	—	0.01	—	—
(*E*)-2-decenal	—	0.01	0.01	—	—	—	—	—	—
neral	0.24	0.08	0.02	0.95	0.19	0.18	4.86	0.09	1.87
dodecanal	—	—	—	—	—	—	0.08	—	—
geranial	0.33	0.10	0.03	1.30	0.27	0.14	8.38	0.13	2.92
(*E*)-2-undecenal	—	0.01	0.01	—	—	—	—	—	—
(*E*,*E*)-2,4-decadienal	—	tr	—	—	—	—	—	—	—
cumin aldehyde	—	—	—	—	—	—	0.01	—	—
perilla aldehyde	0.12	0.28	0.15	0.11	0.08	0.12	0.03	0.03	0.02
tridecanal	—	—	0.01	—	—	—	0.04	—	—
(*E*)-2-dodecenal	—	0.06	0.07	—	0.01	0.14	—	—	—
tetradecanal	—	—	tr	—	—	—	0.04	—	0.05
(*E*)-2-tridecenal	—	0.01	0.01	—	—	—	—	—	—
pentadecanal[t]	—	—	—	—	—	—	0.05	—	—
anisaldehyde	—	—	0.01	—	—	—	—	—	—

TABLE 3.16. *Continued*

Compound	Orange	Mandarin		Pummelo			Lime		
	OXD	MHG	MVL	PVG	PPT	PNR	PEL	DLL	BTL
(*E*)-2-tetradecenal	—	tr	—	—	—	0.05	—	—	—
hexadecanal	—	—	—	—	—	—	0.18	0.05	0.15
octadecanal[t]	—	—	—	—	—	—	0.04	—	—
β-sinensal	0.09	—	—	—	—	—	—	—	—
(*Z*,*E*)-farnesal	0.01	—	—	—	0.01	—	—	—	—
α-sinensal	0.09	0.25	—	—	—	—	—	—	—
nonadecanal	—	—	—	—	—	—	tr	—	—
			Alcohols						
1-heptanol	—	—	—	—	—	—	0.01	—	—
trans-sabinene hydrate	0.03	0.03	0.01	0.01	tr	0.03	0.01	0.10	0.15
2,3-butanediol	—	—	—	—	—	—	0.01	—	—
linalool	0.73	0.26	0.24	0.17	0.14	0.12	0.52	0.15	0.21
cis-sabinene hydrate	tr	0.15	—	—	—	0.12	—	0.14	0.07
1-octanol	0.02	0.02	0.08	—	—	—	—	0.01	—
methyl isoborneol[t]	—	0.01	—	—	—	—	—	—	—
terpinen-4-ol	0.02	0.12	—	0.01	tr	0.11	0.00	0.07	0.01
cis-verbenol[t]	—	—	—	—	—	—	0.01	—	—
trans-*p*-mentha-2,8-dien-1-ol	0.02	0.01	0.02	—	—	—	—	—	—
isopinocampheol	—	—	—	—	—	0.05	—	—	—
nonanol	—	—	tr	—	—	—	0.09	—	—
tetrahydrogeraniol	—	—	0.01	—	—	—	—	—	—
decanol	—	—	0.02	—	—	—	—	—	—
α-citronellol	—	—	—	—	0.19	—	tr	—	—
cis-*p*-mentha-2,8-dien-1-ol	0.03	—	—	—	—	—	—	—	—
α-terpineol	0.26	0.62	0.41	0.26	0.12	0.57	0.08	0.72	0.51
borneol	—	0.01	0.01	—	—	—	—	—	—
thujyl alcohol	—	—	—	—	—	—	—	—	0.02
cis-piperitol	—	—	—	0.03	—	—	—	—	—
decanol	—	—	0.02	—	—	—	—	—	—
β-citronellol	0.06	0.11	0.07	—	tr	0.04	tr	0.06	0.01
7-methyl-3-methylene-6-octen-1-ol	0.01	—	—	—	—	—	—	—	—
nerol	0.03	0.04	0.26	0.12	0.01	0.02	0.04	—	0.02
p-menth-1-en-9-ol	—	—	0.01	—	—	—	—	—	—
(*E*)-carveol	0.02	0.02	0.04	0.02	0.01	0.01	—	0.03	—
geraniol	0.02	0.01	0.02	0.04	tr	tr	0.04	0.00	0.01
p-mentha-1(7),8(10)-dien-9-ol	tr	0.04	—	—	—	—	—	—	—
undecanol	—	—	0.01	—	—	—	—	—	—
(*Z*)-carveol	—	—	—	0.04	—	—	—	—	—
(*R*,*S*)-(+)-*p*-menth-1-en-9-ol	tr	0.02	—	—	—	—	—	—	—
(*S*,*S*)-(+)-*p*-menth-1-en-9-ol	—	tr	—	—	—	—	—	—	—

TABLE 3.16. *Continued*

Compound	Orange	Mandarin		Pummelo			Lime		
	OXD	MHG	MVL	PVG	PPT	PNR	PEL	DLL	BTL
selina-6-en-4-ol	—	0.02	—	—	—	—	—	—	—
p-mentha-1(7),8(10)-dien-9-ol	—	0.04	—	—	—	—	—	—	—
perillyl alcohol	0.03	—	0.02	—	—	—	tr	—	—
p-menth-1-en-9-ol	—	—	0.01	—	—	—	—	—	—
(*Z*)-nerolidol	—	—	0.07	0.01	—	0.05	—	—	—
germacrene D-4-ol[t]	—	0.04	0.01	—	—	—	—	—	—
(*E*)-nerolidol	0.01			tr	0.03	0.03	0.01	—	—
germacradien-4-ol[t]	0.02	0.04	0.01	0.04	0.05	0.02	tr	—	—
β-elemol	0.02	0.03	0.01	—	—	—	tr	0.01	—
α-cedrol	—	—	—	—	—	—	0.01	—	0.03
cedrenol[t]	—	—	—	—	—	—	0.18	—	—
β-bisabolol	—	—	—	—	—	—	0.02	—	0.04
santalol[t]	—	—	—	—	0.02	—	—	—	0.09
thymol	—	0.15	—	—	—	—	tr	—	0.09
α-bisabolol	—	—	—	—	—	—	0.09	0.11	0.24
cinnamyl alcohol	—	—	—	—	—	—	0.05	0.06	—
α-bisabolol	—	—	tr	—	—	—	—	—	—
β-eudesmol	—	—	tr	—	—	—	0.01	—	—
isothymol	—	—	tr	0.01	—	0.02	—	—	—
isoeugenol	—	—	—	0.01	—	—	—	—	—
(*Z*,*E*)-farnesol	—	—	—	—	—	—	tr	—	—
(*E*,*E*)-farnesol	—	—	—	—	0.02	—	0.01	—	—
1-hexadecanol	—	—	—	—	—	—	0.01	—	—
			Esters						
methyl butyrate	—	—	—	—	—	tr	—	—	—
heptyl acetate	—	—	—	—	—	tr	—	—	—
octyl acetate	—	—	—	—	—	—	—	—	—
linalyl acetate	—	tr	tr	—	—	—	—	—	—
β-terpinyl acetate	—	—	0.01	—	—	—	0.01	—	—
nonyl acetate	—	—	—	—	—	0.02	0.38	—	—
citronellyl acetate	tr	0.04	—	0.01	—	0.08	—	0.02	0.01
decyl acetate	tr	0.01	0.01	—	—	—	tr	—	—
α-terpinyl acetate	0.01	—	—	—	—	—	tr	—	—
neryl acetate	0.01	0.11	0.09	—	0.11	0.65	0.04	—	—
carvyl acetate[t]	—	—	0.02	—	0.02	0.17	—	—	—
geranyl acetate	0.01	0.10	—	0.19	—	0.18	0.08	0.23	0.22
dodecyl acetate	—	—	0.02	—	—	—	tr	—	—
perillyl acetate	—	—	—	0.01	—	0.05	—	—	—
cedryl acetate	—	—	—	—	—	—	0.03	—	—
			Ketones						
α-thujone	—	—	tr	—	—	—	—	—	—
menthone	—	—	0.01	—	—	—	—	—	—
δ-camphor	—	tr	—	—	tr	—	—	—	—
solanone	—	—	—	—	—	0.01	—	—	—

TABLE 3.16. *Continued*

Compound	Orange	Mandarin		Pummelo			Lime		
	OXD	MHG	MVL	PVG	PPT	PNR	PEL	DLL	BTL
cis-p-menth-8-en-2-one	0.01	—	—	—	—	—	—	—	—
trans-p-menth-8-en-2-one	0.01	—	—	—	—	—	—	—	—
nootkatone	tr	—	—	0.53	0.03	3.38	—	—	—
(*S*)-carvone	0.02	0.04	0.04	—	—	—	—	0.21	—
p-mentha-1,8-dien-3-one	0.04	0.04	—	—	—	—	—	—	—
l-carvone	—	—	—	—	—	—	tr	—	—
tetrahydro ionone[t]	—	—	—	—	—	—	tr	—	—
piperitone	—	tr	—	—	—	—	—	—	—
p-mentha-1,8-dien-3-one	—	0.04	—	—	—	—	—	—	—
α-ionone	—	—	tr	—	—	—	—	—	—
Oxides									
(*Z*)-limonene oxide	tr	tr	tr	tr	0.01	0.01	tr	0.03	0.01
(*E*)-limonene oxide	0.03	0.01	0.01	0.01	tr	0.01	tr	—	—
(*Z*)-linalool oxide	—	—	0.02	tr	tr	—	nq	0.03	—
(*E*)-linalool oxide	—	—	tr	—	—	0.04	—	—	—
nerol oxide[t]	—	—	tr	—	—	—	—	—	—
(-)-caryophyllene oxide	tr	—	—	—	—	—	0.01	—	0.02
Others									
1,8-cineole	0.01	0.01	0.01	tr	tr	—	0.03	0.32	0.04
perillene[t]	0.01	—	—	—	0.01	—	—	—	—
decanoic acid	—	—	—	—	—	—	0.06	—	—
nonanoic acid	—	0.01	—	—	—	0.04	—	—	—
decanoic acid	—	0.01	—	—	—	—	—	—	—
thymol methyl ether	—	0.50	—	—	—	—	—	—	—
methyl-*N*-methyl anthranilate	—	0.02	0.03	—	—	—	—	—	—
diterpene 1	—	—	—	1.70	—	—	—	—	—
diterpene 2	—	—	—	0.65	—	—	—	—	—

[t]Tentatively identified.
tr: Trace, weight percent quantified less than 0.005%.
nq: Detected but not quantified.

The six esters were identified, accounting for 0.04% of the total oil volatiles. Neryl acetate, geranyl acetate, and α-terpinyl acetate were found at low concentrations as much as 0.01%. In the other minor group of ketones, (*S*)-carvone (a known oxidation product of limonene) was identified at a level of 0.02% and nootkatone (a characteristic compound of grapefruit and pummelo oils) was also detected at trace amounts. The two isomers, *cis*- and *trans*-dihydrocarvone, were present in Xa Doai orange at a concentration of 0.01%, while *p*-mentha-1,8-dien-3-one was quantified to be 0.04%. Xa Doai sweet orange oil also contains (*Z*)- and (*E*)-limonene oxides at a level of 0.03% or less. The two ethers found in this orange were 1,8-cineole and perillene, present at the same amount, at 0.01%.

***Mandarin (Citrus reticulata* Blanco).** The citrus fruits of mandarin (*Citrus reticulata* Blanco) collected from Ha Giang (MHG) and Vinh Long (MVL) provinces, Vietnam, in November 2005 were used. The fresh fruits of Ha Giang and Vinh Long mandarins were of medium size with average weights of 94.3 and 71.4 g, respectively. The yield of cold-pressed oils accounted for 0.07% and 0.15% (w/w), accordingly, of the whole fruit of MHG and MVL. The oils obtained had a greenish-yellow color with green and sharp notes for MHG, whereas MVL oil had green and aldehyde-like notes with milder aroma compared to MHG. A total of 95 and 81 compounds have been identified, constituting about 98.78% and 99.11% of the total oil of MHG and MVL, respectively (Table 3.16). Hydrocarbons were the most extensively identified group in the mandarin oils. A series of homologous alkanes from C_{11} to C_{14}, except for C_{12}, were found in MHG oil at very low quantities of trace amounts. The same result was also observed for MVL oil, with the additional existence of pentadecane. Tetradecane was determined at a higher concentration among this group than the other mandarin oils reported by Lan Phi and Sawamura (2007). A total of 16 monoterpenes were found in MHG oil. The major components found in this group were limonene (74.46%), followed by γ-terpinene (12.65%), myrcene (2.3%), and α-pinene (2.14%). The two monoterpenes, γ-terpinene and β-pinene, were important to mandarin aroma and flavor (Shaw et al., 1981). β-Pinene was present at a rather high content of 0.89% in this mandarin oil. *p*-Cymene accounted for a relatively high amount of 0.48%. This component, however, was considered as an indicator for aging of yuzu oil. α-*p*-Dimethyl styrene, usually found in yuzu oil, was also detected in this mandarin oil at trace amounts. α-Thujene, usually identified in tangerine oil (Shaw, 1979), was also found in these two oils at very low concentrations.

In MVL, monoterpenes presented at higher amounts than those reported for MHG oil, accounting for 96.9%. The content of limonene (91.58%) in MVL seems to cause this difference. The second most abundant compound found in MVL was myrcene (2.79%), followed by α-pinene (0.93%). γ-Terpinene, the second most abundant compound in MHG, was identified at a trace amount in MVL oil, but not detected in Vietnamese tangerine cultivated in Ha Tay as reported by Minh Tu et al. (2002a). δ-3-Carene (trace) and α-terpinene (0.32%), found in MHG, were not detected in MVL oil.

Fourteen sesquiterpenes were identified in MHG, in which germacrene D (0.65%), (*E*,*E*)-α-farnesene (0.17%), bicyclogermacrene (0.14%), and α-copaene (0.11%) were the major components. These compounds made up 75.69% of the total sesquiterpenes quantified. However, only nine sesquiterpenes were identified in MVL oil, amounting to 0.64% of the total oil volatiles with germacrene D (0.30%), δ-cadinene (0.19%), and the other compounds present at 0.07% or less.

Aldehydes are said to be important to mandarin flavor (Shaw, 1979; Chisholm et al., 2003a). Fifteen aldehydes were identified in MHG and MVL oils, accounting for 1.00 and 0.78%, respectively. Among them, perilla aldehyde (0.28%), α-sinensal (0.25%), geranial (0.10%), and neral (0.08%) were predominant in MHG oil, while decanal (0.17%), octanal, and perilla aldehyde (0.15% each) were the major aldehydes in MVL. α-Sinensal, a farnesene-type sesquiterpenoid, has been reported to contribute significantly to the aroma of many sweet orange oils (Shaw, 1979; Sawamura, 2000) and tangerine oil (Moshonas and Shaw, 1974). Its content in this mandarin oil was relatively high, whereas it was not detected in tangerine oil. A series of aliphatic aldehydes ranging from octanal (C_8) to undecanal (C_{11}) in MHG oil and C_8 to C_{14}, except for dodecanal, in MVL oil, were also found. Decanal was the greatest component, with contents of 0.06% and 0.17% in MHG and MVL oils, respectively. The result was in agreement with previous studies that saturated straight-chain aldehydes with even carbon numbers occurred in higher quantities than those with adjacent members with odd carbon numbers (Shaw, 1979). A series of unsaturated fatty aldehydes, (*E*)-2-compounds of decenal to tetradecenal, were also identified and quantified at the amount ranging from trace of (*E*)-2-tetradecenal to 0.06% of (*E*)-2-dodecenal in MHG oil. These compounds were reported as contributors to the aroma of clementine oil (Buettner et al., 2003). (*E*,*E*)-2,4-Decadienal and anisaldehyde were found in MVL oil, but not detected in MHG oil. The other terpene aldehydes existed at 0.07% or less in these mandarin oils.

Twenty and 22 alcohols were identified and quantified in MHG and MVL peel oils, and accounted for 1.69% and 1.30%, respectively. The major alcohols were α-terpineol (0.62% and 0.41%) and linalool (0.26% and 0.24%). Terpinen-4-ol and α-terpineol have been reported at high amounts in Japanese mandarin oil (Choi et al., 2002). In this study, *cis*-sabinene hydrate and thymol (0.15% each) and terpinen-4-ol (0.12%) were found in MHG but not detected in MVL. Thymol, an important flavor compound in mandarin and tangerine (Shaw, 1979), was completely absent from MVL. This compound was also not found in both Japanese and Korean Satsuma mandarin oils (Choi et al., 2002) and Vietnamese tangerine produced from Ha Tay province (Minh Tu et al., 2002a). The two isomers (*R*,*S*) and (*S*,*S*) of (+)-*p*-menth-1-en-9-ol were identified by comparison of MS spectra, and retention indices of chemical references, and confirmed by co-injection with an authentic commercial mixture of (*R*,*S*)- and (*S*,*S*)-isomers. Methylisoborneol and borneol were present at the amount of 0.01% each. Selina-6-en-4-ol and methylisoborneol were tentatively identified for the first time in mandarin oil. The four aliphatic alcohols ranging from octanol (C_8) to undecanol (C_{11}) were present at a low level (less than 0.02%) in MVL.

There are five esters identified, of which neryl (0.11%) and geranyl acetate (0.10%) made up 82%. The main esters are of acetic acid and terpene hydrocarbons, except for decyl acetate (0.01%). This group in MVL oil was composed of 6 components, accounting for 0.15% of the total oil volatiles. Neryl acetate was also the major component in this group (0.09%) as reported for MHG peel oil. The minor group of ketones includes four compounds with the concentration ranging from trace to 0.04%. (*S*)-Carvone and *p*-mentha-1,8-dien-3-one occurred at the level of 0.4% each. Carvone, an oxidation product of limonene, was the prominent compound. The oxides were 1,8-cineole and (*Z*)- and (*E*)-isomers of limonene oxide. These compounds were present at very low concentrations (up to 0.01%) in both mandarin oils. 1.8-Cineole also existed at the same amount (0.01%) in Vietnamese orange oils. (*Z*)- and (*E*)-Linalool oxides were found only in MVL and were not detected in MHG oil. In addition, the remaining group including two acids and one ether was found in MHG oil. Methyl-*N*-methylanthranilate, a contributor of mandarin aroma (Charles, 1981), was identified at quantities of 0.02% and 0.03% in MHG and MVL, respectively. An important component of tangerine flavor, thymol methyl ether, was completely absent from MVL, whereas it was existed at a relatively high amount (0.50%) in MHG oil.

Pummelo (Citrus grandis* (L.) Osbeck*). Pummelo fruits cultivated in Ha Tinh province (Phuc Trach pummelo, PPT), Hung Yen province (Van Giang pummelo, PVG), and Can Tho province (Nam Roi pummelo, PNR) in Vietnam were collected at the end of the mature season in Vietnam on October 26, November 10, and November 28, 2005, respectively. The average weights of PVG, PPT, and PNR were 1400, 1000, and 1200g per fruit, accordingly. The yields of CPOs were 0.07, 0.04, and 0.07% (w/w) of the whole fruit, respectively. The oils possessed a pale-yellow color with fresh and sweet odor. The volatile compounds separated in three pummelo oils are listed in Table 3.16. Ninety-one components were separated and quantified in the peel oil of the three pummelo varieties. Among them, 54 compounds were commonly found in PVG and PPT and 73 in PNR oils. The components amounted to 99.61, 99.87, and 99.26% of the total oil volatiles, respectively.

Monoterpene hydrocarbons constituted the most dominant chemical group among the volatiles of PVG (86.71%), PPT (90.82%), and PNR (87.70%) peel oils. Limonene was the most abundant compound, accounting for 66.35, 85.83, and 70.46% in each of the oils, respectively. The content of limonene in these pummelo oils was lower than that in pummelo oil previously reported (Minh Tu et al., 2002a). The other prominent monoterpene hydrocarbons in each of these pummelo oils were α-pinene (1.69%) and γ-terpinene (11.09%) in PNR, and myrcene (18.00, 2.63, and 1.97%) in PVG, PPT, and PNR oils, accordingly. α-Thujene, which was not detected in previously investigated pummelo oil, was identified in these oils at a trace quantity. PVG could be discriminated from PPT and PNR because the oil contained a higher level of myrcene (18.00%). (*E*)-β-Ocimene (0.65%) isolated PPT from the other pummelos, while NR could be distinguished by its high amount of γ-terpinene (11.09%). The contents of γ-terpinene (0.01–11.09%) and terpinolene (0.02–0.53%) were in agreement with Tosa buntan (*C. grandis* Osbeck forma *Tosa*), Vietnamese pummelo grown in Japan (*C. grandis* Osbeck forma *Vietnam*), and Akano-buntan (*C. grandis* Osbeck) cold-pressed oils (Sawamura et al., 1991). γ-Terpinene was not detected in the Vietnamese pummelo sample reported by Minh Tu et al. (2002a). The NR oil contained δ-3-carene and α-terpinene, which were not detected in the other two oils. *p*-Cymene was found in PNR oil (0.26%) and at a trace quantity in PPT oil, but it was not detected in PVG pummelo oil.

A total of 14 sesquiterpene hydrocarbons were found in each of the PVG and PPT oils, and 20 in NR oil. The amounts of these components were 6.67, 7.67, and 3.90% in PVG, PPT, and PNR oils, respectively. Among the constituents, germacrene D was the most abundant. Its content was 3.56% in PVG, 6.37% in PPT, and 1.81% in PNR oils. These amounts were higher than those reported in literature for most pummelo oils of different origins (Dugo et al., 2002; Minh Tu et al., 2002a). Other components relatively notably present in three oils were β-caryophyllene (0.21–0.53%), α-humulene (0.04–0.20%), δ-cadinene (0.04–0.21%), β-elemene (0.3–0.7%), and (*E*,*E*)-α-farnesene (0.02–0.07%). Several sesquiterpenes that were not identified in NR oil existed at relatively high amounts of 0.34% (RI = 1595), 0.11% (RI 1765), and 0.08% (RI 1465). Bicyclogermacrene, present at 0.30% in PVG and 0.58% in PPT oils, was not detected in PNR oil. The variations in occurrence of these sesquiterpenes could be used to differentiate the respective pummelo oils.

Out of 11 aldehydes identified, 6 compounds were found in PVG, 8 in PPT, and 10 in PNR oil, amounting to 2.37, 0.58, and 1.62% of the total oil, respectively. Geranial, neral, and perilla aldehyde were the major aldehydes. The highest amount was reported for geranial (1.30%), followed by neral (0.95%) in PVG oil. The aliphatic aldehydes, octanal, nonanal, decanal, and undecanal, were present in NR oil, but their contents were 0.02% or less and nonanal and undecanal could not be detected even in the other two oils. Among them, octanal and decanal were the most predominant. These two compounds were also the predominant aldehydes of OHG, OTB, and OXD oils. (*E*,*E*)-Farnesal was present only in PPT pummelo oil. The compositional variations of the aldehydes could be used to distinguish these oils.

Alcohols amounted to 0.75, 0.60, and 1.20% of the PVG, PPT, and PNR oils, respectively. The relatively prominent alcohols in those oils were α-terpineol (0.12–0.57%) and linalool (0.12–0.17%). Nerol in PVG oil (0.11%) and terpinen-4-ol at 0.11% in PNR oil were present at the highest amount among these oils. The two isomers, *cis*- and *trans*-sabinene hydrates, were found in most of the oils investigated in this study. *trans*-Sabinene hydrate more frequently appeared at a rather low concentration of 0.03% or less. Another two isomers of carveol were also found in these pummelo oils. (*Z*)-Carveol was not detected in the PPT and PNR oils. (*Z*)- and (*E*)-Isomers of nerolidol were also found, constituting up to 0.05% in each oil. The former, a compound rarely reported in citrus oils, was absent in PPT oil. In contrast, α-citronellol and (*E*,*E*)-β-farnesol were found only in PPT oil and their contents were 0.19 and 0.02%, respectively. The presence of these two compounds distinguished the PPT oil from the PVG and PNR oils.

A total of nine ester compounds were found, constituting about 0.21, 0.13, and 1.36% in PVG, PPT, and PNR oils, respectively. The most important and frequently used terpene esters in flavors are the acetates of nerol, geraniol, citronellol, linalool, and isoborneol. Citronellyl acetate and geranyl acetate were found in PVG and PNR oils but neither in PPT oil. Neryl and geranyl acetates were predominent in these oils, being constituted of 0.11–0.65%. Neryl acetate could be used to differentiate the PVG oil from PPT and PNR, and geranyl acetate distinguished the PPT oil from the other oils.

Nootkatone is well known as a character-impact compound of grapefruit (Shaw, 1979) and also a significant key compound for defining the identity of the pummelo species (Sawamura et al., 1991). Nootkatone was found at a great amount in PNR oil (3.38%), followed by that in PVG (0.53%) and PPT (0.03%) oils. The content of nootkatone showed considerable differences in the total ketone concentrations of PVG, PPT, and PNR oils: 0.53, 0.04, and 3.39%, accordingly. Oxide group content was less than 0.06% of the total oil volatiles of PVG, PPT, and PNR. The oxides found in these oils were (*Z*)- and (*E*)-isomers of both limonene oxides and linalool oxides. 1,8-Cineol and (*Z*)-linalool oxide were present only in PVG and PPT oils and neither were found in PNR oil. (*E*)-Linalool oxide was detected only in PNR oil, but not in the others. The other compounds found in three pummelo oils were perillene, nonanoic acid, and two diterpene hydrocarbons. Perillene, the terpene ether found in OXD, was detected in PVG and PPT oils at trace to 0.01%. The two diterpenes were detected only in PVG oil, amounting to a total of 2.36% in PVG oil volatiles. Nonanoic acid, the only aliphatic acid, was present at a minor quantity (0.04%) in the PNR sample.

The differences in the volatile compositions among the peel oils of the three pummelos were noted and characterized. The occurrence of nootkatone, one of the most characteristic compounds of grapefruit and pummelo oils, was also demonstrated in those pummelo samples. The results based on the essential oil composition could be useful information applicable to the classification of pummelo cultivars and utilization of their fruit products.

***Lime (C. aurantifolia* Swingle and *C. limonia* Osbeck).** *Citrus aurantifolia* Persa (Persa lime) fruits obtained in September 2004 from the Institute of Fruit and Vegetable Research, Hanoi, *Citrus aurantifolia* Swingle (BT lime), and *Citrus limonia* Osbeck (DL lime) fruits obtained in November 2005 from Ben Tre and Lam Dong provinces (Vietnam), respectively, were used to analyze the composition of essential oils. The yield of the essential oil was 0.02% of total weight of the fresh fruit. The oil has a greenish-yellow color with a pleasant, citrusy aroma.

Ninety-two compounds among 96 volatile components were detected in the Persa lime oil (Table 3.16). These volatile compounds, constituting 97.93% of the lime oil, can be classified into monoterpene hydrocarbons (77.77%), sesquiterpene hydrocarbons (3.26%), aldehydes (15.35%), alcohols (1.19%), esters (0.21%), acids (0.06%), oxides (0.02%), ethers (0.03%), and ketones in trace amounts. Thus, monoterpenes were the major group in this lime oil (77.77%), in which Limonene (73.5%) was the most abundant compound, followed by geranial (8.38%), neral (4.86%), myrcene (2.11%), and β-bisabolene (1.62%). The proportion of limonene was higher than that in the literature reported for distilled lime oil (39–47%) and cold-pressed lime oil (50–71%) (Chisholm et al., 2003b). A series of 12 aliphatic aldehydes ranging from heptanal to nonadecanal, except heptadecanal, were also identified. The straight-chain aldehyde, nonadecanal, was found in lime oil for the first time. It is surprising that citral (neral and geranial) was present at a very high proportion, accounting for 86% of total aldehydes. Germacrene B and D were determined at proportions of 0.03% and 0.10%, respectively.

For the volatile components of lime (*C. aurantifolia* Swingle) oil (BT lime), 67 compounds were identified and quantified in this lime oil (Table 3.16). The monoterpene hydrocarbons were also found to be prominent in BT lime peel oil (77.41%) with Limonene as the most abundant compound (41.40%), followed by β-pinene (18.54%), γ-terpinene (7.13%), sabinene (4.52%), α-pinene (2.87%), and myrcene (1.21%). Limonene in Key lime (*C. aurantifolia* Swingle) cold-pressed oil was reported to have the lowest concentration among citrus essential oils (Dugo et al., 2002). The high content of β-pinene was matched with various studies on Key lime (*C. aurantifolia*) oil cited by Dugo et al. (2002). β-Bisabolene (3.71%), α-farnesene (2.34%), (*E*)-α-bergamotene (2.29%), β-caryophyllene (2.11%), and germacrene B (1.28%) were found to be the major components among sesquiterpene hydrocarbons. Of the 29 oxygenated compounds, 9 aldehydes, 15 alcohols, 2 esters, and 3 oxides were identified, accounting for 5.39, 1.54, 0.23, and 0.07%, respectively. Geranial (2.92%) and neral (1.87%) were found to make up most of the content of the aldehyde group. High levels of geranial and neral were also reported for Vietnam lime oil previously studied (Lan Phi et al., 2006). α-Terpineol (0.51%), α-bisabolol (0.24%), and linalool (0.21%) were principal alcohols and geranyl acetate (0.22%) was the main ester identified. Three oxides—1,8-cineole, (*Z*)-limonene oxide, and caryophyllene oxide—were also detected. (*Z*)-limonene oxide (0.01%) was found in most of the citrus oils investigated in this study.

Fifty-seven compounds were identified and quantified, amounting to 98.51% of DL lime oil volatiles. The monoterpene hydrocarbons were prominent, accounting for 87.38%, higher than that reported for Persa lime (77.77%) and BT lime oil (77.41%). β-Pinene and γ-terpinene were found to be the second most abundant components in the DT lime oil, as in BT oil. However, the ratio of β-pinene to γ-terpinene in DL oil was 1:2.6, while that in BT oil was 2.7:1 and almost the same level was observed from the Persian (*C. latifolia*) cold-pressed lime oils extracted in the laboratory (Njoroge et al., 1996). The result also indicates that (*E*)-α-bergamotene (1.14%), β-bisabolene (1.85%), and α-farnesene (1.52%) were abundant among sesquiterpenes identified. The content of germacrene D (1.28%) was higher than that of BT lime (0.77%), while germacrene B was present at the very small amount of 0.03%. Eight aldehydes, 11 alcohols, 2 esters, 1 ketone, and 2 oxides were also detected and quantified in this lime oil, accounting for 1.41, 1.46, 0.25, 0.21 and 0.35%, respectively. Citronellal (0.77%), α-terpineol (0.72%), geranyl acetate (0.23%), carvone (0.21%), and 1,8-cineole (0.32%) were representatives among those compounds. Three different lime varieties (*C. aurantifolia* Persa, *C. aurantifolia* Swingle, and *C. limonia* Osbeck) were analyzed, and their volatile compositions were identified. The oils were discriminated from each other and other lime varieties investigated by their volatile components and their ratio in a certain oil mixture. It was likely that (*E*)-α-bergamotene might play an important role in lime oil aroma.

3.5 EUROPE

Marco Poiana

The *Citrus* diffusion in Europe includes the Mediterranean countries: France, Portugal, Spain, Italy, and Greece. These countries, located in the EU, produce 10% of the worldwide quantity. Among the different *Citrus* species, European countries account for more than 15% of the world production of lemons. The named minor *Citrus*, such as mandarin, clementine, tangerine, and bergamot, are also important productions in European countries; these *Citrus*, combined in a single class, are nearly 15% of the total world production. The total quantity of citrus fruits yielded and declared in recent years is about 10 million tons. The distribution for the single species or group of species is as follows: lemons nearly 1.5 million tons, oranges and 5–6 minor citrus fruits, previously named, 2.5–3.0. Among the European countries, Spain and Italy produce respectively 45% and 40% of the lemons. Forty-five percent of oranges are produced in Spain, 35% in Italy, 15–16% in Greece, and nearly 5% in Portugal. Mandarins, Satsumas, and tangerines are mainly produced in Spain (more than 70%) and Italy (20%), with only 4% in Greece and less than 1% in Portugal and France. Citrus production in Spain is mainly located in four regions: Catalonia, Comunidad Valenciana, Murcia, and Andalusia. The Comunidad Valenciana is the most important, and in this area the citrus production represents 70% of the Spanish product; it is particularly focused on oranges. Italy has its main production regions in Sicily, Calabria, and Campania; the last one is important for lemon typically harvested in Amalfi-Surrento peninsulae, where a particular and typical liquor is obtained from infusion of parts of this fruit. Apulia and Basilicata are also important, but only for fresh-consumed production. Calabria has a typical and unique product: bergamot. It is cultivated only in the area near Reggio Calabria and it is harvested for the character of its essential oil, long used in perfumery compounds. Sicily is known for lemon and bitter and sweet orange essential oils.

If the market is limited by some types of citrus essential oils, researchers have studied their composition in relation to typical and traditional citrus species and also to new hybrids.

Considering the citrus fruit transformation, only a minor amount is dedicated to essential oil production. In particular, oranges and lemons are harvested for juices and essential oils, but these products show a contraction in their amounts. Only bergamot has its essential oil as the only product from the fruits; in fact the juice is not used in foodstuffs.

The main citrus essential oils currently produced in Europe are:

- Lemon essential oil obtained from the flavedo part of the fruit.
- Bergamot essential oil obtained from the flavedo part of the fruit.
- Orange (sweet and bitter) essential oil obtained from the flavedo part of the fruit.
- Mandarin essential oil obtained from the flavedo part of the fruit (but in some processes the whole fruit is squeezed and subsequently the oil is separated by centrifuge).
- Essences of lemon from the fruit peels by infusion with hydro-alcoholic solvents of food grade.
- Essences of citron from the whole fruit by infusion with hydro-alcoholic solvents of food grade.
- Distilled oils obtained from particular parts of flowers of bitter orange, named neroli, or leaves of bitter orange, named petit grain. At the present time, these distillates are not important.

Table 3.17 shows the cold-pressed essential oil compositions (range) of the main components detected by GC regarding essential oils of some citrus species produced in Europe (Calvarano et al., 1994; Dugo et al., 2002).

3.5.1 Lemon

The most common citrus essential oil is lemon. The main cultivars used in essential oil production (also used in juice production) are: "Femminello commune," "Monachello," "Interdonato," and "Eureka."

Limonene is the main component of the volatile fraction, with a content varying from 60 to 71%. Two other monoterpene hydrocarbon molecules, β-pinene and γ-terpinene, are contained in wide concentration intervals of 10–18% and 7–11%, respectively, while α-pinene, sabinene, and myrcene make up over 1% of the volatile fraction. Aldehydes, in particular neral and citral, are the most representative class of oxygenated compounds, which on average comprise a fraction of 2 to 7%. Variations in the volatile fraction of lemon essential oil are strongly linked to seasonality and consequently connected to the qualitative level of the essential oil produced. Oil obtained from winter lemons is considered to be of higher quality than oil obtained from summer lemons. From a composition aspect, in Italian and particularly Sicilian production, the presence of aldehydes such as neral and citral in the volatile fraction is higher in essential oils produced from fruit harvested during winter compared with summer harvests. The greatest presence of other aldehydes such as citronellal, nonanal, and decanal is observed during summer. Overall, and in particular for lemon essential oil produced in Sicily, there is a minimal content of carbonyl compounds in summer lemon productions, which without doubt results in their inferior quality. There is a significant reduction in limonene during the summer, resulting in minimum content of 60% of the volatile fraction in the essential oils produced, while the opposite

TABLE 3.17. Volatile components of Italian citrus essential oils

Compound	Lemon	Sweet Orange	Bitter Orange	Bergamot	Mandarin	Citron
α-thujene	0.4–0.5			0.2–0.5	0.1–1.1	0.8–1.0
α-pinene	1.5–2.4	0.4–0.7	0.4–0.6	0.7–1.8	2.0–2.8	1.8–2.4
sabinene	1.1–2.8	0.2–1.0	0.3–0.5	0.1–2.0	0.2–0.3	0.2–0.3
β-pinene	9.5–17.8		0.6–1.3	4.4–11.0	1.4–2.1	1.9–2.1
myrcene	1.1–1.9	1.7–2.5	1.7–1.8	0.7–1.8	1.6–2.0	1.4–1.6
octanal		0.1–0.4	0.1–0.2		0.1–0.2	0.2–0.4
δ-3-carene		0.1–0.3				
α-terpinene	0.1–0.3			0.1–1.2	0.3–0.5	0.1–0.5
p-cymene	0.1–0.7			0.1–0.8	0.1–0.8	0.4–0.5
limonene	59.6–71.1	92.7–95.9	92.5–93.8	24.1–54.9	65.3–74.5	51.3–61.2
(*Z*)-β-ocimene	0.1–0.2					0.9–1.5
(*E*)-β-ocimene	0.1–0.3		0.2–0.4	0.1–0.4		1.2–2.1
γ-terpinene	6.6–11.3			5.4–11.4	16.2–22.8	22.4–27.7
terpinolene	0.2–0.4			0.2–0.5	0.7–1.0	0.6–1.1
linalool	0.1–0.2	0.3–0.7	O.2–0.3	1.6–20.3	0.1–0.2	0.1–0.3
nonanal	0.1–0.2					
citronellal	0.1–0.2					0.1–0.5
α-terpineol	0.1–0.3				0.1–0.3	0.2–0.3
decanal		0.1–0.4	0.1–0.2			0.4–0.5
octyl acetate				0.1–0.2		
nerol	0.1					0.1–0.4
neral	0.5–1.3			0.1–0.7		0.7–1.7
geraniol						0.1–0.4
linalyl acetate			0.6–1.2	15.1–40.4		
geranial	0.6–2.3	0.1–0.2		0.2–0.5		1.1–2.7
bornyl acetate						
undecanal						
citronellyl acetate						
neryl acetate	0.2–0.9			0.1–0.7		0.1–0.7
geranyl acetate	0.2–0.8			0.1–0.8		0.1–0.6
N-metyl antranilate					0.3–0.7	
β-caryophyllene	0.1–0.3			0.2–0.6		0.1–0.2
(*E*)-α-bergamottene	0.2–0.6			0.2–0.4		0.2–0.4
valencene		0.1–0.4				
β-bisabolene	0.3–0.9			0.3–0.7		0.2–0.6
α-sinensal					0.1–0.5	

trend is observed in two other important monoterpene hydrocarbons, β-pinene and sabinene (Cotroneo et al., 1988).

Of the variables studied, extraction technology also influences the composition of the volatile fraction. In the main European countries, Spain and Italy, cold-pressed lemon essences are mainly extracted using three types of machines: "pelatrice," "sfumatrice," and a smaller quantity obtained from in-line FMC. There has been a sharp reduction in the use of distillation to obtain essence from the fruit. It has been observed that "pelatrice," which processes more lemons than the other two machines, produces lemon essential oils more highly enriched in oxygenated compounds and with a lower content of monoterpene hydrocarbons (Cotroneo et al., 1986a, 1988; Verzera et al., 1999). With the growth in lemon cultivation, especially in major lemon-producing areas such as Sicily, new hybrids are being introduced whose fruit is also used for the production of essential oil. The oil obtained is not significantly different from that found for traditional cultivars (Starrantino et al., 1997).

Lemons are also used in the preparation of drinks obtained from the infusion of flavedo in hydroalcoholic solvent. In some regions, above all in Italy, production is limited to certain areas. In order to safeguard specificity, it is important to characterize the volatile fraction of the extract obtained from maceration in ethyl alcohol. This practice is widespread with lemons grown on the Amalfi and Sorrento coastline near Naples as well as other areas in southern Italy. Extracts have shown a content of oxygenated compounds ranging from 4 to 8%, higher than that observed in cold-pressed essential oils. The composition of the extract, as already noted for cold-pressed essential oils, is strongly influenced by the harvest season and the variety of the fruit, enabling, in certain cases, a distinction to be made between different productions and identifying a link with the territory (Poiana et al., 2006).

Psoralenic and cumarinic molecules are found in the nonvolatile fraction of cold-pressed lemon essential oils, including among the latter 5-geranyloxy-7-methoxycoumarin, citropten and 5-isopentenyloxy-7-methoxycoumarin, while bergamottin, 8-geranyloxypsoralen, oxypeucedanin, byakangelicol, oxypeucedanin hydrate, byakangelicin, imperatorin, phellopterin, isoimperatorin, and 5-isopent-2′-enyloxy-8-(2′,3′-epoxyisopentyloxy)-psoralen are found in psoralens. The main components are bergamottin (160–291 mg/100 g of oil) and 5-geranyloxy-7-methoxycoumarin (180–250 mg/100 g of oil) (Dugo et al., 1998b).

3.5.2 Bergamot

The bergamot essential oil is very important for its commercial value, particularly in Italian citrus production, where it is used in the perfume industry. Moreover, it has a typically strong characteristic due to the limited area of production as previously noted.

This essential oil has a lower overall variability because extraction for commercial production is carried out exclusively by "pelatrice." There are essentially only three cultivars: "Femminello," "Fantastico," and "Castagnaro," and the productive area is limited. Nevertheless, bergamot oil exhibits a variability linked to the pedoclimatic characteristics of the production area, which, although covering a small area, exhibits diversity due to the harvesting period. In recent years, the chemical-physical and compositional characteristics that distinguish the essence have evidenced a trend showing a worsening of the characteristics. The causes of this phenomenon are due to the reduction in attention to agronomical practices and climatic regions that have shown anomalous temperatures and rainfall in recent years.

The economic importance linked to its use is due to the composition of the volatile fraction. Indeed, the content of hydrocarbon compounds is markedly lower than that present in other citrus essential oils, whereas there is a greater presence of oxygenated compounds, particularly linalool, in the optically active levorotatory form, and its ester, linalyl acetate. These two compounds represent, with very wide composition intervals, 2–20% and 15–40%, respectively, of the volatile fraction. The optical activity of linalool permits the assessment of genuineness of bergamot essential oil (Cotroneo et al., 1992). The period in which the fruit is harvested has a considerable influence on the ratio between linalool and linalool acetate. In December, at the start of the season, there is a higher quantity of alcohol, which tends to decrease during the following months, reaching its minimum values in the March harvest. Linalyl acetate follows the opposite trend (Dugo et al., 1991). The monoterpene hydrocarbon fraction is principally represented by limonene, which varies from 24 to 55%, β-pinene (4–11%), and γ-terpinene (5–11%) (Mazza, 1986).

The nonvolatile fraction is principally made up of psoralens and coumarins, including bergapten, which has greatly conditioned the use of this essential oil due to its photosensitivity. The compounds detected are bergamottin, which ranges between 1.02% and 2.75%, 5-geranyloxy-7-methoxycoumarin (between 0.08 and 0.22%), citropten (between 0.14% and 0.35%), and bergapten (between 0.11 and 0.32%). The mean content of bergamottin and 5-geranyloxy-7-methoxycoumarin did not vary during the production period, while that of citropten and bergapten decreased considerably from January to March (Mondello et al., 1993).

The extraction of the bergamot flavedo carried out using compressed solvents such as supercritical carbon dioxide (CO_2) results in extracts with different chemical compositions compared to essential oils extracted using "pelatrice." Moreover, the composition of both the volatile and nonvolatile fraction is strongly influenced by the solvent characteristics of CO_2, expressed by its density: A higher density increases the solvent capacity. A higher content of bergapten is observed in extracts obtained from CO_2 at high density and for prolonged extraction times, evidencing a lower solubility of the compound in the solvent fluid (Poiana et al., 1999).

3.5.3 Sweet Orange

Sweet orange essential oil is extracted industrially using the "pelatrice" and FMC extractor. The cultivars used can be divided according to the pigmentation of the pulp: pigmented and blonde. The "Tarocco," "Moro," and "Sanguinello" varieties are found in the former, while the latter include the "Comune" or "Biondo comune," "Ovale," "Valencia," "Navel" ("Washington" and "Navelina"), and "Belladonna" varieties. The ratio between volatile and nonvolatile fractions of the essential oil is similar to that of other essential oils derived from citrus fruits. The main component of the volatile fraction is always limonene, which makes up over 90%. Other components present in significant amounts are myrcene (1.7–2.5%), sabinene (0.2–1.0%), and α-pinene (0.4–0.7%). Of the oxygenated compounds, on average linalool (0.4–0.5%), decanal, and octyl aldehyde (0.1–0.5%) are found in quantities above 0.1%, while the other components identified are very often found only at trace levels. Valencene, a sesquiterpene, is present in trace concentrations of up to 0.6% of the volatile fraction. Its presence is linked to the period of harvest, increasing from the start of the season (January) to the end (May). Moreover, a difference in this component was observed between fruit with blonde and pigmented pulp. In the latter, valencene was found in higher quantities compared with the former, while the aldehyde content was lower (Dugo et al., 1994; Verzera et al., 1996). For the purposes of a qualitative evaluation it should be remembered that the characteristics of the essential oil of sweet orange are linked to the aldehyde content, which is an important index of the deterpenated oil yield. Indeed, this process reduces the hydrocarbon content, which makes a minor contribution to the creation of the aroma. The nonvolatile fraction consists above all of flavons.

3.5.4 Bitter Orange

The extraction of bitter oranges to produce essential oil is carried out using "pelatrice," "sfumatrice," "torchio," and FMC machines. The volatile fraction is largely made up of limonene (over 90%) while the other monoterpene hydrocarbons recorded in significant quantities are the same as those found in sweet oranges: myrcene (1.6–1.9%), β-pinene (0.5–1.4%), α-pinene (0.4–0.6%), and sabinene (0.2–0.5%). Of the oxygenated compounds, the linalool acetates and linalool make up over 1% of the volatile fraction (Dugo et al., 1993; Lota et al., 2001).

Four coumarins (osthol, meranzin, isomeranzin, and meranzin hydrate), three psoralens (bergapten, epoxybergamottin, and epoxybergamottin hydrate), and four polymethoxyflavones (tangeretin, 3,3′,4′,5,6,7,8-heptamethoxyflavone, nobiletin, and *tetra-O*-methylscutellarein) were identified in the nonvolatile fraction. Italian essential oils usually exhibited a higher content of oxygen heterocyclic compounds than the Spanish oils (Dugo et al., 1996).

3.5.5 Mandarin

Essential oils obtained from mandarins exhibit a high degree of variability in their composition due to the characteristics of the different species that make up this group of citrus fruit, the ripening phase in which the fruit is harvested, as well as the technology used in obtaining the essential oil. The "King," "Satsuma," "Mandarini Avana," "Tangerini," and "Fortune" varieties are widespread in European cultivations. Mandarin essential oil may be obtained by pressing followed by separation from the juice or using FMC machines or "pelatrice." The volatile fraction mainly consists of monoterpene hydrocarbons such as limonene (65–75%) and γ-terpinene (16–23%). Other monoterpene hydrocarbons present in smaller quantities include α-pinene (1.9–2.9%), β-pinene (1.3–2.2), myrcene (1.4–2.0%), and terpinolene (0.6–1.1%) (Mazza, 1987; Dugo et al., 1992). Genuineness of the essential oil is defined as having a presence of (+)-limonene in a range of between 97.4 and 98.2% compared with the total of the two optical isomers (Dugo et al., 1992). Among the oxygenated compounds it was found that the esters were mainly made up of *N*-methyl anthranilate of methyl, which, in small concentrations of 0.2–0.7% of the volatile fraction, may be considered a typical marker of this essential oil. With regard to the influence of the harvest period on the quality of the essential oil, it was found that it is closely linked to the botanic heterogeneity, which permits harvest over a very wide period of time. In any case, in Italian production, the content of limonene increases as the season progresses while that of other components, both monoterpene hydrocarbons and characteristic components such as the already-mentioned *N*-methyl anthranilate of methyl and the sesquiterpene α-sinensal in the volatile fraction, decrease.

The nonvolatile fraction is principally made up of methoxyflavons, which contribute toward characterizing it from a chemical-physical as well as constituent viewpoint.

In recent years there has been an increase in clementine cultivation in the citrus-growing areas of Italy and Spain, which include the "Monreal," "Comune," "Oroval," and "Nules" varieties. Therefore, the essential oil obtained from these citrus is becoming more important. Its composition is principally made up of limonene, which forms 92–96% of the volatile fraction; other monoterpene hydrocarbons present in significant quantities are α-pinene and sabinene (Verzera et al., 1997).

The heterocyclic compounds present in the nonvolatile fraction of clementine essential oil are mainly represented by polymethoxylated flavones. Six components were identified: tangeretin, 3,3′,4′,5,6,7,8-heptamethoxyflavone, nobiletin, *tetra-O*-methylscutellarein, sinensetin, and 3,3′,4′,5,6,7-hexamethoxyflavone (Verzera et al., 1997).

3.5.6 Grapefruit

Grapefruit is not particularly predisposed for the extraction of essential oil, which is mainly obtained by pressing or from FMC machines; the most widespread cultivars are "Marsh" and "Duncan." The composition of the volatile fraction consists above all of limonene and other terpene hydrocarbons. There is also a modest quantity of the nootkatone compound, which may be considered as a marker for grapefruit essence.

Applying technologies that use solvents to extract its components in the extraction of grapefruit essential oil results in obvious differences in the composition. Indeed, when using an unpolar solvent such as pentane or a supercritical fluid, a lower content of monoterpene hydrocarbons and higher content of sesquiterpenes and oxygenated compounds are observed in the oleoresin extract. The extracts also evidence a high content of nootkatone. The solvent effect of the fluid in supercritical phase increases with its density, resulting in a greater extraction of compounds such as sequiterpenes, alcohols, aldehydes, esters, and nootkatone (Poiana et al., 1998a).

3.5.7 Citron

The extraction of citron essential oil is not particularly developed owing to the anatomic characteristics of the fruit, with its spongy albedo, which has a retentive effect on the essential oil; the shape of the fruit, which is often irregular; and also the markets, which tend to sell the fruit whole. Among the most widespread cultivars are "Digitato," "Diamante," "Etrog," and "Cedro della Corsica." The essential oil is often confused with lemon oil as a result of the blends carried out as well as their characteristic compositional similarities. Studies were carried out on the composition of essential citron oil obtained by hydrodistillation, hydrocarbon solvent extraction, and using supercritical CO_2 as solvent. The hydrodistillate had the highest content of monoterpene hydrocarbons, whereas the lowest content was observed in those extracts obtained with the highest density of the supercritical fluid (Poiana et al., 1998b). The main component of the volatile fraction is limonene (55–60%), followed by γ-terpinene (22–24%), α-pinene (1.9–2.4%), β-pinene (1.9–2.1%), myrcene (1.5–1.6%), (*Z*)-β-ocimene (0.8–1.6%), and (*E*)-β-ocimene (1.1–2.2%) (Cotroneo et al., 1986b). Significant sesquiterpenes include *trans*-α-bergamottene and β-bisabolene, which, in extracts obtained with supercritical fluids, reach up to 3 and 6% of the volatile fraction, respectively.

REFERENCES

ACIAR. (2008). Market development for citrus from eastern Indonesia. http://www.aciar.gov.au.

Agilent 6890 GC and ChemStation Operation. (2004). Agilent Technologies.

Agro. 2006. Actual situation and sustainable development strategy of edible fruit production up to 2015. http://www.agro.gov.vn.

Ahmed, E.M., Dennison, R.A., Shaw, P.E. (1978). Effect of selected oil and essence volatile components on flavor quality of pump out orange juice. *Journal of Agricultural and Food Chemistry* **26**: 368–372.

Anonim. 2009. Citrus hystrix. http://zipcodezoo.com/Plants/C/Citrus_hystrix/Default.asp.

Ashoor, S.H.M., Bernhard, R.A. (1967). Isolation and characterization of terpenes from *Citrus* reticulata Blanco and their comparative distribution among other *Citrus* species. *Journal of Agricultural and Food Chemistry* **15**: 1044–1047.

Azzouz, M.A., Reineccius, G.A., Moshonas, M.G. (1976). Comparison between cold-pressed and distilled lime oils through the application of gas chromatography and mass spectrometry. *Journal of Food Science* **41**: 324–328.

Baik, J.S., Kim, S.S., Lee, J.A., Oh, T.H., Kim, J.Y., Lee, N.H., Hyun, C.G. (2008). Chemical composition and biological activities of essential oils extracted from Korean endemic citrus species. *Journal of Microbiology and Biotechnology* **18**: 74–79.

Biro Pusat Statistik. (2002). *Statistik pertanian*. Jakarta: BPS.

Boelens, M.H. (1991). A critical review on the chemical composition of citrus oils. *Perfumer and Flavorist* **16**: 17–34.

Buettner, A., Schieberle, P. (2001). Evaluation of aroma differences between hand squeezed juices from Valencia late and navel oranges by quantitation of key odorants and flavour reconstitution experiments. *Journal of Agricultural Food Chemistry* **49**: 2387–2394.

Buettner, A., Mestres, M., Fischer, A., Guasch, J., Schieberle, P. (2003). Evaluation of the most odour-active compounds in the peel oil of clementines (*Citrus reticulata* Blanco cv. *clementine*). *European Food Research and Technology* **216**: 11–14.

Calvarano, M., Cotroneo, A., Crispo, F., Di Giacomo, A., Dugo, G., Lezzi, U., Mincione, B., Poiana, M. (1994). Gli oli essenziali agrumari. In: Di Giacomo, A., Mincione, B. (ed.), *Gli oli essenziali agrumari in Italia*. Italy: Laruffa Editore, pp. 71–185.

Chamblee, T.S., Clark, B.C., Brewster, G.B., Radford, T., Iacobucci, G.A. (1991). Quantitative analysis of the volatile constituents of lemon peel oil: Effects of silica gel chromatography on the composition of its hydrocarbon and oxygenated fractions. *Journal of Agricultural and Food Chemistry* **39**: 162–169.

Charles, W.W. (1981). Thymol, methyl-*N*-methylanthranilate and monoterpene hydrocarbons to the aroma and flavour of mandarin cold-pressed oils. *Journal of Agricultural and Food Chemistry* **29**: 494–496.

Chisholm, M.G., Jell Ja, Jr., D.M.C. (2003a). Characterization of the major odorants found in the peel oil of *Citrus reticulata* Blanco cv. *Clementine* using gas chromatography–olfactometry. *Flavour and Fragrance Journal* **18**: 275–281.

Chisholm, M.G., Wilson, M.A., Gaskey, G.M. (2003b). Characterization of aroma volatiles in key lime essential oils (*Citrus aurantifolia* Swingle). *Flavour and Fragrance Journal* **18**: 106–115.

Choi, H.S., Sawamura, M. (2000). Composition of the essential oil of *Citrus tamurana* Hort. ex Tanaka (Hyuganatsu). *Journal of Agricultural and Food Chemistry* **48**: 4868–4873.

Choi, H.S., Kondo, Y., Sawamura, M. (2001). Characterization of the odor-active volatiles in citrus hyuganatsu (*Citrus tamurana* Hort. ex Tanaka). *Journal of Agricultural and Food Chemistry* **49**: 2404–2408.

Choi, H.S., Sawamura, M., Kondo, Y. (2002). Characterization of the key aroma compounds of *Citrus flaviculpus* Hort. ex Tanaka by aroma extraction dilution analysis. *Journal of Food Science* **67**: 1713–1718.

Choi, H.S., Sawamura, M. (2002). Comparison of cold-pressed peel oils composition between Korean and Japanese Satsuma mandarin (*Citrus unshu* Marcov. forma *Miyagawa-wase* by GC, GC-MS, and GC-O. *Journal of Food Science and Nutrition* **7**: 5–11.

Choi, H.S. (2003). Character impact odorants of Citrus Hallabong [(*C. unshiu* Marcov. × *C. sinensis* Osbeck) × *C. reticulata* Blanco] cold-pressed peel oil. *Journal of Agricultural and Food Chemistry* **51**: 2687–2692.

Choi, H.S., Min, K.C. (2004). Headspace-SPME analysis of *Citrus* hybrid, Hallabong. *Food Science and Biotechnology* **13**: 126–129.

Choi, H.S. (2005). Characteristic odor components of Kumquat (*Fortunella japonica* Swingle) peel oil. *Journal of Agricultural and Food Chemistry* **53**: 1642–1647.

Cotroneo, A., Dugo, G., Licandro, G., Ragonese, C., Di Giacomo, G. (1986a). On the genuineness of citrus essential oils. Part XII: Characteristics of sicilian lemon essential oil produced with the FMC extractor. *Flavour and Fragrance Journal* **1**: 125–134.

Cotroneo, A., Verzera, A., Alfa, M., Dugo, G. (1986b). Sulla genuinità delle essenze agrumarie. Nota XIV. L'olio essenziale di cedro. *Essenze—Derivati Agrumari* **56**: 105–120.

Cotroneo, A., Verzura, A., Dugo, G., Dugo, G., Licandro, G. (1988). Sulla genuinità delle essenze agrumarie. Nota XXII: La composizione dell'essenza di limone siciliana prodotta industrialmente nell'annata 1984–85. *Industria delle bevande* **17**: 209–224.

Cotroneo, A., Stagno d'Alcontres, I., Trozzi, A. (1992). On the genuineness of *Citrus* essential oils. Part XXXIV: Detection of added reconstituted bergamot oil in genuine bergamot essential oil by high resolution gas chromatography with chiral capillary columns. *Flavour and Fragrance Journal* **7**: 15–17.

Dellacassa, E., Lorenzo, D., Moyna, P., Verzera, A., Mondello, L., Dugo, P. (1997). Uruguayan essential oils. Part VI. Composition of lemon oil. *Flavour and Fragrance Journal* **12**: 247–255.

Dharmawan, J., Kasapis, S., Curran, P., Johnson, R.J. (2007). Characterization of volatile compounds in selected citrus fruit from Asia. Part I: Freshly squeezed juice. *Flavour and Fragrance Journal* **22**: 228–232.

Dharmawan, J., Kasapis, S., Curran, P. (2008). Characterization of volatile compounds in selected citrus fruits from Asia. Part II: Peel oil. *Journal of Essential Oil Research* **20**: 21–24.

Dharmawan, J., Kasapis, S., Sriramula, P., Lear, M.J., Curran, P. (2009). Evaluation of aroma-active compounds in Pontianak orange peel oil (*Citrus nobilis* Lour. var. *Microcarpa* Hassk.) by gas chromatography–olfactometry, aroma reconstitution, and omission test. *Journal of Agricultural and Food Chemistry* **57**: 239–244.

Dugo, G., Cotroneo, A., Verzera, A., Donato, M.G., Del Duce, R., Licandro, G., Crispo, F. (1991). Genuineness characters of Calabrian bergamot oil. *Flavour and Fragrance Journal* **6**: 39–56.

Dugo, G., Stagno d'Alconres, I., Cotroneo, A., Dugo, P. (1992). On the genuineness of *Citrus* essential oils. Part XXXV. Detection of added reconstituted mandarin oil in genuine cold-pressed mandarin essential oil by high-resolution–gas chromatography with chiral capillary columns. *Journal of Essential Oil Research* **4**: 589–594.

Dugo, G., Verzera, A., Stagno D'Alcontres, I., Cotroneo, A., Ficarra, R. (1993). On the genuineness of citrus essential oils. Part XLI: Italian bitter orange essential oils: Composition and detection of contamination and additions of oils and terpenes of sweet orange and lemon. *Flavour and Fragrance Journal* **8**: 25–33.

Dugo, G., Verzera, A., Stagno d'Alcontres, I., Cotroneo, A., Trozzi, A., Mondello, L. (1994). On the genuineness of citrus essential oils. Part XLIII: The composition of the volatile fraction of Italian sweet orange oils (*Citrus sinensis* (L.) Osbeck). *Journal of Essential Oil Research* **6**: 101–137.

Dugo, P., Mondello, L., Cogliandro, E., Verzura, A., Dugo, G. (1996). On the genuineness of citrus essential oils. Part 51: Oxygen heterocyclic compounds of bitter orange oil (*Citrus aurantium* L.). *Journal of Agricultural and Food Chemistry* **44**: 544–549.

Dugo, P., Mondello, L., Lamonica, G., Dugo, G. (1997). Characterization of cold-pressed Key and Persian lime oils by gas chromatography, gas chromatography/mass spectroscopy, high-performance liquid chromatography, and physicochemical indices. *Journal of Agricultural and Food Chemistry* **45**: 3608–3616.

Dugo, P., Cotroneo, A., Bonaccorsi, I., Mondello, L. (1998a). On the genuineness of citrus essential oils. Part LVII: The composition of distilled lime oil. *Flavour and Fragrance Journal* **13**: 93–97.

Dugo, P., Mondello, L., Cogliandro, E., Cavazza, A., Dugo, G. (1998b). On the genuineness of citrus essential oils. Part LIII: Determination of the composition of the oxygen heterocyclic fraction of lemon essential oils (*Citrus limon* (L.) Burm. f.) by normal-phase high performance liquid chromatography. *Flavour and Fragrance Journal* **13**: 329–334.

Dugo, G., Cotroneo, A., Verzera, A., Bonaccorsi, I. (2002). Composition of the volatile fraction of cold-pressed citrus peel oils. In: Dugo, G., Di Giacomo, A. (eds.), *Citrus: The genus Citrus*. London: CRC Press, Taylor & Francis Group, pp. 201–317.

Dugo, G., Giacomo, A.D. (2002). In: Dugo, G., Di Giacomo, A. (eds.), *Citrus: The genus Citrus*. New York: Taylor & Francis.

El-Shazly, A., Doral, G., Wink, M. (2002). Chemical composition and biological activity of the essential oils of *Senecio aegyptius* var. *discoideus Boiss. Zeitschrift Naturforschung* **57c**: 434–439.

Feger, W., Brandauer, H., Ziegler, H. (2001). Analytical investigation of Sweetie peel oil. *Journal of Essential Oil Research* **13**: 309–313.

Fellers, P.J. (1985). *Citrus: Sensory quality as related to rootstock, cultivar, maturity, and season: Evaluation of quality of fruit and vegetables*. Westport, CT: AVI, pp. 83–128.

Fischer, A., Grab, W., Schieberle, P. (2008). Characterization of the most odor-active compounds in a peel oil extract from Pontianak oranges (*Citrus nobilis* Lour. var. *Microcarpa* Hassk.). *European Food Research Technology* **227**: 735–744.

Frizzo, C.D., Lorenzo, D., Dellacassa, E. (2004). Composition and seasonal variation of the essential oils from two mandarin cultivars of southern Brazil. *Journal of Agricultural and Food Chemistry* **52**: 3036–3041.

Fujita, S., Inoue, Y., Nonaka, A. (2005). Constituents of the essential oil of *Citrus tachibana* Tanaka. *Proceedings of Symposium on the Chemistry of Terpenes, Essential Oils, and Aromatics (TEAC)*, Fukui, Japan, pp. 21–23.

Gancel, A.L., Olle, D., Ollitrault, P., Luro, F., Brillouet, J.M. (2002). Leaf and peel volatile compounds of an interspecific citrus somatic hybrid [*Citrus aurantifolia* (Christm.) Swing. + *Citrus paradisi* Macfadyen]. *Flavour and Fragrrance Journal* **17**: 416–424.

Giacomo, A.D., Mincione, B. (1994). Olio essenziale di arancia dolce. In: *Gli olii essenziali agrumari in Italia*. Reggio Calabria: Laruffa Editore, pp. 115–129.

Gonzalez de, C.N., Sanchez, F., Quintero, A., Usubillaga, A. (2002). Chemotaxonomic value of essential oil in *Citrus* species. *Proceedings of the International Conference on Medicinal and Aromatic Plants. Acta Horticulturae* **576**: 49–51.

Guenther, E.S., Langenau, E.E. (1943). An investigation of the chemical constituents of distilled lime oil (*Citrus medica*, L. var. *Acida*, Brandis) (*Citrus aurantifolia*, Swingle). *Journal of the American Chemical Society* **65**: 959–963.

Hadiyanto, Sulasmi, E.S., Mujiarto, E. (2007). Kekerabatan genetik beberapa spesies jeruk berdasarkan taksonometri. *Journal Hortikultura* **17**: 203–216.

Herout, V. (1971). Biochemistry of sesquiterpenoids. In: Goodwin, T.W. (ed.), *Aspects of terpenoid chemistry and biochemistry*. London: Academic Press, pp. 53–90.

Hodgson, R.W. (1967). Horticultural varieties of *Citrus*. In: Reuther, W., Bachelor, L.D., Webber, H.J. (eds.), *The citrus industries, volume 1*. Berkeley, CA: University of California, pp. 431–591.

Hugo, B., Treatt, P.L.C., Bury, S.E. (1996). Natural aroma chemicals from orange and other botanical sources. *Perfumer and Flavorist* **21**: 9–11.

Jantan, I., Ahmad, A.S., Ahmad, A.R., Ali, N.A.M., Ayop, N. (1996). Chemical composition of some citrus oil from Malaysia. *Journal of Essential Oil Research* **8**: 627–632.

Jeong, J.W., Lee, Y.C., Jung, S.W., Lee, K.M. (1994). Flavour components of citron juice as affected by the extraction method. *Korean Journal of Food Science and Technology* **26**: 709–712.

Jung, J.H. (1975). Studies on the processing and the storage of *Citrus junos*. *Rural Development Review* **9**: 107–110.

Kang, S.K., Jang, M.J., Kim, Y.D. (2006). A study on the flavor constituents of the citron (*Citrus junos*). *Korean Journal of Food Preservation* **13**: 204–210.

Katayama, S., Imayoshi, Y., Iwabuchi, H. (2002). Study on the volatiles of Banpeiyu. *Proceedings of International Symposium on the Chemistry of Essential Oils, Terpenes and Aromatics*, Tokushima, Japan, pp. 1–3.

Katzer, G. (1998). Kaffir lime (*Citrus hystrix* DC.). http://www.-ang.khfunigraz.ac.at/-katzer/engl/Citr_hys.html.

Kim, T.H., Lee, S.M., Kim, Y.S., Kim, K.H., Oh, S.S., Lee, H.J. (2003). Aroma dilution method using GC injector split ratio for volatile compounds extracted by headspace solid phase microextraction. *Food Chemistry* **83**: 151–158.

Kim, Y.E., Kim, I.H., Kim, H.M., Lee, Y.C. (1996). Volatile compounds of citron (*Citrus junos*) peel extracted by supercritical carbon dioxide. *Korean Journal of Food Preservation* **9**: 500–503.

Ko, Y.H., Kim, J.H. (2001). Storage of citrus orange Hallabong after γ-ray irradiation. *Applied Radioisotope Research Bulletin* **15**: 29–33.

Kwang, J.J., Kim, D.Y., Lee, K.H. (1992). Volatile components of kumquat (*Fortunella margarita*). *Korean Journal of Food Science and Technology* **24**: 423–427.

Lan-Phi, N.T., Minh Tu, N.T., Nishiyama, C., Sawamura, M. (2006). Characterisation of the odour volatiles in *Citrus aurantifolia* Persa lime oil from Vietnam. In: Bredie, W.L.P., Petersen, M.A. (eds.), *Flavour science: recent advances and trends*. Amsterdam: Elsevier, pp. 193–196.

Lan-Phi, N.T., Sawamura, M. (2007). Recent studies on citrus essential oils from East Asia. In: Jirovetz, L., Dung, J.N.X., Varshney, V.K. (eds.), *Aromatic plants from Asia: Their chemistry and application in food and therapy*. India: Har Krishan Bhalla & Sons, pp. 127–153.

Lan-Phi, N.T., Sawamura, M. (2008). Characteristic aroma composition profile of mature stage *Citrus junos* (Yuzu) peel oil from different origins. *Food Science and Technology Research* **14**: 359–366.

Lan-Phi, N.T., Shimamura, T., Ukeda, H., Sawamura, M. (2009). Chemical and aroma profiles of yuzu (*Citrus junos*) peel oils of different cultivars. *Food Chemistry* **115**: 1042–1047.

Lawrence, B.M., Hogg, J.W., Terhune, S.J., Podimuang, V. (1971). Constituents of the leaf and peel oil of *Citrus hystrix* DC. *Phytochemistry* **10**(6): 1404–1405.

Lawrence, B.M. (1993). Progress in essential oil. *Perfumer and Flavourist* **18**: 43–68.

Lee, H.Y., Hawer, W.D., Shin, D.H., Chung, D.H. (1987a). Analysis of the aroma constituents of Korean mandarin (*Citrus reticulata*) and orange juices by capillary GC and GC/MS. *Korean Journal of Food Science and Technology* **19**: 346–354.

Lee, H.Y., Kim, Y.M., Shin, D.H., Sun, B.K. (1987b). Aroma components in Korean Citron (*Citrus medica*). *Korean Journal of Food Science and Technology* **19**: 361–365.

Lee, K.M., Lee, M.S., Hwang, J.B., Jeong, J.W. (1997). Quality evaluation of extracted citron juice by long term storage. *Korean Journal of Food and Nutrition* **10**: 145–150.

Lee, S.H., Park, H.J., Back, O.H., Chun, H.K., Rhie, S.G., Lee, G.S. (2005). Comparison of the nutritional composition of 3 kinds of citrus produced on Jeju Island, Korea. *Korean Journal of Community Living Science* **16**: 15–20.

Lee, S.J., Chun, B.S. (2002). Extraction of volatile essential oil from *Citrus junos* peel by supercritical carbon dioxide. *Korean Journal of Biotechnology and Bioengineering* **17**: 148–152.

Lota, M.-L., de Rocca Serra, D., Jacquemonod, C., Tomi, F., Casanova, J. (2001). Chemical variability of peel and leaf essential oils of sour orange. *Flavour and Fragrance Journal* **16**: 89–96.

Lota, M.-L., Serra, Dd.R., Tomi, F., Jacquemond, C., Casanova, J. (2002). Volatile components of peel and leaf oils of lemon and lime species. *Journal of Agricultural and Food Chemistry* **50**: 796–805.

Maryoto, A. (2004). Kita memiliki ratusan varietas Jeruk. Kompas Daily, October 26. http://air.bappenas.go.id/doc/pdf/kliping/Kita%20Ratusan%20Varietas%20Jeruk.pdf.

Masyarakat Jeruk Indonesia. (2008). Satu Jeruk banyak olahan. http://www.citrus-indonesian.com.

Matsumoto, R. (2001). Shiranui: A late-maturing citrus cultivar. *Bulletin of National Institute of Fruit Tree Science* **35**: 115–120.

Mazza, G. (1986). Gas chromatographic and mass spectrometric study of the aromatic composition of bergamot (*Citrus aurantium* subsp. *bergamia* Risso et Poiteau Engler) essential oil. *Journal of Chromatography* **362**: 87–99.

Mazza, G. (1987). Gas chromatography and mass spectrometry study of the aromatic composition of mandarine essential oil. *Sciences des Aliments* **7**: 459–479.

Minh Tu, N.T., Thanh, L.X., Une, A., Ukeda, H., Sawamura, M. (2002a). Volatile constituents of Vietnamese pummelo, orange, tangerine and lime peel oils. *Flavour and Fragrance Journal* **17**: 169–174.

Minh Tu, N.T., Onishi, Y., Choi, H.S., Kondo, Y., Mitiku, S.B., Ukeda, H., Sawamura, M. (2002b). Characteristic odor components of *Citrus sphaerocarpa* Tanaka (Kabosu) cold-pressed peel oil. *Journal of Agricultural and Food Chemistry* **50**: 2908–2913.

Minh Tu, N.T. (2003). Studies on the characteristic aroma of citrus essential oils. PhD Thesis, Ehime University, Japan.

Ministry of Agriculture, Animal Industry and Fisheries. (2001). *Report on production trends of major fruits in Uganda*. Kampala, Uganda.

Mitiku, S.B., Sawamura, M., Itoh, T., Ukeda, H. (2000). Volatile components of peel cold-pressed oils of two cultivars of sweet orange (*Citrus sinensis* (L.) Osbeck) from Ethiopia. *Flavour and Fragrance Journal* **15**: 240–244.

Mitiku, S.B., Sawamura, M., Njoroge, S.M., Koaze, H. (2002). Analytical discrimination of cold-pressed oils of mandarins and their hybrids. *Journal of Essential Oil Research* **14**: 196–202.

Miyazato, H., Hashimoto, S., Hayashi, S. (2008). Investigation on potent aroma compound in Yuzu (*Citrus junos* Tanaka) (II). *Proceedings of Symposium on Chemistry of Terpenes, Essential Oils and Aromatics*, Gunma, Japan, pp. 69–71.

Miyazawa, M., Shindo, M., Shimada, T. (2001). Oxidation of 1,8-cineole, the monoterpene cyclic ether originated from *Eucalyptus polybractea*, by cytochrome P450 3A enzyme in rat and human liver microsomes. *Journal of Drug Metabolism and Digestion* **29**: 200–205.

Miyazawa, N., Tomita, N., Kurobayashi, Y., Nakanishi, A., Ohkubo, Y., Maeda, T., Fujita, A. (2009). Novel character impact compounds in yuzu (*Citrus junos* Sieb. ex Tanaka) peel oil. *Journal of Agricultural and Food Chemistry* **57**: 1990–1996.

Mohammad, N.O. (1992). Development and application of *Citrus hystrix* flavor for food. *Proceedings of ASEAN Workshop on the Production of Natural Flavors for Food*, Kuala Lumpur, Malaysia.

Mondello, L., Stagno d'Alcontres, Del Duce, R., Crispo, F. (1993) On the genuineness of citrus essential oils. Part XL: The composition of the coumarins and psoralens of Calabrian bergamot essential oil (*Citrus bergamia* Risso). *Flavour and Fragrance Journal* **8**: 17–24.

Mondello, L., Dugo, P., Cavazza, A. (1996). Characterization of essential oil of pummelo (cv. *Chandler*) by GC/MS, HPLC and physicochemical indices. *Journal of Essential Oil Research* **8**: 311–314.

Moshonas, M.G. (1971). Analysis of carbonyl flavor constituents from grapefruit oil. *Journal of Agricultural and Food Chemistry* **19**: 769–770.

Moshonas, M.G., Shaw, P.E. (1974). Quantitative and qualitative analysis of tangerine peel oil. *Journal of Agricultural and Food Chemistry* **22**: 282–284.

Moshonas, M.G., Shaw, P.E. (1979). Composition of essence oil from overripe oranges. *Journal of Agricultural and Food Chemistry* **27**: 1337–1339.

Mwasaru, M.A., Mathooko, F.M., Onyango, C.A., Kiiyukia, C., Njoroge, S.M., Kenji, G.M., Koaze, H., Ueda, Y. (1998). Production and utilization of food commodities in Kenya. *Food Preservation Science* **24**: 255–266.

Njoroge, S.M., Ukeda, H., Kusunose, H., Sawamura, M. (1994a). Volatile components of Japanese yuzu and lemon oils. *Flavour and Fragrance Journal* **9**: 159–166.

Njoroge, S.M., Ukeda, H., Kusunose, H., Sawamura, M. (1994b). Volatile components of the essential oils from Kabosu, Daidai, and Yuko, Japanese sour *citrus* fruits. *Flavour and Fragrance Journal* **9**: 289–297.

Njoroge, S.M., Ukeda, H., Kusunose, H., Sawamura, M. (1995). Japanese sour *Citrus* fruits. Part III: Volatile constituents of sudachi and mochiyuzu oils. *Flavour and Fragrance Journal* **10**: 341–347.

Njoroge, S.M., Ukeda, H., Kusunose, H., Sawamura, M. (1996a). Japanese Sour *Citrus* Fruits. Part IV: Volatile compounds of naoshichi and Tahiti lime essential oils. *Flavour and Fragrance Journal* **11**: 25–29.

Njoroge, S.M., Ukeda, H., Sawamura, M. (1996b). Changes in the volatile composition of yuzu (*Citrus junos* Tanaka) cold-pressed oil during storage. *Journal of Agricultural and Food Chemistry* **44**: 550–556.

Njoroge, S.M., Koaze, H., Karanja, P.N., Sawamura, M. (2005a). Essential oil constituents of three varieties of Kenyan sweet oranges (*Citrus sinensis*). *Flavour and Fragrance Journal* **20**: 80–85.

Njoroge, S.M., Mwaniki, M., Minh Tu, N.T., Sawamura, M. (2005b). Essential oils of Kenyan citrus fruits: Volatile components of two varieties of mandarins (*Citrus reticulata*) and a tangelo (*C. paradisi* x *C. tangerina*). *Flavour and Fragrance Journal* **20**: 74–79.

Njoroge, S.M., Koaze, H., Karanja, P.N., Sawamura, M. (2005c). Volatile constituents of redblush grapefruit (*Citrus paradisi*) and pummelo (*Citrus grandis*) peel essential oils from Kenya. *Journal of Agricultural and Food Chemistry* **53**: 9790–9794.

Njoroge, S.M., Mungai, H.N., Koaze, H., Lan Phi, N.T., Sawamura, M. (2006). Volatile constituents of mandarin (*Citrus reticulata* Blanco) peel oil from Burundi. *Journal of Essential Oil Research* **18**: 659–662.

Njoroge, S.M., Karanja, P.N., Sawamura, M. (2008). Essential oil components of common mandarins (*Citrus reticulata* Blanco) from Uganda. *Journal of Essential Oil Bearing Plants* **11**: 609–614.

Njoroge, S.M., Lan Phi, N.T., Sawamura, M. (2009). Chemical composition of peel essential oils of sweet oranges (*Citrus sinensis*) from Uganda and Rwanda. *Journal of Essential Oil Bearing Plants* **12**: 26–33.

Nugroho, S.A. (1995). Ekstraksi dan Karakterisasi Minyak Kulit Jeruk Pontianak (*Citrus nobilis* var. *microcarpa*), Navel (*Citrus sinensis*) serta Valencia (*Citrus sinensis*). Undergraduate final year project, Faculty of Agriculture, Bogor Agricultural University, Indonesia.

Nursten, H.E. (1977). The important volatile flavour components of foods. In: Birch, G.G., Brennan, J.G., Parker, K.J. (eds.), *Sensory properties of foods*. London: Applied Science, pp. 151–166.

Owusu-Yaw, J., Matthews, R.F., West, P.E. (1986). Alcohol deterpenation of orange oil. *Journal of Food Science* **51**: 1180–1182.

Poiana, M., Sicari, V., Mincione, B. (1998a). Supercritical carbon dioxide (SC-CO_2) extraction of grapefruit flavedo. *Flavour and Fragrance Journal* **13**: 125–130.

Poiana, M., Sicari, V., Mincione, B. (1998b). A comparison between the chemical composition of the oil solvent extract and supercritical carbon dioxide extract of *Citrus medica* cv. *Diamante*. *Journal of Essential Oil Research* **10**: 145–152.

Poiana, M., Fresa, R., Mincione, B. (1999). Supercritical carbon dioxide extraction of bergamot peels: Extraction kinetics of oil and its components. *Flavour and Fragrance Journal* **14**: 358–366.

Poiana, M., Attanasio, G., Albanese, D., Di Matteo, M. (2006). Alcoholic extracts composition from lemon fruits of the Amalfi-Sorrento peninsula. *Journal of Essential Oil Research* **18**: 432–437.

Pudil, F., Wijaya, H., Janda, V. (1996). Chemical composition of *Citrus hystrix* oil. In: Sandra, P., Devos, G. (eds.), *XVIII: International Symposium on Capillary Chomatography, Vol. II, 20.5–24.5*, Riva del Garda, pp. 1027.

Pudil, F., Wijaya, H., Janda, V., Volfova, J., Valentova, H., Pokorny, J. (1998). Changes in *Citrus hystrix* oil during autooxidation. In: Contis, E.T. et al. (eds.), *Food flavors:*

Formation, analysis and packaging influences. Amsterdam: Elsevier Science B.V., pp. 707–718.

Raymond, P., Scott, W. (2003a). *Gas chromatography*. Library for Science, LLC, pp. 23–46.

Raymond, P., Scott, W. (2003b). *Gas chromatography detector*. Library for Science, LLC, pp. 1–10, 33–42.

Raymond, P., Scott, W. (2003c). *Principle and practice of gas chromatography*. Library for Science, LLC, pp. 34–55.

Rocha, S.F.R., Ming, L.C. (1999). *Piper hispidinervum*: A sustainable source of safrole. In: Janick, J. (ed.), *Perspectives of new crops and new uses*. Alexandria, VA: AHS, pp. 479–481.

Rodríguez, G.O., Godoy, V.M., Colmenares, N.G., Salas, L.C., Ferrer, B.Sd. (1998). Composition of venezuelan lemon essential oil *Citrus limon* (L.) Burm.f. *Revista de la Facultad de Agronomía* **15**: 343–349.

Rodríguez, G.O., Ysambertt, F., Ferrer, B.S., Cabrera, L. (2003). Volatile fraction composition of Venezuelan sweet orange essential oil (*Citrus sinensis* (L.) Osbeck). *CIENCIA* **11**: 55–60.

Rukmana, R. (2000). *Jeruk Nipis* (10th ed). Yogyakarta: Penerbitan Kanisius.

Sarwono, B. (1994). *Jeruk dan Kerabatnya* (7th ed). Jakarta: Penebar Swadya.

Sato, A., Asano, K., Sato, T. (1990). The chemical composition of *Citrus hystrix* DC (Swangi). *Journal of Essential Oil Research* **2**: 179–183.

Sawamura, M., Kuriyama, T. (1988). Quantitative determination of volatile constituents in the pummelo (*Citrus grandis* Osbeck forma *Tosa-buntan*). *Journal of Agricultural and Food Chemistry* **36**: 567–569.

Sawamura, M., Tsuji, T., Kuwahara, S. (1989). Changes in the volatile constituents of pummelo (*Citrus grandis* Osbeck forma Tosa-buntan) during storage. *Agricultural and Biological Chemistry* **53**: 243–246.

Sawamura, M., Kuwahara, S., Shichiri, K., Aoki, T. (1990). Volatile constituents of several varieties of pummelos and comparison of the nootkatone levels in pummelos and other citrus fruits. *Agricultural and Biological Chemistry* **54**: 803–805.

Sawamura, M., Shichiri, K., Ootani, Y., Zheng, X.H. (1991). Volatile constituents of several varieties of pummelos and characteristics among citrus fruits. *Agricultural Biology and Chemistry* **55**: 2571–2578.

Sawamura, M., Sun, S.H., Ozaki, K., Ishikawa, J., Ukeda, H. (1999). Inhibitory effects of citrus essential oils and their components on the formation of *N*-nitrosodimethylamine. *Journal of Agricultural and Food Chemistry* **47**: 4868–4872.

Sawamura, M. (2000). Volatile components of essential oils of the *Citrus* genus. In: Pandalai, S.G. (ed.), *Recent research development in agricultural and food chemistry, volume 4*. Trivandrum: Research Signpost, pp. 131–164.

Sawamura, M. (2001). Citrus fruits and their aroma and function properties. *Koryo* **211**: 81–92.

Sawamura, M., Song, H.-S., Choi, H.-S., Sagawa, K., Ukeda, H. (2001). Characteristic aroma components of Tosa-buntan (*Citrus grandis* Osbeck forma *Tosa*) Fruit. *Food Science and Technology Research* **7**: 45–49.

Sawamura, M., Minh Tu, N.T., Onishi, Y., Ogawa, E., Choi, H.S. (2004). Characteristic odor component of *Citrus reticulata* Blanco (Ponkan) cold-pressed oil. *Bioscience Biotechnology and Biochemistry* **68**: 1690–1967.

Sawamura, M. (2005). *Citrus junos* Sieb. ex Tanaka (yuzu) fruit. In: Dris, R. (ed.), *Fruits: Growth, nutrition and quality*. Helsinki, Finland: WFL, pp. 1–24.

Sawamura, M., Lan Phi, N.T., Furukawa, A., Taguchi, K. (2006). Flavor characteristics of seedling and grafted yuzu. *Proceedings of Symposium on the Chemistry of Terpenes, Essential Oils, and Aromatics*, Yokohama, Japan, pp. 319–321.

Shaw, P.E. (1979). A review of quantitative analysis of citrus essential oils. *Journal of Agricultural and Food Chemistry* **27**: 246–257.

Shaw, P.E., Wilson, C.W., Berry, R.E. (1981). Some important flavor compounds in mandarin, grapefruit and orange juices and peel essential oils. *Proceedings of 4th International Citrus Congress*, Tokyo, Japan, pp. 911–914.

Shaw, P.E. (1991). Fruits, II. In: Maarse, H. (ed.), *Volatile compounds in foods and beverages*. New York: Marcel Dekker, pp. 305–327.

Shaw, P.E. (1997). Essential oils. In: Nagy, S., Shaw, P.E., Veldhuis, M.K. (eds.), *Citrus science and technology, volume 1*. Westport, CT: AVI, pp. 427–462.

Song, H.S., Sawamura, M., Ito, T., Ukeda, H. (1999). Chemical compositions of the volatile part of yuzu (*Citrus junos* Tanaka) peel cold-pressed oils from Japan and Korea. *Flavour and Fragrance Journal* **14**: 383–389.

Song, H.S., Sawamura, M., Ito, T., Kawashimo, K., Ukeda, H. (2000). Quantitative determination and characteristic flavour of *Citrus junos* (yuzu) peel oil. *Flavour and Fragrance Journal* **15**: 245–250.

Song, H.S., Park, Y.H., Moon, D.G. (2005). Volatile flavor properties of Hallabong grown in open field and green house by GC/GC-MS and sensory evaluation. *Journal Korean Society of Food Science and Nutrition* **34**: 1239–1245.

Song, H.S., Lan Phi, N.T., Park, Y.H., Sawamura, M. (2006). Volatile profiles in cold-pressed peel oil from Korean and Japanese Shiranui (*Citrus unshiu* Marcov. × *C. sinensis* Osbeck × *C. reticulata* Blanco). *Bioscience Biotechnology and Biochemistry* **70**: 737–739.

Song, H.S., Sawamura, M. (2007). Volatile profile of the peel oil of Setoka, a new hybrid sweet citrus fruit. *Abstract of International Symposium of the Korean Society of Food Science and Nutrition*, Muju Resort, Korea, p. 192.

Song, H.S. (2008). The volatile composition of Kiyomi peel oil (*Citrus unshiu* Marcov. × *C. sinensis* Osbeck) cultivated in Korea. *Journal of Food Science and Nutrition* **13**: 292–298.

Starrantino, A., Terranova, G., Dugo, P., Bonaccorsi, I., Mondello, L. (1997). On the genuineness of citrus essential oils. Part IL: Chemical characterization of the essential oil of new hybrids of lemon obtained in Sicily. *Flavour and Fragrance Journal* **12**: 153–161.

Sugisawa, H., Yamamoto, M., Tamura, H., Takagi, N. (1989). The comparison of volatile components in peel oil from four species of navel orange. *Nippon Shokuhin Kogyo Gakkaishi* **36**: 455–462.

Sunarjono, H. (2008). *Berkebun 21 Jenis Tanaman Buah* (7th ed). Jakarta: Penebar Swadaya.

Tajima, K., Tanaka, S., Yamaguchi, T., Fujita, M. (1990). Analysis of green and yellow yuzu peel oils (*Citrus junos* Tanaka): Novel aldehyde components with remarkably low odor thresholds. *Journal of Agricultural and Food Chemistry* **38**: 1544–1548.

Tatum, J.H., Nagy, S., Berry, R.E. (1967). Some compounds formed during nonenzyme browning of orange powder. *Journal of Agricultural and Food Chemistry* **15**: 773–775.

Tim Penulis, P.S. (2007). *Peluang Usaha dan Pembudidayaan Jeruk Siam*. Jakarta: Penebar Swadaya.

Tirado, C.B., Stashenko, E.E., Combariza, M.Y., Martinez, J.R. (1995). Comparative study of Colombian citrus oils by high-resolution gas chromatography and gas chromatography–mass spectrometry. *Journal of Chromatography A* **697**: 501–513.

Ubukata, Y., Hanafusa, M., Hayashi, S., Hashimoto, S., Honda, K., Kujo, M. (2002). Essential oil constituents of the Ukon-no-tachibana (*Citrus tachibana*) in Heian-Jingu Shrine. *Proceedings of International Symposium on the Chemistry of Essential Oils, Terpenes and Aromatics*, Tokushima, Japan, pp. 7–9.

Umano, K., Hagi, Y., Tamura, T., Shoji, A., Shibamoto, T. (1994). Identification of volatile compounds isolated from round kumquat (*Fortunella japonica* Swingle). *Journal of Agricultural and Food Chemistry* **42**: 1888–1890.

UNCTAD. (2004). http://www.unctad.org/infocomm/anglais/orange/market.htm.

Usai, M., Arras, G., Fronteddu, F. (1992). Effects of cold storage on essential oils of peel of Thomson navel orange. *Journal of Agricultural and Food Chemistry* **40**: 271–275.

Verzera, A., Trozzi, A., d'Alcontres, I.S., Cotroneo, A. (1996). On the genuineness of citrus essential oils. XLVIII: The composition of volatile fraction of some varieties of sweet orange oils. *Journal of Essential Oil Research* **8**: 159–160.

Verzera, A., Mondello, L., Trozzi, A., Dugo, P. (1997). On the genuineness of citrus essential oils. Part LII: Chemical characterization of essential oil of three cultivars of *Citrus clementine* Hort. *Flavour and Fragrance Journal* **12**: 163–172.

Verzera, A., Trozzi, A., Mondello, L., Dellacassa, E., Lorenzo, D. (1998). Uruguayan essential oils. Part X: Composition of the oil of *Citrus clementine* Hort. *Flavour and Fragrance Journal* **13**: 189–195.

Verzera, A., Cotroneo, A., Dugo, P., Mondello, L. (1999). Extraction technology and lemon oil composition [*Citrus limon* (L.) Burm.]. *Italian Journal of Food Sciences* **11**: 361–370.

Verzera, A., Trozzi, A., Cotroneo, A., Lorenzo, D., Dellacassa, E. (2000). Uruguayan essential oil. Part 12: Composition of Nova and Satsuma mandarin oils. *Journal of Agricultural and Food Chemistry* **48**: 2903–2909.

Webber, H.J., Reuther, W., Lawton, H.W. (1967). History and development of the citrus industry. In: Reuther, W., Webber, H.J., Batchelor, L.D. (eds.), *The citrus industry, vol. 1*. Berkeley: Division of Agricultural Science, University of California, pp. 1–39.

Wijaya, C.H. (1995). Oriental natural flavour: Liquid and spray-dried flavor of "Jeruk Purut" (*Citrus hystrix* DC) leaves. In: Charalambous, G. (ed.), *Food flavors: Generation, analysis and process influence*. Amsterdam: Elsevier Science B.V., pp. 235–248.

Wijaya, C.H., Sandra, S., Hidayat, F.K. (2000). Ekstraksi minyak astiri dari daun jeruk purut (*Citrus hystrix* D.C) pada skala pilot-plant. *Jurnal Teknologi Industri Pertanian* **9**: 164–171.

Wijaya, C.H., Apriyantono, A. (2003). Aroma volatiles of several unique tropical fruits and spices. In: Le Quere, J.L., Etievant, P.X. (eds.), *Flavour research at the dawn of the twenty-first century*. Paris: Intercept, pp. 749–752.

Wolford, R.W., Kesterson, J.W., Attaway, J.A. (1971). Physicochemical properties of citrus essential oils from Florida. *Journal of Agricultural and Food Chemistry* **19**: 1097–1105.

Xiaoyu, H., Xiuyin, Z., Yi, S. (1998). Extraction and identification of volatile oil in fingered citron. *Journal of South China Agricultural University* **19**: 101–106.

4

ENANTIOMERIC AND STABLE ISOTOPE ANALYSIS

Nguyen Thi Thao
Hanoi University of Technology
Hanoi, Vietnam

Adulteration of cold-pressed citrus essential oils has been practiced for commercial oils for a long time, since these valuable oils provide a natural and important source of flavor and fragrance (McHale, 2002). Nowadays, there are two main types of adulterations for cold-pressed oils. One is rough addition of some natural and/or synthetic products of low value. In such cases, the aim is not to try to get a composition of the oil exactly similar to the genuine one; what is important is "passing certain examinations" like percentage of residue, density and optical rotation, citral content, ester number, UV absorbance, and so forth. Some conventional techniques can be useful in detecting these kinds of adulteration. One method is thin-layer chromatography (TLC). The second type of adulteration includes the sophisticated adulterations that make the oil very similar to a genuine one. In such cases, addition of natural and/or synthetic products of low value is used to obtain an economic profit while attempting to maintain the qualitative or even the quantitative composition of the natural oil, making the detection of the adulteration very difficult.

Several analytical methods have been developed for authenticity control of flavors and essential oils. High-resolution gas chromatography (HRGC), either with conventional stationary phases or with the relatively new chiral phases, is the

Citrus Essential Oils: Flavor and Fragrance, Edited by Masayoshi Sawamura

technique that best helps the analyst in detecting citrus oil adulteration. The information obtained on the volatile fraction of the oils is enough to ascertain whether an oil is genuine, and sometimes it is also possible to know what kind of product has been added, and to estimate the level of adulteration. Two phenomena, enantioselectivity and isotope discrimination, during biosynthesis may both serve as endogeneric parameters in the authenticity control of natural flavor and fragrance compounds, if suitable methods and comprehensive data from authentic sources are available (Mosandl, 2004). Enantioselective capillary gas chromatography (enantio-cGC) and isotope ratio mass spectrometry (IRMS), coupled online with capillary gas chromatography (cGC), are reported as important tools in the authenticity control of flavor and essential oils. Recently, a new analytical method for determining the isotope ratio in citrus essential oil by using gas chromatography–mass spectrometry (GC-MS) was also developed (Sawamura et al., 2001). This is a promising technique in the authenticity control of essential oil.

4.1 ENANTIOMERIC ANALYSIS

Nguyen Thi Thao

Chiral compounds contain one or more asymmetric carbon atoms and exhibit optical activity. Flavor and fragrance research frequently deals with the phenomenon of chirality because many flavor and fragrance components are chiral. Chiral flavor and fragrance components of natural origin generally have a characteristic distribution of enantiomers that is attributable to stereoselectively controlled biogenetic formation mechanisms. Thus an excess of one or the other enantiomer occurs in a variety of essential oils and natural flavor extracts. Enantiomers differ in their qualitative organoleptic properties and also exhibit differences in their threshold values. Therefore, the character and intensity of flavor and fragrance compounds are often related to stereochemistry. Chirospecific determinations of optically and organoleptically active compounds point out new possibilities in structure–function relationships and biogenesis of chiral volatiles. This growing awareness of the importance of chirality in flavor and fragrance chemistry has resulted in considerable efforts to develop GC methods for the analysis of chiral components. Chiral fruit flavor compounds have been detected with characteristic size of enantiomeric ratios, defined as fruit-specific enantiomeric distributions. In enantiomer analysis, cGC is currently the method of choice.

In the early 1980s, stereoanalysis of chiral flavor compounds was rather difficult because of the lack of suitable stationary GC phases. A real breakthrough in this field occurred as enantio-cGC became more and more available. In particular, since 1988, selectively modified cyclodextrins have been synthesized, serving as chiral stationary phases in enantio-cGC. Derivatized cyclodextrins (CDs) are now the most popular chiral selector in the direct GC enantiomer separation of volatile racemates. The use of CDs in routine enantiomer recognition is a well-established and fast approach because the high enantioselectivity of CDs and the high stability and reproducibility of capillary GC columns prepared with CDs permit reliable analysis of a very large number of racemates. Moreover, more than 90% of racemates are separated without derivatization (Bicchi et al., 1999). Because of the high complexity of natural essential oil, reliable chirality evaluation needs highly efficient sample cleanup procedures. The online GC-GC coupling, the so-called *enantioselective multidimentional GC (enantio-MDGC) systems*, has proven to be the method of choice.

Enantiomeric purity and enantiomeric excess are usual terms used in the determination of enantiomers. Enantiomeric purity is defined as the measured ratio (expressed as a percentage) of the detected enantiomers, whereas enantiomeric excess values describe the relative difference of the separated enantiomers (expressed as percentage). Usually quantifications are given in enantiomeric excess values. Enantiomer separation and enantiomeric ratio determination are of great importance in the fields of flavors and essential oils. It is important to characterize an extract, to provide a valuable criterion for differentiating natural flavor compounds from those of synthetic origin, and/or to identify possible adulterations.

A comprehensive review on the chiral compounds of citrus essential oils has been done by Mondello et al. (2002), and data present in literature on the enantiomeric distribution of some components of the volatile fraction of citrus oils such as lemon oil, mandarin oil, sweet orange oil, bitter orange oil, lime oils, bergamot oil, neroli, and petitgrain oils have been reported. The data on enantiomeric distribution of various components such as α-pinene, β-pinene, limonene, sabinene, linalool, terpinen-4-ol, α-terpineol, α-copaene, δ-cadinene, carvone, citronellal, linaly acetate, and (*E*)-nerolidol for different citrus essential oils were obtained by using a double-oven system of GC using pre-column and β-cyclodextrin derivative main column; or by using two multidimensional gas chromatography (MDGC) systems. Specifically, the high-performance liquid chromatography–high-resolution gas chromatography (HPLC-HRGC) system permits the transfer and subsequent GC analysis of LC fractions that contain compounds of the same polarity. When possible, a direct enantiomeric cGC analysis can be applied for analyzing simple matrix. The variations of enatiomeric ratio of volatile components in several citrus essential oils were also monitored during the production season. Complete data on chiral compounds can be obtained for authenticity control of natural citrus essential oils.

In a systematic study on analytical methods for discrimination of cold-pressed citrus peel oils of several cultivars, species, and hybrids, Mitiku et al. (2001) analyzed as much as possible the enantiomeric distribution of α-pinene, β-pinene, sabinene, and linalool. Eighty different self-prepared *Citrus* oils, which belong to 37 varieties of 12 *Citrus* species cultivated in Ethiopia, Kenya, Italy, and Japan, were investigated. Depending on the citrus oil, the enantiomeric distribution of α-pinene, β-pinene, sabinene, limonene, linalool, citronellal, and α-terpineol was studied by simple and reliable enantioselective GC methods involving either a chiral capillary column or an online coupling of non-chiral and chiral capillary columns. This online system provided effective separation and sufficient quantitative determination of some of the major enantiomers. In addition, volatile compositions of the cold-pressed peel oils of Satsuma mandarin cultivar from Japan, and four other cultivars of mandarin hybrids such as Temple, Orlando, Kara, and Minneola obtained from Ethiopia and Kenya, were analyzed by GC and GC/MS, without prior separation. With this chiral analysis study, a broad range of enantiomeric distribution of components in volatile fraction of citrus essential oil could be determined. This enantiomeric distribution is characteristic for each citrus variety or species.

4.2 STABLE ISOTOPE RATIO ANALYSIS

Nguyen Thi Thao and Atsushi Satake

Among the developed techniques, the determination of the isotope values of constituents is increasing in importance, especially in view of the increased demand for authenticity control and origin determination of food products. Stable isotope analysis is considered to be an excellent tool for origin assessment. It is known that the natural abundance of the isotopes of each element is distributed in given ratios. Atmospheric carbon dioxide contains about 1.1% of the heavier carbon isotope ^{13}C and 98.9% of the lighter isotope ^{12}C. Plants on the Earth first convert solar energy into biochemical energy and higher plants fix CO_2 by the Calvin-Benson cycle to biosynthesize various organic compounds for their constituents. It is apparent that one of the important steps in the carbon cycle that contributes both directly and indirectly to $^{13}C/^{12}C$ variation of carbon-containing materials in nature is the photosynthetic fixation of carbon by marine and terrestrial plants. Plants discriminate against ^{13}C during photosynthesis in ways that reflect plant metabolism and environment. It is known that enzyme ribulose-1,5-diphosphate carboxylase differentiates a small mass difference between $^{12}CO_2$ and $^{13}CO_2$ when it fixes CO_2 from atmosphere (Park and Epstein, 1960). This function is the so-called "isotope effect." In addition, this effect could be achieved by every step involved in the biosynthetic and metabolic pathways of plants, resulting in a small but appreciable difference in isotopic content. The principal components that will affect the overall isotope discrimination during photosynthesis are diffusion of CO_2, interconversion of CO_2 and HCO_3^-, incorporation of CO_2 by phosphoenolpyruvate carboxylases (C_4 plants) or ribulose bisphosphate carboxylase (C_3 plants), and respiration (O'Leary, 1981). It is therefore reasonable to suggest that the isotopic content in citrus essential oils would be influenced by the isotope effect of plants.

Water, mainly water pool of soil, supplies hydrogen and oxygen for photosynthesis. Oxygen can be obtained from other sources such as atmospheric oxygen and carbon dioxide. Fractionation of hydrogen and oxygen isotopes takes place along with the evaporation and condensation processes of the water cycle. Water passing from its liquid state in the ocean to that of the vapor in the atmospheric moisture undergoes a strong isotope fractionation resulting in depletion of the heavier isotopes (^{2}H or ^{18}O) in vapor and clouds. The effect of the climatic geographic and topographic conditions results in a worldwide distinctive isotope pattern of meteoric water (Craig, 1961; Dansgaard, 1964). Consequently, the stable isotope ratios of water (oxygen and hydrogen) can yield unique geographic information (Asche et al., 2003). This spatial variation in precipitation composition is recorded in plant material since plants take up soil water that is derived generally from local precipitation and incorporate those hydrogen and oxygen atoms into the products of photosynthesis (Dawson et al., 2002). This distinction of isotope content can be transferred to plants, creating an isotopic "fingerprint" for geographical characteristics of the vegetation. This notion is also applied to the authenticity of foods such as milk and dairy products (Manca et al., 2006), meat (Franke et al., 2008), and beverages (West et al., 2007; Calderone and Guillou, 2008).

There is also a difference in ^{15}N content of atmospheric nitrogen and that of the biosphere and soil. This probably results from the isotope discrimination in the reactions involved in the biological nitrogen cycle. Nitrogen isotope fractionation is based on kinetic isotope effects, which tend to favor the lighter isotope ^{14}N and enriches the unreacted starting material in the heavier isotope. Isotope effects that occur during biological process (nitrification and denitrification) account for the $\delta^{15}N$ values of soils that mostly show a ^{15}N abundance higher than atmospheric nitrogen (Delwiche and Steyn, 1970). The uptake and assimilation of nitrogen by plants are accompanied by the isotope effect, too. Normally, the $\delta^{15}N$ value of plant nitrogen is slightly depleted in ^{15}N compared with the nitrogen source (Yoneyama et al., 1991). In addition, fertilizers, soil characteristics, and climatic factors also have an influence on the $\delta^{15}N$ values of plants. As a result of these factors, which influence the $\delta^{15}N$ value of plants, the ^{15}N abundance could depend on the location of plants.

The stable isotope ratio of carbon, hydrogen, oxygen, or nitrogen of components can be used for verification of the origin of flavors and fragrances. The combination of multiple isotope values could give more information than one value alone. The two main techniques used to determine the isotope ratios of natural products are isotope ratio mass spectrometry (IRMS) and site-specific natural isotope fractionation studied by nuclear magnetic resonance (SNIF-NMR).

4.2.1 GC-IRMS

IRMS is a technique that can distinguish chemically identical compounds based on their isotope content. A specially designed mass spectrometer is used to accurately measure the isotope ratio and is able to separate gases with a different isotopic composition such as $^{1}H_2$ and $^{1}H^{2}H$ (or $^{12}CO_2$ and $^{13}CO_2$, $^{16}O_2$ and $^{18}O^{16}O$). Complex molecules have to be converted into a gas prior to measurement. Thus, to measure the isotope ratio in ^{2}H of a compound, it has to be reacted to yield H_2O. The isotope ratio of ^{13}C of an organic compound, on the other hand, involves the combustion to CO_2 and direct measurement of IRMS. This technique has become more and more important in food authenticity assessment since GC coupled online via a suitable combustible/pyrolysis interface with IRMS has been realized. Moreover, the components can be detected in the nanomole range with high precision (Mosandl, 2004). IRMS is the reliable instrument for determination of isotope ratio and this technique is considered to be the standard method to measure δ value. Such a procedure permits the isotope ratio of individual components of essential oils to be determined (Frank et al., 1995; Faulhaber et al., 1997; Nhu-Trang et al., 2006). IRMS, however, is not always available in the flavor and food laboratories.

The isotope ratio analysis method can be used to determine the isotope content of the main components in the volatile fraction. But often it is used for the determination of the δ values of minor components, which play an important role in the characteristic flavor of the investigated essential oil. For example, methyl *N*-methylanthranilate is a characteristic flavor compound of mandarin essential oil, so it can be added to reconstituted mandarin oils. In a study on $\delta^{13}C_{PDB}$ and $\delta^{15}N_{AIR}$ values of methyl *N*-methylanthranilate in mandarin essential oils using capillary gas chromatography, online coupled with isotope ratio mass spectrometry (GC-IRMS), it was shown that the combination of the $\delta^{13}C$ and $\delta^{15}N$ values is useful in the authenticity control of mandarin oils (Faulhaber et al., 1997).

4.2.2 NMR

Nuclear magnetic resonance (NMR) can be also used to determine stable isotope ratios and affords a means of measuring isotopic patterns within molecules. NMR is based on the measurement of absorption of radiofrequency radiation by atomic nuclei with non-zero spins in a strong magnetic field. Although it is possible to determine $^{13}C/^{12}C$ ratios at particular sites in a molecule, the majority of the work to date has been directed at establishing the $^{2}H/^{1}H$ ratios at specific sites. The method is known as *site-specific natural isotope fractionation (SNIF-NMR)*. Unlike the IRMS technique, which can determine the average $^{2}H/^{1}H$ ratio only of the whole molecule, SNIF-NMR can determine the isotope ratio of $^{2}H/^{1}H$ at a specific site in a molecule. Consequently, the nonstatistical pattern of the distribution of $^{2}H/^{1}H$ in organic molecules was observed (Martin and Martin, 1981) by using SNIF-NMR. It is shown that very large differences exist in the internal distribution of natural deuterium, and the ^{2}H quantitative NMR method is proposed as an efficient tool for characterizing the chemical and geographical origin of a molecule and for investigating chemical and biochemical mechanisms. In a nonsymmetric molecule like glucose or terpene, ^{2}H atoms (and analogously the other heavy isotopes) are introduced into each C–H group by specific reactions with specific ^{2}H isotope effects. Because of that, the distribution of the light and the heavy isotope(s) of an element in a given compound is nonrandom and is determined by the synthesis processes of that particular compound (Rossmann et al., 1991; Martin et al., 2004). This means that the relative abundance of a heavy isotope at each position in a compound is determined by the (bio)chemical and physical history of that compound. NMR has the advantage over IRMS that the natural abundance of ^2H isotopomers may be precisely and accurately quantified by SNF-NMR (Martin and Martin, 1991), whereas IRMS gives only a mean value of the deuterium content of a given chemical species. It gives more specific isotopic information about a molecule, thereby permitting natural and synthetic molecules to be clearly differentiated (Martin et al., 1990; 1996a; 1996b; Martin and Martin, 1999). However, the disadvantages are that the equipment is very expensive, data acquisition times are long, and relatively large quantities of pure compound are needed for analysis.

4.2.3 Isotope Ratio of Monoterpene Hydrocarbons by GC-MS

Gas chromatography–mass spectrometry (GC-MS) is currently the most convenient instrumental technique for analyzing volatile compounds in food and flavor. It comprises a gas chromatograph (GC) coupled to a mass spectrometer (MS) to separate the components of a mixture, and MS characterizes each of the components individually. In this way, one can both qualitatively and quantitatively analyze complex mixtures containing numerous compounds. In order for a compound to be analyzed by GC-MS it must be sufficiently volatile and thermally stable. In GC-MS, the ions required for mass analysis are generally formed by electron impact ionization. In the mass spectra it is important to remember that the atomic weight of an element is a weighted average of the naturally occurring isotopes. Mass spectrometers separate these isotopes and are even used to measure their relative abundance. Although this complicates the mass spectrum, it also provides useful information for identifying the elements in an ion.

In the search for a common analytical method for flavor authentication and food quality assessment, recently a new isotope ratio method using gas chromatography–mass spectrometry (GC-MS) has been developed by Sawamura et al. (2001). It has been thought that ordinary GC-MS is not proper for isotope analysis, because its sensitivity and accuracy are not sufficient for the analysis. It may be difficult to measure the stable isotope ratio based on the molecular ion peak and its isotope peak of $^2H/^1H$, of which isotope ratio is low, or $^{18}O/^{16}O$, of which proportion is relatively low in organic compounds. However, the measurement of the $^{13}C/^{12}C$ ratio is successful, because the isotope ratio and abundance in organic compounds are quite high. By using the selected ion monitoring (SIM) acquisition mode, the mass spectrometry offers accurate data for the isotope ratio value. In the application for the citrus essential oils, the isotope ratio m/z 137/136 of monoterpene hydrocarbons is used because monoterpene hydrocarbons are the main component that accounts for more than 90% in the volatile fraction of the citrus essential oil. In the following sections, a systematic review on the development of analytical methods for the determination of isotope ratio in citrus essential oils will be presented.

Isotope Ratio of Monoterpene Hydrocarbons in Citrus Essential Oils

SAMPLE PREPARATION. All of the citrus fruits samples were collected at the ripening stage and were of the best commercial quality. Cold-pressed peel oil

(CPO) was prepared in such a way that there is almost no influence on the quality of natural essential oil (Sawamura and Kuriyama, 1988). The fruit mesocarp and the albedo layers were peeled off using a sharp knife and discarded, to expose the flavedo and its oil ducts. The prepared flavedo was pressed manually to crack the oil ducts and express the essential oil. The crude essential oil was collected on ice; it was saturated with brine and centrifuged at 4000 *g* for 15 min at 4°C. It was decanted, dried with anhydrous sodium sulfate for 24 h at 5°C, and filtered to obtain the cold-press oil for the study. Each CPO sample was stored at –25°C until needed for analysis. Analytical reference compounds used in identification of the essential oil components (authentic compounds) for mass spectrometry were purchased from different sources.

Gas Chromatography—Mass Spectrometry (GC-MS). The analysis was carried out with a GC-6890N instrument (Agilent Technologies) coupled with JMS-Q1000 GTA mass spectrometer (Jeol Datum) (Thao et al., 2007) or with Shimadzu GC-17A linked to a Shimadzu QP-5000 (Sawamura et al., 2001), or Shimadzu QP-5500 (Satake et al., 2003). The GC column was a DB-Wax fused-silica capillary type and the column temperature was programmed for the best separation of monoterpene hydrocarbons.

Determination of the Isotope Ratio. The following 10 monoterpene compounds were examined for the isotope ratios: α-pinene, β-pinene, sabinene, myrcene, α-phellandrene, α-terpinene, limonene, β-phellandrene, γ-terpinene, and terpinolene. The isotope ratio was calculated on the bases of the intensity of molecular peak (*m/z* 136) and isotope peak (*m/z* 137). The isotope ratio of fragments that had been generated during mass bombardment was evaluated on the basis of the intensity of the fragment peak (m) and its isotope peak (m + 1). The SIM mode was employed to carry out the MS analysis in order to increase the sensitivity (Meier-Augenstein, 2002). The isotope ratio (Ir) was calculated by the following equation:

$$\text{Ir}\ (\%) = ((\text{Intensity of } m/z\ (\text{m}+1) \text{ isotope peak})/(\text{Intensity of } m/z\ (\text{m}) \text{ peak})) \times 100$$

where the intensity is the mean value from triplicate measurements.

Standard Repeatability and Analytical Precision of Isotope Ratio Analysis by GC-MS. For the isotope ratio analyses by ordinary GC-MS method with practical applications, the acquisition mode of SIM was set for two ions of each monoterpene hydrocarbon: the *m/z* 136 ion and *m/z* 137 ion for the molecule and its isotope peaks, respectively. The performance of the instrument for isotope ratio analysis by GC-MS was accessed by repeated measurement of authentic α-pinene solution at different concentrations in acetone (n = 15). The concentrations of α-pinene solutions ranged from 0.1 to 50%, which is in accordance with the natural range of monoterpene hydrocarbons in volatile fractions of essential oils. According to this observation, the maximum relative standard deviation (RSD) of the isotope value for each solution was 1.59%, indicating good instrument performance and analytical method stability. A solution with 0.1% concentration had a statistically lower isotope ratio. This can be explained by the fact that when the proportion of investigated compound is present in a small or trace amount, it will lead to a weak signal isotope peak in the mass spectra. In order to get stable isotope ratio data, each ion peak has to be adjusted for the total intensity higher than 10^6 IC (ion concentration) of MS (Satake et al., 2003). This small signal, therefore, was not the linear range of the instrument analysis. However, the analytical method for determination of isotope ratio *m/z* 137/136 using GC-MS showed high repeatability over a wide range of concentrations of the investigated compounds; this is applicable to the determination of monoterpene hydrocarbon in essential oils.

Accuracy of the Isotope Ratio by Ordinary GC-MS. The repeatability of the isotope ratio (Ir) values for various monoterpene hydrocarbons was examined (Satake et al., 2003). In principle, it is possible to obtain the isotope ratio from MS data. However, more detailed analytical conditions need to be found to achieve more precise measurement. The intensity of each molecular ion peak is not very strong. In addition, the isotope peak is approximately 10% of that of the molecular ion peak in the case of monoterpene hydrocarbons in citrus essential oils. The concentrations of the standard samples for GC-MS of α-pinene, β-pinene, sabinene, α-phellandrene, α-terpinene, and terpinolene were within the range of 0.5–1.8% (w/w). The Ir value for each monoterpene hydrocarbon was plotted in Figure 4.1 where the coefficient of variation (CV) is also presented.

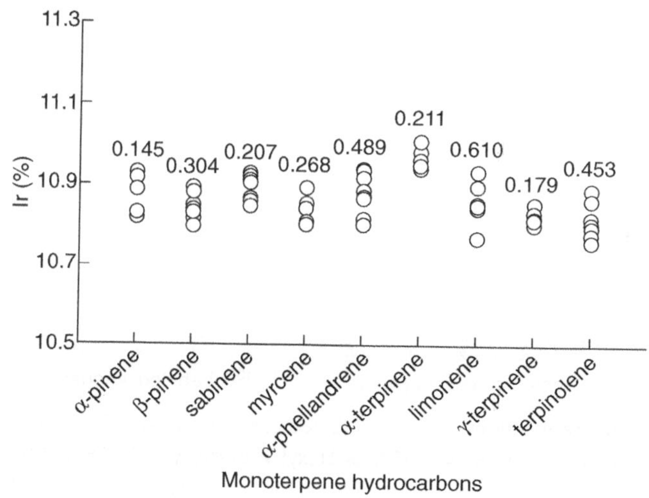

Figure 4.1. Isotope ratio values of the monoterpene hydrocarbon standards. The figures above the symbols show the coefficient of variation.

These Ir values seem to vary only over a narrow range, since their CVs were not more than 0.61% (limonene).

4-Acetyl-1-methylcyclohexene had a purity of 95% by GC, and contained 5% 1-methyl-3(1-methy-(2-^{13}C)-ethenyl)-cyclohexene. It was confirmed that the δ 108.30 (C-10) signal was increased. The *m/z* and peak intensity (%) data for the fragment in the mass spectrum were as follows: MS (nonlabeled limonene) *m/z* 136 (18, M^+), 107 (19), 94 (27), 93 (67), 92 (23), 78 (30), 68 (100), 52 (29); MS (^{13}C-labeled limonene) *m/z* 137 (18, M^+), 108 (19), 95 (24), 94 (35), 93 (51), 79 (19), 68 (100), 67 (52), 52 (27). The δ values from the ^{13}C-NMR spectrum of each carbon in the ^{13}C-labeled limonene were as follows: δ 133.75 (C-1), δ 27.92 (C-2), δ 30.59 (C-3), δ 41.18 (C-4), δ 30.18 (C-5), δ 120.67 (C-6), δ 23.45 (C-7), δ 150.25 (C-8), δ 20.80 (C-9), δ 108.30 (C-10).

The relationship of the ratio of the isotope peak intensity to the molecular mass peak intensity (Ir) and the isotopic ratio of ^{13}C were then examined. ^{13}C-Labeled esters and limonene were added to nonlabeled compounds, and the Ir values were measured. As shown in Figure 4.2, a strong linear relationship was observed between the Ir value and the ^{13}C isotopic ratio. The R^2 value for the esters was greater than 0.96, except for decyl acetate. The accuracy with decyl acetate was rather low (R^2 = 0.85), because the intensity of the molecular ion peak tended to decrease with increasing molecular weight. The difference in the intercept and gradient between octyl acetate and the other acetates may be explained by the difference between the isotope ratio of octanol and those of the other alcohols.

These results show that the reproducibility for determining the peaks of the molecular ion and its isotope by ordinary GC-MS is satisfactory and applicable for practical use. It is expected that this method of isotope analysis can also be applied to organic compounds that have a wide range of molecular weight.

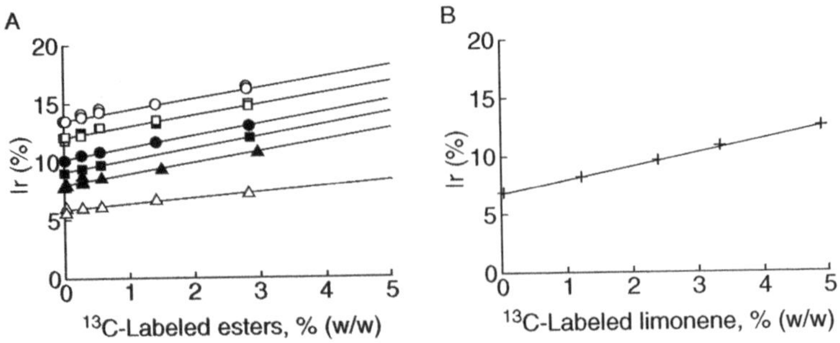

Figure 4.2. Isotope ratio values of the ^{13}C-labeled compounds. **A**: ^{13}C-Labeled esters. ▲ Pentyl acetate: y = 8.053 + 0.961x, R^2 = 0.958; ■ Hexyl acetate, y = 9.196 + 1.016x, R^2 = 0.984; ● Heptyl acetate, y = 10.224 + 1.000x, R^2 = 0.992; △ Octyl acetate, y = 5.871 + 0.484x, R^2 = 0.980; □ Nonyl acetate, y = 12.19 + 0.949x, R^2 = 0.976; ○ Decyl acetate, y = 13.63 + 0.917x, R^2 = 0.849. **B**: ^{13}C-Labeled limonene. + Limonene, y = 10.047+0.866x, R^2 = 1.000.

4.2.4 Effects of Variable Factors on the Isotope Ratio

The isotope ratio analysis was developed and shows rather good performance by using ordinary GC-MS. However, there remain some questions about samplings from the fundamental scope. In order to normalize this method, the variations or individual differences that each material substantially owns should be further investigated. There are therefore several variable factors in sampling incidental to any food analysis where investigated for yuzu fruit (*Citrus junos* Sieb. ex Tanaka), an important sour citrus fruit in Japan.

Effects of Annual Variations and Tree Variation on the Isotope Ratio Values in Yuzu Essential Oils. The sampling was done in November 2001 and 2002. Fruits of each fruit position were collected from three trees to prepare cold-pressed oil from individual years. The weight percent measurement of the 10 monoterpene hydrocarbons in an oil sample for each fruiting position was triplicate, and then the data of each position were analyzed by *t*-test between the two years. Finally, the results of the *t*-test were applied for the sign test (Sawamura et al., 2004). It was shown that there was no significant difference in the isotope ratio values between the trees ($P < 0.05$). This suggests that any tree in a given area can be sampled without significant variation.

Effects of Fruiting Position on the Isotope Ratio Values in Yuzu Essential Oils. The six fruiting positions on each tree were as follow: top, inside, and the four sides of east, west, south, and north around the equatorial canopy of the tree. The isotope ratio values of 10 monoterpene hydrocarbons from each fruiting position on the trees were analyzed by the least significant difference test. No significant difference ($P < 0.05$) was seen.

Effects of Maturity on the Isotope Ratio m/z 137/136 of Monoterpene Hydrocarbons in Yuzu Essential Oil. For the practical use of the isotope ratio analysis method by GC-MS, the isotope ratio *m/z* 137/136 of nine monoterpene hydrocarbons, α-pinene, β-pinene, sabinene, myrcene, α-terpinene, limonene, β-phellandrene, γ-terpinene, and terpinolene, were measured in the essential oils of yuzu fruits collected at different stages of fruit maturity. The samples were collected on November 2, November 14, and November 29, representing different degrees of maturity of yuzu fruits. No significant variation during the ripening period was observed and harvest dates of yuzu fruit had no noticeable effect on the isotopic data of yuzu essential oils.

Influence of Storage on the Isotope Ratio m/z 137/136 of Monoterpene Hydrocarbon in Yuzu Essential Oil. The yuzu CPO was stored at different temperatures, −25°C, 5°C, and 25°C, during the 12-month period starting from the time of CPO preparation. The CPO was then analyzed every three months for isotope ratio change using ordinary GC-MS. Moreover, when using the selected ion monitoring (SIM) acquisition mode, the intensity of *m/z* 136 and *m/z*

137, representing molecular and isotope peak of all monoterpene hydrocarbons, could be determined at the same time. Accordingly, the relative change in isotope ratio of the investigated monoterpene hydrocarbons is evaluated on the basis of modified isotope ratio value. The relative standard deviations of the multifold determinations of isotope ratio *m/z* 137/136 were less than 2%. The modified isotope ratios of three monoterpene hydrocarbons from yuzu essential oil after 0, 3, 6, 9, and 12 months of storage were monitored. There were no remarkable changes in the isotope ratio of these values, even when the CPO samples were stored under different conditions during long-term storage. Actually, at room temperature, the relative percentage of monoterpene hydrocarbons in yuzu essential oil decreased from 95.6% to 37.7% after storage for 12 months (Njoroge et al., 1996), and each of the individual components exhibited a decreasing trend. Of the observable relative losses of the individual monoterpene hydrocarbons after 12 months at 20°C, those of limonene (from 78.1 to 31.2%), myrcene (from 2.1 to 0.6%), and α-pinene (from 1.8 to 0.7%) were prominent. In the isotope ratio analysis, on the other hand, the variation of the modified isotope ratios of these monoterpene hydrocarbons was less than 7%. A profound change was observed in the relative percentage of the investigated monoterpene hydrocarbons in the yuzu essential oil stored at ambient temperature, but the modified isotope ratio showed insignificant change. If it were independent of other variables, the isotope ratio *m/z* 137/136 by GC-MS would be useful in the application for quality control and authentication of essential oil origin.

4.2.5 Isotope Analysis by GC-TOFMS

The employed gas chromatography–time-of-flight mass spectrometry (GC-TOFMS) essentially has a high mass accuracy and therefore calibration can be carried out correctly using the one-point calibration method. That is, the TOFMS needs only one ion whose exact mass is known (internal standard ion) to measure accurate masses, whereas a magnetic-field mass spectrometer needs two or more internal standard ions of known masses before and after the unknown peak (Ubukata, 2005). In this experiment, acetone was used as an internal standard for mass calibration. Three monoterpene hydrocarbons, α-pinene, myrcene, and limonene from cold-pressed lime peel oil (CPO) and authentic chemicals were chosen for the isotope ratio analysis because they are representative of the different structures of monoterpene hydrocarbons. By high-resolution mass spectrometry of GC-TOFMS, the isotope ratios of the selected monoterpene hydrocarbons were determined by the intensities of two ions: the molecular ion, which has a theoretical mass of 136.12520 atomic mass unit (*amu*); and the isotope ion, whose mass was 137.12860 *amu*. This exact measurement of ion masses affords an opportunity to calculate the isotope ratio of only the M+ ion, $^{12}C_{10}{}^{1}H_{16}$, and its isotope (M + 1)+ ion, $^{12}C_{9}{}^{13}CH_{16}$. Table 4.1 shows the calculated mass of each monoterpene hydrocarbon in lime CPO and in authentic chemicals for which the ion intensity was determined. The differences from theoretical masses of both molecular ion and isotope ion in the analysis were within the

TABLE 4.1. Measurement of Atomic Mass Unit of the Molecule and Its Isotope Peaks by GC-TOFMS

	Ion $(M)^{+a}$		Ion $(M + 1)^{+b}$	
Compounds	Authentic Chemicals	Lime Oil	Authentic Chemicals	Lime Oil
α-Pinene	136.12268	136.12373	137.12807	137.12920
Myrcene	136.12520	136.12564	137.13241	137.13173
Limonene	136.12580	136.12440	137.13187	137.12957

[a]The molecular ion has a theoretical mass of *m/z* 136.12520 *amu*.
[b]The isotope ion has a theoretical mass of *m/z* 137.12860 *amu*.

TABLE 4.2. Isotope Ratio of *m/z* 137/136 of Monoterpene Hydrocarbons from Authentic Chemicals and Lime Essential Oil by GC-TOFMS

	Isotope Ratio (%)	
Compounds	Authentic Chemicals	Lime Oil
α-Pinene	13.53	9.28
Myrcene	9.98	9.56
Limonene	12.05	12.12

acceptable error of the instrument (less than 0.005 *amu*). This accordingly confirmed that analysis by GC-TOFMS can determine isotope ratio on the basis of the desired ions.

Table 4.2 shows the isotope ratio of α-pinene, myrcene, and limonene from authentic chemicals and from lime essential oil. It is obvious that the isotope ratios were not identical among the monoterpene hydrocarbons. The isotope ratio of myrcene was 9.98% in authentic chemicals and 9.56% in lime oil. The isotope ratio of limonene, on the other hand, in authentic chemicals and in lime oil was 12.05% and 12.12%, respectively. This supports the conclusion of our previous studies that the isotope ratios of different compounds are not identical, and it serves to establish the characteristic isotope fingerprint of essential oils belonging to the same citrus species. Calculation of the modified isotope ratio of each compound will characterize the specific pattern of each plant species based on secondary metabolites. This specific pattern of isotope ratios of main compnents or so-called characteristic fingerprint curves was also determined for several genuine oils, including yuzu (Sawamura et al., 2001), bergamot (Juchelka and Mosandl, 1996), lemon (Braunsdorf et al., 1993), and coriander (Frank et al., 1995).

4.2.6 Isotope Ratio of Oxygenated Compounds by GC-MS

In the essential oils of citrus species, the oxygenated compounds account for a small but important fraction of odor-active compounds. Among the oxygenated compounds, linalool is quite abundant in the citrus essential oil (Choi and Sawamura, 2000). It is characterized by the fresh flowery odor, and is very important among the monoterpenes for the flavor and fragrance industry. The authenticity control of essential oil–based isotope ratio of linalool has been reported by SNIF-NMR and IRMS (Hanneguelle et al., 1992; Hor et al., 2001). Naturally, linalool is synthesized from universal precursor geranyl pyrophosphate (GPP), catalyzed by a membrane-bound enzyme, linalool synthase (Sawamura, 1994). During this biosynthesis process, water is attached to the frame of 10 carbon atoms, and therefore it is expected that this brings in the isotope ratio of carbon, hydrogen, oxygen and thus the geographical information of linalool isotope ratio. However, the determination of the isotope ratio of oxygenated compounds by current methods is difficult due to the weak signal strength of the isotope and molecular peaks. A new analytical method that is sensitive enough for the determination of isotope ratio of oxygenated compound is developed in order to find an additional analytical parameter for the discrimination of essential oils and of fruits from different origins.

4.2.7 Determination of Isotope Ratio Of Linalool

The isotope ratio (Ir) is defined as the ratio of the ion concentration of isotope and molecular peak, directly determined by the signal area of ions' peak in the mass spectrometry (MS). Three ions of linalool were determined for ion concentrations by SIM mode of MS: the molecular ion (M^+): *m/z* 154, the isotope ion $(M + 1)^+$: *m/z* 155, and $(M + 2)^+$: *m/z* 156. Ir was calculated using the following equation:

$$\text{Ir } (\%) = (\text{Intensity of isotope peak})/(\text{Intensity of molecular peak}) \times 100$$

where the isotope peaks were *m/z* 155 and *m/z* 156, respectively, and the molecular peak was *m/z* 154.

4.2.8 Accuracy of the Isotope Ratio by Ordinary GC-MS

In principle, it is possible to obtain the isotope ratio from MS data (McLafferty and Turecek, 1993) because the isotope peak contains total isotopic abundance. However, the determination of isotope ratio in oxygenated compounds was often difficult since (1) oxygenated compounds account for small proportion in citrus essential oils; (2) the intensity of each molecular ion peak is rather weak after having undergone the fragmentation due to ionization process of MS; (3) linalool easily splits under high temperature of ion source; and (4) the isotope peak $(M + 1)$ is approximately 10%, whereas the isotope peak $(M + 2)$ is approximately

1%, respectively, of that of the molecular ion peak in the case of linalool in citrus essential oils. Therefore, several experimental conditions have been developed to achieve the sensitivity of the analytical method for determining Ir value. The Ir of linalool was determined at different ionization energies of MS. It is noted that there was no increase in the signal strength of molecular and isotope peak of linalool when using lower ionization energy.

4.2.9 Softer Ionization

By choosing the softer ionization energy (50 eV), suitable detector voltage and scanning rate of the monitored ions, the desired ion peaks were enabled since optimization of the analysis device and the analysis condition were attempted in the actual experiment. By employing quadrupole-type MS with resolution power of 1000, the mass peaks observed in the mass spectrum are m/z 154 $(M)^+$, m/z 155 $(M + 1)^+$, and m/z 156 $(M + 2)^+$. When taking the ratio of those peak intensities, the Ir m/z 155/154 accordingly gives total ratio of $^{13}C/^{12}C$, $^{2}H/^{1}H$, and $^{17}O/^{16}O$; and the Ir m/z 156/154 gives information on $^{18}O/^{16}O$ and $^{13}C/^{12}C$.

The repeatability of the Ir values for linalool was examined by different solutions of authentic linalool. The concentrations of standard linalool solutions were 0.5 to 3% (v/v). The standard linalool solutions were prepared to have a concentration similar to the range of linalool concentration in real yuzu essential oil. The linalool content of yuzu samples from different producing areas varied from 1.18 to 3.58% in the volatile fraction of yuzu essential oil. For each standard linalool solution, the isotope ratio was measured in triplicate in the same way as yuzu essential oils. The isotope ratio m/z 155/154 varied from 11.50 to 11.64%, whereas the Ir values m/z 156/154 were from 1.06 to 1.11%. These Ir values varied in a narrow range and in accordance with the theoretical calculation from natural abundance isotope of carbon, hydrogen, and oxygen. The standard deviation of the measurement was from 0.01 to 0.06%, indicating a good performance of the instrument. The results obtained from the authentic linalool solution showed that the reproducibility for determining the peaks of the molecular ion and its isotope by ordinary GC-MS was satisfactory and applicable for practical use. It is expected that this method can also be applied for other organic compounds.

4.3 APPLICATION IN AUTHENTICITY CONTROL OF ESSENTIAL OIL FROM DIFFERENT ORIGINS

Nguyen Thi Thao

Monoterpene hydrocarbons always contribute to the largest fraction in citrus essential oils, accounting for more than 90% of total volatile components (Choi and Sawamura, 2000). They are the C_{10} representatives of the terpenoid group and are considered to be derived from two isoprene residues (Loomis, 1967) that have chemical formula $C_{10}H_{16}$.

4.3.1 Isotope Ratio of Monoterpene Hydrocarbons by GC-MS

Citrus fruits are among the easily hybridized species. It is natural that the composition of citrus essential oils often varies according to species, variety, ripening stage, growing place, and other conditions. However, the isotope ratio of compounds in a plant is a result of the isotope effect, genealogy, and geological origin (O'Leary, 1981; Faulhaber et al., 1997). In addition, the isotope ratio, which is calculated on the basis of the intensities of the molecular peak (*m/z* 136) and its isotope peak (*m/z* 137) of monoterpene hydrocarbons, gives information about both carbon isotopes and hydrogen isotopes in the whole molecule of essential oil components. It is therefore reasonable to assume that this value would be characteristic for citrus species and that the distribution of isotope ratio in monoterpene hydrocarbon molecules among different citrus species would have a characteristic pattern.

Isotope Ratio of Monoterpene Hydrocarbons in Citrus Essential Oils from Vietnam. The isotope ratio of the monoterpene hydrocarbons in essential oils of Vietnamese pummelo (*C. grandis* Osbeck), lime (*C. aurantifolia* Swingle), orange (*C. sinensis* Osbeck), mandarin (*C. reticulata* Blanco), and their hybrids was determined by using GC-MS (Thao et al., 2007). The relative abundance of ^{13}C and ^{2}H over ^{12}C and ^{1}H in certain monoterpene hydrocarbon molecules was determined by the ratio of the ion intensity of the two masses at *m/z* 137 and *m/z* 136. This ratio reflects the difference in distribution ratio within one molecule of a monoterpene hydrocarbon. When analyzing in the SIM mode, the difference of ion intensities from the molecular and isotope peaks can be estimated at high accuracy. The isotope ratios of each molecular peak (*m/z* 137/136) of the monoterpene hydrocarbons are shown in Table 4.3. The isotope values for α-pinene in lime essential oils were higher than the others and did not vary very much (from 10.50% to 10.67%). Orange and pummelo had lower values (from 10.26% to 10.49% for orange and 10.14% to 10.63% for pummelo). In addition, the isotope ratio of limonene was from 11.03% to 11.30%, which is lower than the theoretically calculated value from natural abundance of carbon and hydrogen (11.42%). This lower value (depleted heavier carbon and hydrogen isotopes) is a result of isotope fractionation and isotope effect, which occurs along the biosynthetic pathway for plant materials (Sawamura et al., 2001).

Isotope Ratio Analysis by GC-MS of Monoterpene Hydrocarbons in Yuzu Essential Oils from Japan. Yuzu fruits were collected from 41 local wholesale markets from northern to southern Japan and the cold-pressed peel oil was prepared (Sawamura et al., 2001). The 10 selected monoterpene hydrocarbons were completely separated on a gas chromatogram (Figure 4.3). The result of the SIM analysis of all essential oils is summarized by the Ir ratio of *m/z* 137/136. The Ir data given as the mean of triplicate values were so stable and reliable that the coefficient of variance was less than 0.5% overall. This demonstrates that the Ir values were different among the 10 monoterpene compounds

TABLE 4.3. Isotope Ratio (%) of the Molecular Peak (*m/z* 137/136) of Monoterpene Hydrocarbons from Vietnamese Citrus Essential Oils

Samples	α - Pinene	β - Pinene	Sabinene	Myrcene	α - Phellandrene	α - Terpinene	Limonene	β - Phellandrene	γ - Terpinene	Terpinolene
Lime LDL	10.50	10.87	10.72	10.09	9.21	10.43	11.06	10.39	10.98	10.68
Lime LBT	10.61	11.03	10.91	9.92	8.90	10.21	11.03	10.63	10.90	10.53
Lime LV5	10.60	10.77	10.60	10.23	9.30	10.46	11.16	10.43	10.99	10.72
Lime LV6	10.67	11.06	10.88	10.25	9.53	10.58	11.17	10.63	11.05	10.74
Pummelo PVG	10.14	10.13	9.97	10.97	9.14	nd	11.13	10.55	nd	nd
Pummelo PBN	10.19	9.67	9.80	10.19	8.12	nd	11.18	10.47	nd	nd
Pummelo PNR	10.63	10.57	10.63	10.24	10.92	10.59	11.23	11.02	11.11	10.78
Pummelo PPT	10.31	9.22	9.79	10.26	8.41	nd	11.10	10.63	9.18	nd
Mandarin MHG	10.55	10.37	10.01	10.22	9.17	10.34	11.21	10.38	11.00	10.66
Mandarin MVL	10.41	10.21	10.20	10.41	10.60	nd	11.30	10.52	nd	nd
Orange OXD	10.31	nd	10.67	10.44	9.48	nd	11.25	10.62	nd	9.62
Orange OVL	10.47	nd	9.66	10.24	8.60	nd	11.14	10.44	nd	nd
Orange OHG	10.26	nd	9.93	10.39	9.12	nd	11.27	10.57	nd	nd

nd: Not detected.

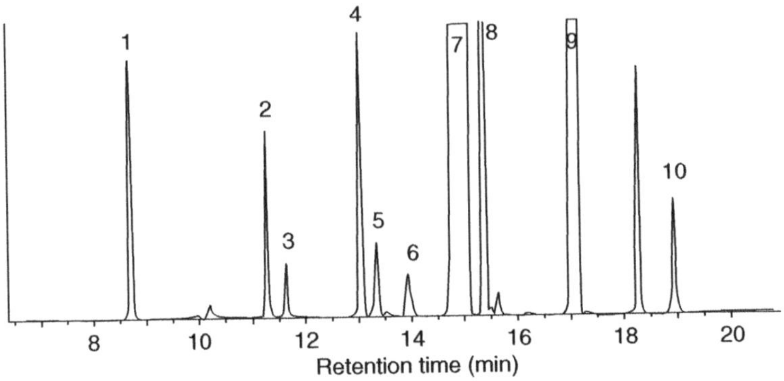

Figure 4.3. Gas chromatogram of yuzu essential oil. **1**: α-pinene, **2**: β-pinene, **3**: sabinene, **4**: myrcene, **5**: α-phellandrene, **6**: α-terpinene, **7**: limonene, **8**: β-phellandrene, **9**: γ-terpinene, **10**: terpinolene.

with the same molecular weight of 136. The 10 monoterpene hydrocarbons in yuzu peel oil had unique Ir values. The range of Ir variation of compound in yuzu oil was as follows: 11.08–11.34 for α-pinene; 11.13–11.35 for β-pinene; 11.47–11.52 for sabinene; 11.01–11.30 for myrcene; 10.99–11.29 for α-phellandrene; 11.17–11.39 for α-terpinene; 11.26–11.52 for limonene; 11.07–11.26 for β-phellandrene; 11.18–11.37 for γ-terpinene; and 11.08–11.32 for terpinolene. Most of these Ir values are lower than the theoretical Ir value for a monoterpene hydrocarbon. All the $C_{10}H_{16}$ monoterpene hydrocarbons should theoretically show an Ir ratio of 11.42 from a calculation of the natural abundance ratio of the hydrogen and carbon isotopes. Even though there would be a considerable deviation from the theoretical value as a result of mechanical factors, the low coefficient of variance indicates high reliability.

4.3.2 MS Fragment Isotope Ratio Analysis of Monoterpene Hydrocarbons

For the isotope ratio analysis using ordinary GC-MS, sometimes it is difficult to measure the isotope ratio when the molecular ion peak is very small or not detected. In GC-IRMS specialized for the measurement of isotope ratios, the value is determined as the whole molecule isotopic ratio. In ordinary GC-MS, on the other hand, the collectable data are not only the molecular ion peak but also various peak fragments resulting from the cleavage of molecules. Thus, the isotope ratio of the fragment ion peaks $m/z = \mathrm{m} + 1$ of a compound, $\mathrm{m} + 1/\mathrm{m}$ (m/z) (MS fragment ratio), can be measured in addition to that of the molecular ion peak. In addition, for a given molecular species, significant differences have been observed as a function of the plant source (Martin et al., 2004). There is a non-statistical distribution of ^{13}C and ^{2}H inside the monoterpene molecules. This results from genealogy and the isotope effect, so that there is a pattern that can be characteristic of the plant material. Consequently, the isotope ratio that was calculated by the intensity of the major fragment peaks was investigated in order to differentiate the essential oils from different citrus species (Satake et al., 2004; Thao et al., 2007).

MS Fragment Isotope Ratio Analysis of Monoterpene Hydrocarbons in Citrus Essential Oil from Japan. MS fragment isotope ratio analysis was done on various kinds of Japan citrus essential oils in Section 4.2.3. The MS fragment isotope ratios for α-pinene, β-pinene, α-terpinene, β-phellandrene, γ-terpinene, and terpinolene are shown in Table 4.4. The ratio of m/z = 137, 122, and 108 isotope fragments corresponding to m/z = 136, 121, and 107 were measured for each compound. The isotope effect was influenced by exogenous factors such as differences in location, climate, and cultivation conditions. When the isotope ratio of monoterpene hydrocarbons is divided by the ratio of one compound, limonene, in each essential oil, the influence of isotope discrimination of CO_2 fixation is eliminated (Faulhaber et al., 1997). This calculation will result in an isotope ratio pattern based on secondary metabolites, showing the specific pattern of each plant species. In this study, this calculation was applied to two MS fragment peaks, m/z 121 and 107, cleaved from the molecule (m/z = 136).

The fragment ratio patterns for citrus species were similar, but those for monoterpene hydrocarbons were quite different. The lime samples were characterized by MS fragment ratios of m/z 107 for β-phellandrene, m/z = 121 for γ-terpinene, and m/z = 107 for terpinolene. Regarding yuzu, the MS fragment ratios of m/z = 107 for α-pinene, m/z = 121 for β-pinene, m/z = 107 for myrcene, and m/z = 121 for β-phellandrene were noteworthy. The lemon samples were also characterized by MS fragment ratios of m/z = 107 for β-pinene, m/z = 107 for myrcene, and m/z = 107 for β-phellandrene.

Isotope Ratio of the Base Peak (m/z 94/93) for Monoterpene Hydrocarbons in Citrus Essential Oils from Vietnam. The isotope ratio of the base peak was estimated for the citrus essential oil samples from Section 4.2.3. Measurement of the base peak gives a greater sensitivity and more accurate results as well as better repeatability. For most of monoterpene hydrocarbons, the m/z 93 fragment is the base peak in their mass spectrum, accounting for 100% of relative intensity in the total ion chromatogram. Only limonene had a different base peak (m/z 68) in the mass spectrum. Table 4.5 displays the isotope ratio of the base peak and its isotope peak (m/z 94/93) of eight monoterpene hydrocarbons from citrus essential oils.

It can be seen from this result that there was a great difference in the isotope ratio values among the monoterpenes. The highest isotope ratio value of all the citrus essential oils can be seen in limonene (around 42%), and the lowest value in α-phellandrene (from 7.33 to 8.23%). On the other hand, the isotope ratio of the whole molecule (m/z 137/136) varied around 11% for all the samples. The highest value that was observed for limonene might have resulted from not only the isotope ratio, but also the addition of other fragments. Fortunately, the isotope

TABLE 4.4. MS Fragment Isotope Ratio of the Monoterpene Hydrocarbons from Citrus Oils

		MS Fragment Isotope Ratio																				
		α-Pinene			β-Pinene			Myrcene			α-Terpinolene			β-Phellandrene			γ-Terpinene			Terpinolene		
		107	121	136	107	121	136	107	121	136	107	121	136	107	121	136	107	121	136	107	121	136
Lime	A	0.84	0.99	1.00	0.82	1.09	1.04	0.92	1.01	0.92	1.64	1.01	1.01	1.73	0.91	0.98	0.75	1.01	0.99	1.10	1.02	0.99
Lime	B	0.82	0.99	0.99	0.76	1.07	1.03	0.96	1.00	0.97	1.64	1.00	1.01	1.77	0.93	0.98	0.75	1.01	0.99	1.09	1.02	0.99
Lime	C	0.84	1.00	1.00	0.85	1.00	1.05	1.01	1.00	1.01	1.65	1.00	1.01	1.72	1.00	0.98	0.75	1.01	1.00	1.09	1.02	0.99
Lime	D	0.86	1.01	0.99	0.91	1.08	1.02	1.01	1.08	0.89	1.63	1.00	1.01	1.49	0.94	0.99	0.75	1.02	0.99	1.09	1.03	0.99
Lime	E	0.82	0.99	1.00	0.84	1.08	1.02	0.99	0.98	0.99	1.63	1.01	1.01	1.71	0.94	1.00	0.75	1.01	1.00	1.10	1.02	0.99
Yuzu	A	0.79	0.99	0.98	0.89	0.97	0.99	0.99	0.99	0.99	1.57	0.99	0.98	1.44	1.02	0.99	0.75	1.03	0.99	1.13	1.04	0.99
Yuzu	B	0.79	0.99	0.97	0.93	0.97	0.99	1.01	0.99	1.00	1.66	0.99	0.97	1.41	1.02	0.99	0.76	1.03	0.99	1.17	1.03	0.98
Yuzu	C	0.79	1.00	0.98	0.89	0.95	0.99	0.99	0.99	0.96	1.53	1.02	0.87	1.43	1.03	0.99	0.76	1.03	0.99	1.16	1.04	0.99
Yuzu	D	0.80	1.00	0.99	0.82	0.98	1.02	1.02	0.99	0.99	1.58	0.99	0.97	1.53	1.01	0.99	0.74	1.03	0.99	1.13	1.03	0.99
Yuzu	E	0.79	0.99	0.98	0.92	0.97	1.01	1.02	0.98	0.99	1.67	0.98	0.99	1.40	1.03	0.98	0.74	1.02	0.99	1.12	1.04	0.99
Yuzu	F	0.79	1.00	0.97	0.86	0.96	1.01	1.00	0.99	0.97	2.02	0.99	0.99	1.52	1.03	0.98	0.75	1.04	0.99	1.12	1.03	0.98
Yuzu	G	0.80	0.99	0.98	0.87	0.98	1.00	1.02	0.99	0.99	1.75	1.01	0.98	1.48	1.01	0.98	0.75	1.03	0.99	1.14	1.04	0.97
Yuzu	F	0.81	0.99	0.98	0.89	0.96	0.99	1.02	1.00	0.99	1.68	0.98	0.96	1.47	1.03	0.98	0.75	1.03	0.99	1.14	1.04	0.98
Yuzu	I	0.80	0.99	0.97	0.88	0.98	1.01	1.02	0.99	0.99	1.60	0.99	0.99	1.47	1.01	0.98	0.76	1.04	0.99	1.15	1.04	0.98
Lemon	A	0.79	1.00	0.98	0.66	0.97	1.02	1.02	0.98	0.99	1.50	1.03	0.97	1.87	1.04	0.97	0.77	1.03	0.99	1.16	1.03	0.99
Lemon	B	0.81	1.00	0.98	0.69	0.98	1.02	1.03	1.00	0.98	1.64	0.99	0.99	1.78	1.02	0.98	0.76	1.02	0.99	1.17	1.03	0.98
Lemon	C	0.81	1.00	0.98	0.66	0.95	1.01	1.04	1.00	1.01	1.62	0.98	0.98	1.89	1.05	0.99	0.75	1.02	0.99	1.14	1.03	0.98
Lemon	D	0.82	0.99	0.99	0.68	1.00	1.01	1.06	0.99	0.98	1.48	0.99	0.95	1.81	1.00	0.99	0.76	1.01	0.99	1.16	1.04	0.98
Lemon	E	0.81	0.99	0.99	0.72	0.98	1.02	1.03	1.01	0.98	1.72	1.01	1.02	1.71	1.03	0.98	0.76	1.02	0.99	1.14	1.01	0.98

Note: The MS fragment ratio of $m/z = 108, 122$, and 137 fragments was measured for each compound. The isotope ratio of each compound was divided by the isotope ratio of one compound, limonene, of each essential oil. Thus, the isotope ratio of limonene comes to 1.00.

TABLE 4.5. Isotope Ratio (%) of Base Peak (*m/z* 94/ 93) of Monoterpene Hydrocarbons from Vietnamese Citrus Essential Oils

No.	Samples	α-Pinene	β-Pinene	Sabinene	Myrcene	α-Phellandrene	Limonene	β-Phellandrene	γ-Terpinene
1	Lime LDL	9.43	13.76	13.96	10.11	7.66	41.67	14.63	9.36
2	Lime LBT	9.43	13.99	14.11	10.08	7.33	42.15	14.64	9.42
3	Lime LV5	9.27	13.79	14.04	10.14	7.65	41.54	14.79	9.46
4	Lime LV6	9.36	14.15	14.18	10.14	7.84	41.24	14.79	9.68
5	Pummelo PVG	9.57	13.35	13.39	11.84	7.91	42.62	14.18	11.24
6	Pummelo PBN	9.61	13.31	13.31	10.16	7.77	42.83	14.19	11.16
7	Pummelo PNR	9.47	13.40	13.48	10.17	8.23	42.40	14.39	9.55
8	Pummelo PPT	9.59	13.26	13.31	10.17	8.10	42.65	14.42	11.34
9	Mandarin MHG	9.35	13.35	13.35	9.82	7.76	42.45	14.13	9.38
10	Mandarin MVL	9.61	13.35	13.40	10.17	7.58	42.72	14.28	11.09
11	Orange OXD	9.59	13.07	13.45	10.20	8.06	43.07	14.19	11.93
12	Orange OVL	9.63	12.65	13.28	10.17	7.58	42.53	14.14	12.75
13	Orange OHG	9.57	12.79	13.34	10.18	7.68	43.07	14.18	11.35

ratio of the other monoterpene hydrocarbons did not show the same behavior as limonene. Moreover, there was little variation in these values from one monoterpene of the same species. The isotope ratio for α-pinene in lime essential oils, for example, varied from 9.27 to 9.36%, whereas this value for pummelo was in the range of 9.47 to 9.59%. These results suggest the different distribution of ^{13}C and ^{2}H at a different carbon position inside the monoterpene molecule. Considering the ratio of $^{13}C/^{12}C$ and $^{2}H/^{1}H$ at different sites in the monoterpene molecule, the isotope ratio values may be increased at certain carbon positions and depleted at others. This notion is illustrated by the study on the fellowship of natural abundance ^{2}H-isotopomers of monoterpenes, for which Martin has reported that the value of $^{2}H/^{1}H$ differed at each carbon position (Martin et al., 2004). On the other hand, going back to the biosynthetic pathway to monoterpenes, glucose is one of the main photosynthetic precursors, and there is evidence for a nonstatistical carbon isotope distribution in natural glucose. The relative carbon isotope content at each position of glucose has been determined by revealing a defined and reproducible ^{13}C distribution in glucose from different origins (Rossmann et al., 1991). Therefore, there should be different isotope ratios in monoterpenes from different citrus essential oils resulting from the characteristic distribution of an isotope within one molecule. In addition, variation in the form of a cleavage fragment according to individual compounds among monoterpene hydrocarbons will give more information for the differentiation of citrus essential oils.

4.3.3 Isotope Fingerprint of Citrus Essential Oil

Because of the characteristic distribution of isotope ratios, a fingerprint of the main components in essential oil from the genuine source can be used in the authenticity control (Frank et al., 1995; Faulhaber et al., 1997). The profile is used to prove the genuineness of commercially available oils. Compared with the authentic samples, the suspected oil can be revealed by showing a difference from the isotope fingerprint.

Isotope Fingerprint of Yuzu Essential Oil. An isotope fingerprint of yuzu essential oils was created for yuzu essential oils from 41 different producing areas in Japan. Experimentation was also conducted on the following additional citrus fruits: *Citrus unshiu* Marcov. (unshu), *C. natsudaidai* Hayata (natsudaidai), *C. limon* Burmann (lemon), and *C. hanaju* Hort. ex Shirai (hanayu). All of these additional samples were harvested during the same season as yuzu.

The $\delta^{13}C_{PDB}$ value induced from the isotope effect is influenced by such exogenous factors as location, climate, and harvest time. The isotope ratio of endogenous biosynthesized compounds is also affected by exogenous factors including differences in cultivars. The isotope ratio of the yuzu essential oil components varied among the yuzu samples to some extent. When the Ir value of one compound in a series of the 10 selected compounds was reduced to zero and its difference was taken from the Ir values of the other 9 compounds, the

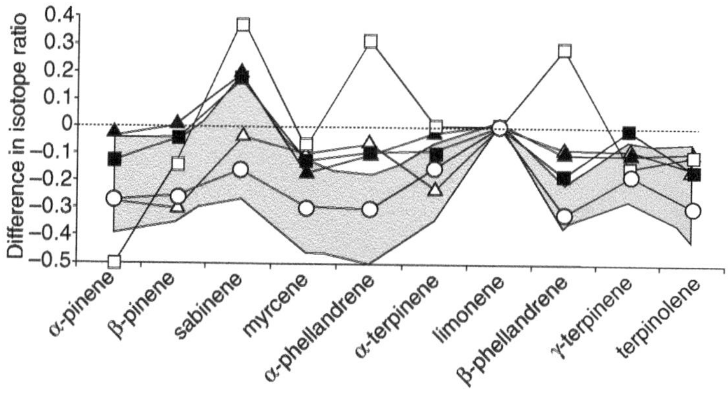

Figure 4.4. Isotope fingerprint of yuzu essential oils and isotope ratio of other citrus essential oils. The shaded band shows the fingerprint of yuzu essential oils. ○ Korean yuzu, □ natsudaidai, △ unshu, ■ lemon, ▲ hanayu.

influence of the isotope discrimination on CO_2 fixation was eliminated. This calculation will result in an Ir pattern based on secondary metabolites, showing the specific pattern of each species of plants.

As shown in Figure 4.4, a shaded band designates the fingerprint of yuzu with >95% probably of significance. Several citrus essential oils other than those of yuzu (i.e., unshu, natsudaidai, lemon, and hanayu) were also analyzed. All samples' plotted patterns were clearly distinct from the yuzu fingerprint. These citrus fruits, except for hanayu, are different species from yuzu according to the taxonomy systems of both Swingle and Tanaka. Hanayu is said to be comparatively close to yuzu, but is obviously different from yuzu in Tanaka's taxonomy. Its aroma is similar to that of yuzu, although not as strong. Hanayu is sometimes used as a substitute for or as an imitation of genuine yuzu, and maybe confused with yuzu. However, the fingerprint analysis based on the isotope ratio demonstrates a distinct difference between yuzu and hanayu. On the other hand, a yuzu sample from Korea fitted perfectly within the Japanese yuzu fingerprint band for the 10 compounds tested. These results suggested that this method could be applied to evaluate the genuineness of essential oils in addition to an enantiomeric analysis.

Isotope Fingerprint of Citrus Essential Oil from Vietnam. Isotope fingerprint was created by the isotope ratio value (*m/z* 137/136) of six monoterpene hydrocarbons—α-pinene, sabinene, myrcene, α-phellandrene, limonene, and β-phellandrene—from different citrus species from Vietnam such as Vietnamese pummelo (*C. grandis* Osbeck), lime (*C. aurantifolia* Swingle), orange (*C. sinensis* Osbeck), mandarin (*C. reticulata* Blanco), and their hybrids (Sawamura and Thao, 2008). Figures 4.5 to 4.8 show the isotope fingerprint of those citrus essential oils in dark band. The oil that is not the investigated oil shows a deviation from the band in the figure. Lime has a narrow isotope range and is distinguishable from the other species. The other species had wider isotope range, probably because

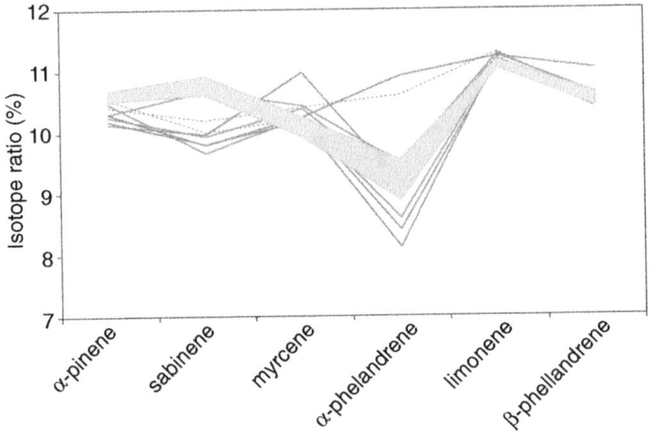

Figure 4.5. Isotope fingerprint of lime essential oils.

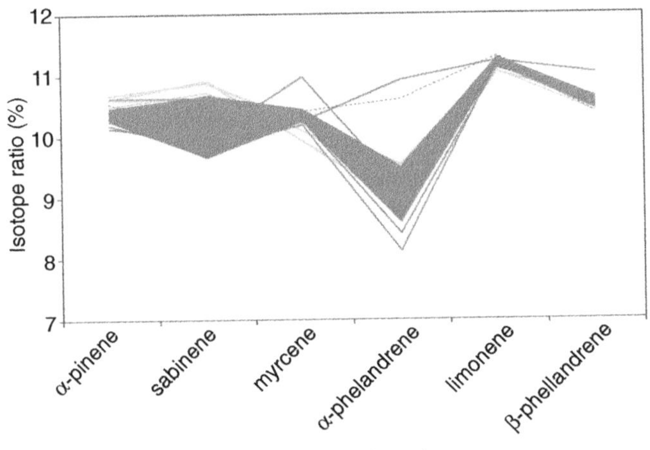

Figure 4.6. Isotope fingerprint of orange essential oils.

they are hybrids from different species. From this result, we can construct a fingerprint that characterizes the citrus species by analyzing as many as possible of the genuine products. In order to verify the origin of a suspect product, we can analyze for the isotope ratio values of main components and compare with the isotope fingerprint created by the authenticity profile for each genuine product.

Isotope Fingerprint of Citrus Essential Oil Based on Modified Isotope Ratio. The isotope ratio analysis was carried out on various kinds of citrus essential oils, including commercial CPO of five lemon oils and five lime oils, an

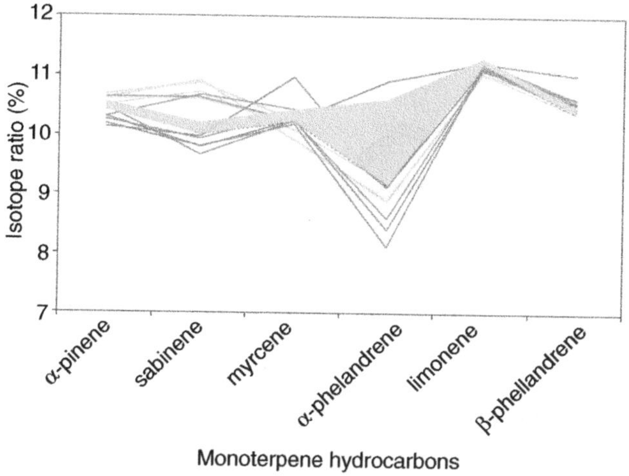

Figure 4.7. Isotope fingerprint of mandarin essential oils.

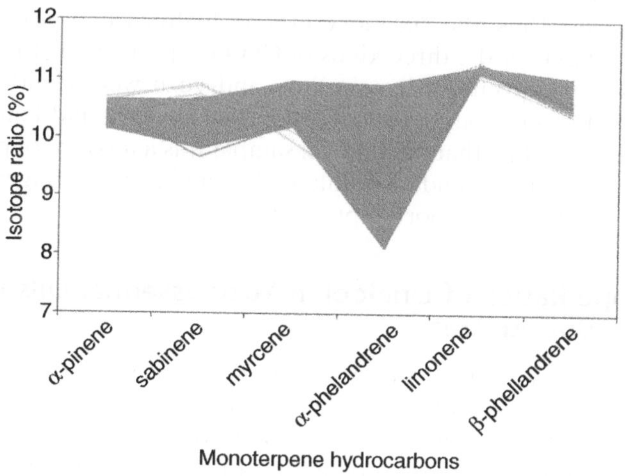

Figure 4.8. Isotope fingerprint of pummelo essential oils.

artificial lemon flavor product, a lemon CPO, and 10 yuzu CPOs from Japan. The isotope effect was found to be influenced by exogenous factors such as differences in location, climate, and cultivation condition. When the isotope ratio of monoterpene hydrocarbons was divided by the Ir value of one compound, limonene, of each essential oil (modified Ir), the influence on isotope discrimination by CO_2 fixation was eliminated. This calculation will result in Ir patterns based on secondary metabolites, showing the specific pattern of each plant species.

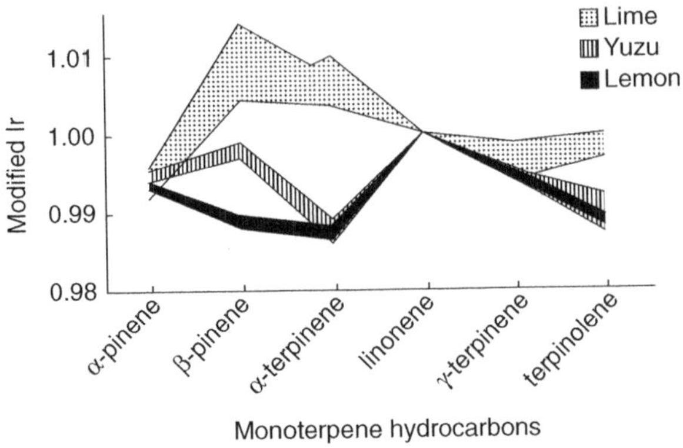

Figure 4.9. Modified isotope ratio values of the monoterpene hydrocarbons from lime, yuzu, lemon oils.

As shown in Figure 4.9, a characteristic fingerprint was obtained for each citrus species. The composition of citrus essential oils generally depends on the variety or species. Thus, the six monoterpene hydrocarbons were selected as common constituents of the three kinds of CPO for performing the isotope ratio analysis. These fingerprints of lemon, lime, and yuzu were clearly distinct, the fingerprint band of lime being broader than that of yuzu and lemon. This may have been due to the fact that the lime oil sample was a mixture of products from various localities, varieties, and/or distillate oil from juice. The fingerprint of yuzu CPO agreed with the one reported previously.

4.3.4 Isotope Ratios of Linalool in Yuzu Essential Oils from Different Producing Areas

Thirty-three samples of yuzu collected from different producing areas in Japan and Korea were analyzed for the isotope ratios by means of GC-MS. Authentic linalool was used for preparing standard solutions at different concentrations with purified acetone. A proper separation of linalool from other volatile compounds of the essential oil by capillary column in practical GC conditions is prerequisite to the determination of isotope ratio value. The linalool fraction was well separated from the other volatile compounds in the yuzu essential oil by employing an appropriate column and oven temperature program.

The isotope ratio *m/z* 156/154 of linalool from authentic chemical (AU) in standard solutions and in yuzu CPO from different producing areas is plotted in the boxplot in Figure 4.10. It is obvious that the authentic linalool had a significantly higher Ir value (1.09%) than those from yuzu essential oils. The Ir values of linalool from yuzu samples grown in Kochi (KC), Ehime (EH), Oita (OT), Tokushima (TK), and Wakayama (WK) prefectures were not statistically different from one another; the average Ir value ranged from 0.96 to 1.02%. The Irs

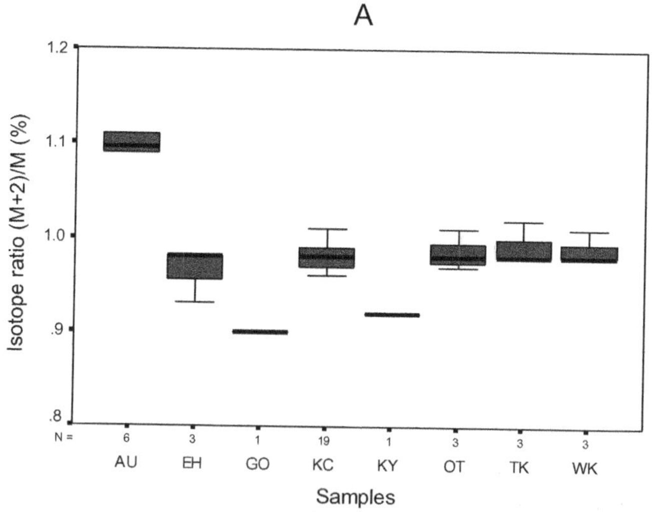

Figure 4.10. Boxplot of isotope ratio (M + 2)/M of linalool from authentic chemicals and yuzu essential oils from different producing areas. Samples from different areas are marked as: Authentic chemicals, AU; Ehime, EH; Goheung, GO; Kochi, KC; Kyoto, KY; Oita, OT; Tokushima, TK; Wakayma, WK.

of linalool in Kyoto (KY) in Japan and Goheung (GO) in Korea samples were 0.91 and 0.89%, respectively. They were, on the other hand, lower than those from the other yuzu samples. The same behavior was also observed for the isotope ratio *m/z* 155/154. The Ir of authentic linalool was significantly higher than the other samples (Figure 4.11), whereas these values were almost equal among the samples from EH, KC, OT, TK, and WK. The Ir *m/z* 155/154 of KY and GO was lower than that of the other yuzu samples.

The latitudes of sampling sites of Kochi, Oita, Ehime, Wakayama, and Tokushima were similar, while those of Kyoto and Goheung were almost similar to each other. The isotope ratio values of linalool in these samples were divided into two distinct groups according to the difference of sampling-site latitudes. There are many factors that influence the isotope ratio value, however, the lower isotope ratio *m/z* 156/154 observed in the yuzu samples from KY and GO probably resulted from the lower isotope ratio in the precipitation in the area of higher latitude and the lower annual temperature in the northern hemisphere (Dansgaard, 1964). In addition, the heavier isotope concentrations in fresh water decrease with increasing latitude and altitude (Dansgaard, 1953). It is suggested that the isotope ratio of linalool may be reflected by the spatial distribution of oxygen, hydrogen, and carbon isotopic content. Although there are several factors that influence the isotope ratio values, we can see the trend of differentiating yuzu from different producing areas. This finding suggests the possibility of the application of GC-MS to authenticity control by means of component isotope ratio.

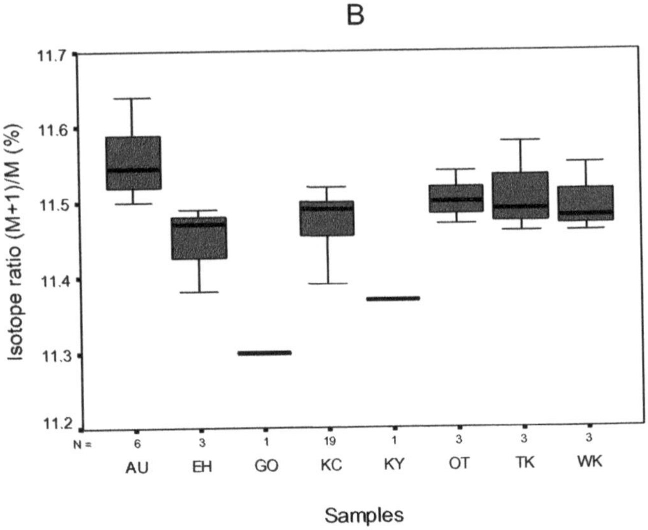

Figure 4.11. Boxplot of isotope ratio (M + 1)/M of linalool from authentic chemicals and yuzu essential oils from different producing areas. Samples from different areas are marked as: Authentic chemicals, AU; Ehime, EH; Goheung, GO; Kochi, KC; Kyoto, KY; Oita, OT; Tokushima, TK; Wakayma, WK.

4.3.5 Discrimination of Citrus Essential Oils from Different Species and Hybrids

Multivariate Analysis of Isotope Ratio of Monoterpene Hydrocarbons. The study of authenticity control of food origin cannot be completed without the interpretation of datasets by appropriate chemometrics or statistical methods. The multivariate analysis of multicomponents is a promising tool for this recognition (Tzouros and Arvanitoyannis, 2001; Kelly et al., 2005). The modified Ir data for monoterpene hydrocarbons from the three species of citrus oils in Japan were subjected to a multivariate analysis. According to principal component analysis, the citrus essential oils examined were clearly discriminated, with 93.3% of the accumulation contribution ratio of both PC1 and PC2 (Figure 4.12A). As shown in Figure 4.12B, β-pinene, α-terpinene, and β-phellandrene were large for the absolute value of the eigenvector of monoterpene system hydrocarbons, followed by terpinolene. These compounds greatly contributed to the modified Ir discrimination of the citrus essential oils.

The cluster analysis is shown in Figure 4.13; all of the essential oils, except for lime oil E, were classified into the species clusters. Regarding the yuzu oils, it is noteworthy that the essential oils from Yamagata, Kochi, Shizuoka, and Tokushima prefectures, which each had a high sensory evaluation, were classified into the same cluster, which is in accordance with the findings in our previous report. The artificial lemon flavor essence and the lemon CPO from Wakayma prefecture in Japan were classified into the same cluster as the commercial lemon samples.

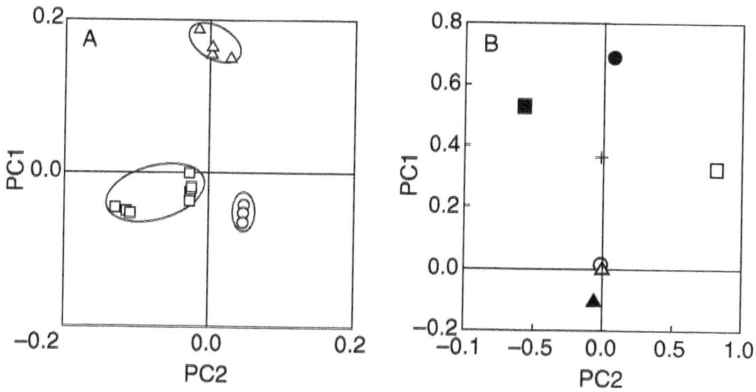

Figure 4.12. Principal component analysis of the modified Ir values of the monoterpene hydrocarbons from citrus oils. **A**: Principal component scores of citrus oils. △ lime, ○ yuzu, □ lemon. **B**: Characteristic vectors of monoterpene hydrocarbons. ▲ α-pinene, ■ β-pinene, ● α-terpinene, △ limonene, □ β-phellandrene, ○ γ-terpinene, + terpinolene.

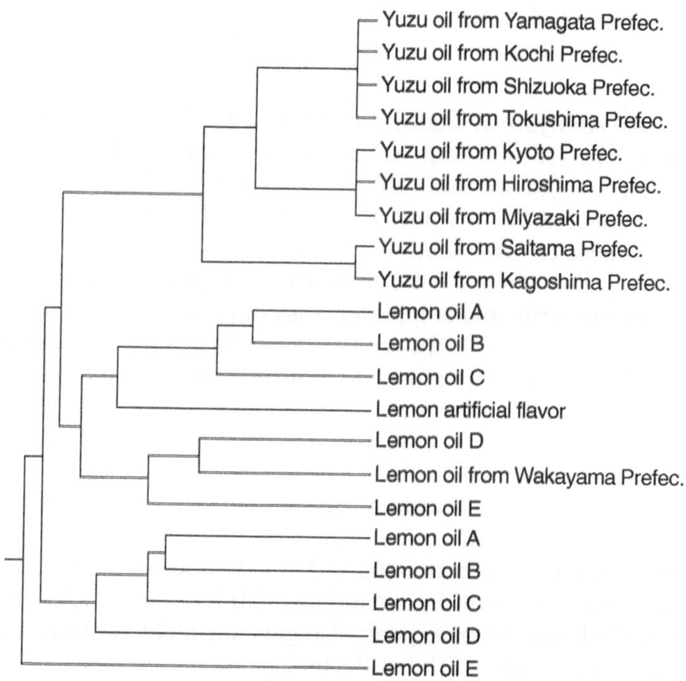

Figure 4.13. Cluster analysis of the modified isotope ratio values of monoterpene hydrocarbons from yuzu, lime, and lemon essential oils.

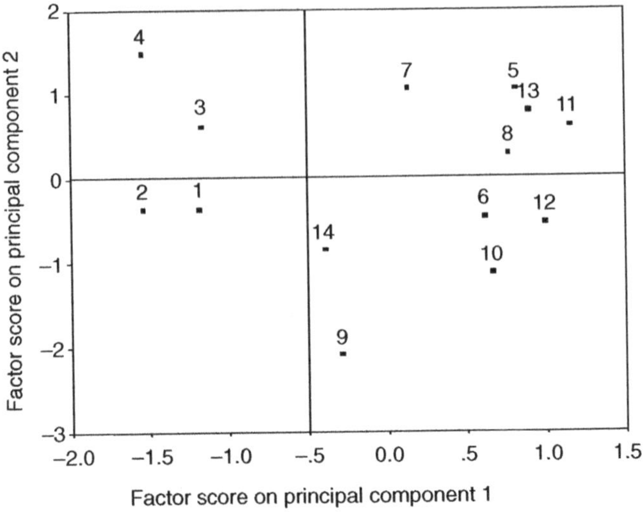

Figure 4.14. Principal component analysis of isotope ratio *m/z* 94/93 of the monoterpene hydrocarbons. Numbers are denoted according to Table 4.5. 1–4: lime; 5–8: pummelo; 9, 10: mandarin; 11–13: orange; 14: Naruto orange.

Multivariate Analysis of Isotope Ratio of Base Peak from Monoterpene Hydrocarbons. The isotope ratio values for the base peaks (*m/z* 94/93) with eight monoterpene hydrocarbons (Table 4.5) from 14 citrus essential oils in Vietnam were subjected to a principal component analysis in order to find a relationship for these citrus essential oils. The result of the principal component analysis is displayed in Figure 4.14, in which each point represents one citrus sample. The first two principal components accounted for 72% of the total variance of isotope ratio for the eight monoterpene hydrocarbons. In this analysis, lime oils could be clearly distinguished from the other oils by having a distinct location on the graph. Although orange and pummelos were placed in proximity, they could be differentiated in this analysis. ONR was the only example from Japan in this study and it is said to be a hybrid between pummelo and mandarin. The great distance between ONR and the same hybrid groups, OVL and OHG, from the PCA analysis might have been caused by the factor of geographical difference. In addition, mandarin sample MVL was located far from the other citrus samples, while the hybrid of mandarin (MHG) was at a location near to orange. This analysis for the base peak also gave a similar result to that from an analysis of the isotope ratio of the molecular peak.

Multivariate Analysis of Isotope Ratio of MS Fragment from Monoterpene Hydrocarbons. The MS fragment ratios for monoterpene hydrocarbons from the three species of citrus oils were subjected to principal component analysis. The PC number with an eigenvalue greater than 1 was 6.

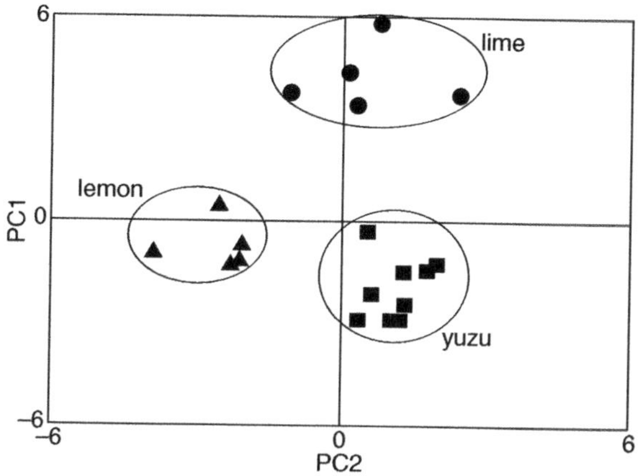

Figure 4.15. Principal component analysis of MS fragment isotope ratios of the monoterpene hydrocarbons from citrus oil. ● lime, ■ yuzu, ▲ lemon.

The contribution ratio was 36.8%, 14.9%, and 11.4% for PC1, PC2, and PC3, respectively; thus both PC1 and PC2 explained 51.7% of the information regarding those essential oils, as shown in Figure 4.15. The lemon essential oils were distinguished from the other essential oils by PC1, and the lime essential oils were distinguished from the other oils by PC2.

The cluster analysis is shown in Figure 4.16; all of the essential oils were classified according to species. In the cases of lemon and lime, the result based on the MS fragment ratio agreed almost perfectly with the result based on the ratio of the intensity of isotope peak to its molecular peak. In the case of yuzu, these two results were different, and four clusters of locality in which the isotope ratio was common were obtained. The lemon CPO from Wakayama prefecture in Japan (Lemon D) and artificial lemon flavor essence (Lemon E) were classified into the lemon species cluster including the commercial essential oils. This suggests that the MS fragment isotope ratio analysis method can be also applied to the evaluation of monoterpene hydrocarbons from essential oils in addition to the isotope ratio analysis of molecular ion peaks.

4.3.6 Discrimination of Citrus Essential Oils from Different Producing Areas

In a study on the isotope ratio of yuzu essential oils of different producing areas from northern to southern Japan, Sawamura et al. (2001) analyzed 41 cold-pressed yuzu oils and compared those data by the following procedures: The significant difference between the two Ir values of each compound from different yuzu samples was checked by the *t*-test ($P < 0.05$). The sign test was then performed on the following basis: The results of each sample were classified as positive, negative, or no significant difference. If one Ir value was greater than the other, the former was given a plus and the latter a minus. If there was no

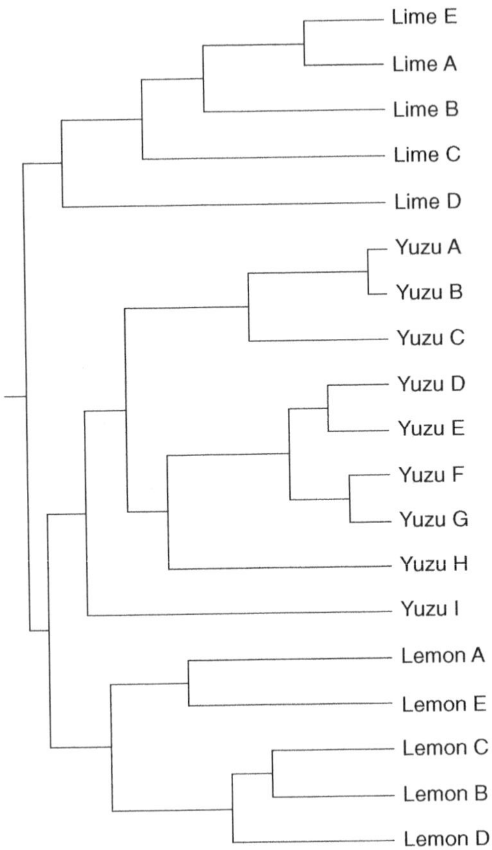

Figure 4.16. Cluster analysis of MS fragment isotope ratio of the monoterpene hydrocarbons from citrus oil.

significant difference, both were given zero. A database of these values was constructed for the 10 compounds of each of the 41 samples and revealed several predominant cultivation regions. Out of 41 samples, only eight samples were not significantly different as indicated by the low shaded value. This was also the first time that a substantial difference among yuzu fruits from different production areas has been detected. This isotope ratio method seems to be more relevant in comparison to other parameters for evaluating citrus fruit quality such as fruit weight, soluble-solid, acidity, and color index (L, a, and b). Those common factors may not be relevant to a determination of the quality and characterization of the production area. These results suggest that, in addition to an enantiomeric analysis, this analytical method can be applied to evaluate the genuineness of essential oils. Furthermore, it is expected that this technique of isotope ratio analysis will be applicable to evaluate the origin of citrus essential oils and their products, and also to specify organic compounds from natural resources.

Closing Remarks. The characteristics and quality of citrus flavors have commonly been evaluated on the basis of their essential oil components. Citrus flavors or their essential oils, on the other hand, are apt to vary in composition as a result of maturity, storage, or cultivation conditions. Moreover, it may be difficult to clearly distinguish characteristic differences among the same cultivars from different production districts solely by means of an essential oil component analysis, since their compositions are quite similar. The isotope analyses by GC-MS provide new information about these matters. It was confirmed that the isotope ratio of the investigated monoterpene hydrocarbon in citrus essential oils was not influenced by the compositional change taking place during the storage period, or by the fruit harvest date. These results lend support to the validity of the isotope ratio analysis method by ordinary GC-MS in the authenticity control of essential oils. In addition, it is suggested that the data obtained from the isotope ratio analysis method, which is used for discriminating producing districts or genuineness of crops, are independent on common variations incidental to samplings as long as the samples are collected in the same area. Many common components of foods usually fluctuate among individual samples. It is expected that this analysis will be widely used for judgment of the characteristics of agricultural products.

REFERENCES

Asche, S., Michaud, A.L., Brenna, J.T. (2003). Sourcing organic compounds based on natural isotopic variations measured by high precision isotope ratio mass spectrometry. *Current Organic Chemistry* **7**: 1527–1543.

Bicchi, C., D'Amato, A., Rubiolo, P. (1999). Cyclodextrin derivatives as chiral selectors for direct gas chromatographic separation of enantiomers in the essential oil, aroma and flavour fields. *Journal of Chromatography A* **843**: 99–121.

Braunsdorf, R., Hener, U., Stein, S., Mosandl, A. (1993). Comprehensive cGC-IRMS analysis in the authenticity control of flavours and essential oils. Part I: Lemon oil. *Zeitschrift fur Lebensmittel-Untersuchung und Forschung* **197**: 137–141.

Calderone, G., Guillou, C. (2008). Analysis of isotopic ratios for the detection of illegal watering of beverages. *Food Chemistry* **106**: 1399–1405.

Choi, H.S., Sawamura, M. (2000). Composition of the Essential Oil of *Citrus tamurana* Hort. ex Tanaka (Hyuganatsu). *Journal of Agricultural and Food Chemistry* **48**: 4868–4873.

Craig, H. (1961). Isotopic variations in meteoric waters. *Science* **133**: 1702–1703.

Dansgaard, W. (1953). The abundance of ^{18}O in atmospheric water and water vapour. *Tellus* **5**: 461–469.

Dansgaard, W. (1964). Stable isotopes in precipitation. *Tellus* **16**: 436–468.

Dawson, T.E., Mambelli, S., Plamboeck, A.H., Templer, P.H., Tu, K.P. (2002). Stable isotopes in plant ecology. *Annual Review of Ecology and Systematics* **33**: 507–559.

Delwiche, C.C., Steyn, P.L. (1970). Nitrogen isotope fractionation in soils and microbial reactions. *Environmental Science & Technology* **4**: 929–935.

Faulhaber, S., Hener, U., Mosandl, A. (1997). GC/IRMS analysis of mandarin essential oils. 1. $^{13}C_{PDB}$ and $^{15}N_{AIR}$ Values of Methyl *N*-Methylanthranilate. *Journal of Agricultural and Food Chemistry* **45**: 2579–2583.

Frank, C., Dietrich, A., Kremer, U., Mosandl, A. (1995). GC-IRMS in the authenticity control of the essential oil of *Coriandrum sativum* L. *Journal of Agricultural and Food Chemistry* **43**: 1634–1637.

Franke, B.M., Koslitz, S., Micaux, F., Piantini, U., Maury, V., Pfammatter, E., Wunderli, S., Gremaud, G., Bosset, J.O., Hadorn, R., Kreuzer, M. (2008). Tracing the geographic origin of poultry meat and dried beef with oxygen and strontium isotope ratios. *European Food Research and Technology* **226**: 761–769.

Hanneguelle, S., Thibault, J.N., Naulet, N., Martin, G.J. (1992). Authentication of essential oils containing linalool and linalyl acetate by isotopic methods. *Journal of Agricultural and Food Chemistry* **40**: 81–87.

Hor, K., Ruff, C., Weckerle, B., Konig, T., Schreier, P. (2001). Flavor authenticity studies by $^{2}H/^{1}H$ ratio determination using on-line gas chromatography pyrolysis isotope ratio mass spectrometry. *Journal of Agricultural and Food Chemistry* **49**: 21–25.

Juchelka, D., Mosandl, A. (1996). Authenticity profiles of bergamot oil. *Pharmazie* **51**: 417–422.

Kelly, S., Heatonb, K., Hoogewerff, J. (2005). Tracing the geographical origin of food: The application of multi-element and multi-isotope analysis. *Trends in Food Science & Technology* **16**: 555–567.

Loomis, W.D. (1967). Biosynthesis and metabolism of monoterpenes. In: Pridham, J.B. (ed.), *Terpenoids in plants*. London and New York: Academic Press, pp. 59–82.

Manca, G., Franco, M.A., Versini, G., Camin, F., Rossmann, A., Tola, A. (2006). Correlation between multielement stable isotope ratio and geographical origin in Peretta cows' milk cheese. *Journal of Dairy Science* **89**: 831–839.

Martin, G.G., Hanote, V., Lees, M., Martin, Y.L. (1996a). Interpretation of combined ^{2}H SNIF/NMR and ^{13}C SIRA/MS analyses of fruit juices to detect added sugar. *Journal of AOAC International* **79**: 62–72.

Martin, G.J., Martin, M.L. (1981). Deuterium labelling at natural abundance level as studied by high field quantitative ^{2}H NMR. *Tetrahedron Letters* **22**: 3525–3528.

Martin, G.J., Danho, D., Guillou, C. (1990). NMR and MS stable isotope studies of fruit juice adulteration. *Abstracts of Papers of the American Chemical Society* **200**: 154–AGFD.

Martin, G.J., Martin, M.L. (1991). Deuterium labelling at the natural abundance level as studied by high field quantitative ^{2}H-NMR. *Tetrahedron Letters* **22**: 3525–3528.

Martin, G.J., Koziet, J., Rossmann, A., Dennis, J. (1996b). Site-specific natural isotope fractionation in fruit juices determined by deuterium NMR: A European inter-laboratory comparison study. *Analytica Chimica Acta* **321**: 137–146.

Martin, G.J., Lavoine-Hanneguelleb, S., Mabonc, F., Martina, M.L. (2004). The fellowship of natural abundance ^{2}H-isotopomers of monoterpenes. *Phytochemistry* **65**: 2815–2831.

Martin, M.L., Martin, G.J. (1999). Site-specific isotope effects and origin inference. *Analysis* **27**: 209–213.

McHale, D. (2002). Adulteration of citrus oils. In: Dugo, G. (ed.), *Citrus: The genus Citrus*. Taylor & Francis, CRC Press, pp. 496–517.

McLafferty, F.W., Turecek, F. (1993). *Interpretation of mass spectra*. Sausalito, CA: University Science Books, p. 371.

Meier-Augenstein, W. (2002). Stable isotope analysis of fatty acids by gas chromatography-isotope ratio mass spectrometry. *Analytical Chimica Acta* **465**: 63–79.

Mitiku, S.B., Ukeda, H., Sawamura, M. (2001). Enantiomeric distribution of α-pinene, β-pinene, sabinene and limonene in various citrus essential oils. In: Spanier, A.H. (ed.), *Food flavors and chemistry: Advances of the new millenium*. Cambridge, UK: Royal Society of Chemistry, pp. 216–232.

Mondello, L., Dugo, P., Dugo, G. (2002). The chiral compounds of citrus essential oils. In: Dugo, G. (ed.), *Citrus: The genus Citrus*. Taylor & Francis, CRC Press, pp. 461–495.

Mosandl, A. (2004). Authenticity assessment: a permanent challenge in food flavor and essential oil analysis. *Journal of Chromatographic Science* **42**: 440–449.

Nhu-Trang, T.T., Casabianca, H., Grenier-Loustalot, M.F. (2006). Authenticity control of essential oils containing citronellal and citral by chiral and stable-isotope gas-chromatographic analysis. *Analytical and Bioanalytical Chemistry* **386**: 2141–2152.

Njoroge, S.M., Ukeda, H., Sawamura, M. (1996). Changes in the volatile composition of yuzu (*Citrus junos* Tanaka) cold-pressed oil during storage. *Journal of Agricultural and Food Chemistry* **44**: 550–556.

O'Leary, M.H. (1981). Carbon isotope fractionation in plants. *Phytochemistry* **20**: 553–567.

Park, R., Epstein, S. (1960). Carbon isotope fractionation during biosynthesis. *Geochimica et Cosmochimica Acta* **21**: 110–126.

Rossmann, A., Butzenlechner, M., Schmidt, H.-L. (1991). Evidence for a nonstatistical carbon isotope distribution in natural glucose. *Plant Physiology* **96**: 609–614.

Satake, A., Une, A., Ueno, T., Ukeda, H., Sawamura, M. (2003). Isotope ratio analysis by HRGC-MS of monoterpene hydrocarbons from citrus essential oils. *Bioscience, Biotechnology, and Biochemistry* **67**: 599–604.

Satake, A., Furukawa, K., Ueno, T., Ukeda, H., Sawamura, M. (2004). MS fragment isotope ratio analysis for evaluation of citrus essential oils by HRGC-MS. *Bioscience, Biotechnology, and Biochemistry* **68**: 312–316.

Sawamura, M., Kuriyama, T. (1988). Quantitative determination of volatile constituents in the pummelo (*Citrus grandis* Osbeck forma Tosa-buntan). *Journal of Agricultural and Food Chemistry* **36**: 567–569.

Sawamura, M. (1994). Citrus flavor. *Kagaku to Seibutsu* **32**: 114–119.

Sawamura, M., Ito, T., Une, A., Ukeda, H., Yamasaki, Y. (2001). Isotope ratio by HRGC-MS of *Citrus junos* Tanaka (yuzu) essential oils: *m/z* 137/136 of terpene hydrocarbons. *Bioscience, Biotechnology, and Biochemistry* **65**: 2622–2629.

Sawamura, M., Satake, A., Ueno, T., Une, A., Ukeda, H. (2004). Effects of several variable factors on the isotope ratio by HRGC-MS. *Bioscience, Biotechnology, and Biochemistry* **68**: 215–217.

Sawamura, M., Thao, N.T. (2008). *Development* of analytical method for identification and differentiation of citrus fruits by GC-MS. *Journal of Chemistry* **T46**: 432–436.

Thao, N.T., Kashiwagi, T., Sawamura, M. (2007). Characterization by GC-MS of Vietnamese citrus species and hybrids based on the isotope ratio of monoterpene hydrocarbons. *Bioscience, Biotechnology, and Biochemistry* **71**: 2155–2161.

Tzouros, N.E., Arvanitoyannis, I.S. (2001). Agricultural produces: Synopsis of employed quality control methods for the authentication of foods and application of chemometrics for the classification of foods according to their variety or geographical origin. *Critical Reviews in Food Science and Nutrition* **41**: 287–319.

Ubukata, M. (2005). Features and applications of newly-developed GC-TOFMS: "The AccuTOF GC." *JEOL News* **40**: 38–45.

West, J.B., Ehleringer, J.R., Cerling, T.E. (2007). Geography and vintage predicted by a novel GIS model of wine $\delta^{18}O$. *Journal of Agricultural and Food Chemistry* **40**: 7075–7083.

Yoneyama, T., Omata, T., Nagata, S., Yamasaki, J. (1991). Fractionation of nitrogen isotopes during the uptake and assimilation of ammonia by plants. *Plant Cell Physiology* **32**: 1211–1217.

5

GAS CHROMATOGRAPHY–OLFACTOMETRY AND AROMA-ACTIVE COMPONENTS IN CITRUS ESSENTIAL OILS

Nguyen Thi Lan-Phi

Ho Chi Minh City University of Technology
Ho Chi Minh City, Vietnam

Since the 1960s, with the developing of GC and GC-MS equipment and informatics, essential oils of numerous citrus species and hybrids have been extensively identified. Hundreds of volatile compounds have been found as both common and novel components in different citrus peel oils. It was understood, however, that only a small number of identified compounds was really important to a certain citrus flavor. These are called *odor/aroma key compounds*, *aroma-impact compounds*, *character-impact compounds*, *aroma-characteristic compounds*, *potent odorants*, or *aroma/odor-active compounds*. Identification of the compounds responsible for "character-impact odorants" in essential oils is of particular interest to the perfume and flavor industry. GC and GC-MS can detect and identify the volatile components but these instruments cannot determine the aroma-impact compounds and their odors.

Gas chromatography–olfactometry (GC-O) and its techniques were approved as valuable tools in characterizing the key odorants in food and essential oils. This chapter provides an overview of GC-O and its derivative techniques, and focuses on the odorants that are important to the pleasant and distinctive citrus aroma.

Citrus Essential Oils: Flavor and Fragrance, Edited by Masayoshi Sawamura

5.1 GAS CHROMATOGRAPHY–OLFACTOMETRY

Gas chromatography–olfactometry (GC-O) has been reviewed by many researchers worldwide (Acree, 1993; Delahunty et al., 2006; van Ruth, 2001). It has been widely applied in food (Blank and Grosch, 1991; Christensen and Reineccius, 1995; Counet et al., 2002; Curionia and Bosset, 2002; d'Acampora et al., 2008; Gurbuz et al., 2006; Guth, 1997; Le Guen et al., 2000; Marin et al., 1992; Miranda-Lopez et al., 1992; Ott et al., 1997; Poisson and Schieberle, 2008; Rychlik and Grosch, 1996; Schnermann and Schieberle, 1997; Semmelroch and Grosch, 1996) and essential oils (Buchbauer et al., 1996; Buettner et al., 2003; Eyres et al., 2007; Kamath et al., 2001; Lan-Phi et al., 2009; Sawamura et al., 2006).

GC-Olfactometry is a combination of human perception of odor and chromatographic separation of compounds. This method, proposed by Fuller (Fuller et al., 1964), has been successfully used to estimate the contribution of single-odor compounds in an odorous mixture. This method refers to the use of the human nose as a sensor detector to detect and evaluate the volatile compounds in the eluted gas stream from the GC via a specific odor port. A description of the odor is given for each retention time recorded from the GC integrator. Results of GC-O analysis can give information about the presence or absence of odor in a compound, measure the duration of odor activity, describe the quality of the odor perceived, and quantify the intensity of that odorant. GC-O is not only used to investigate the odor-active compounds and their quality but also to locate the odor-active regions in the chromatogram and generate an odor profile for the whole essential oil sample (Eyres et al., 2007).

5.1.1 Performance of GC-O

The odorants were separated by GC and transfered from the GC column through a purified, humidified, thermally moderated air stream to a human nose (Figure 5.1). The sniffer recorded the exact moment an odor were first detected at the sniff port, associated it with a descriptor, and then recorded the moment the odor was no longer detectable. The sensory data produced with the GC-O can be recorded by different methods such as simply interrupting a strip chart recorder, creating macros for spreadsheet programs, creating scripts for database programs, or purchasing specialized software to record both detection times and sensory perceptions (van Ruth, 2004).

The classical GC-O analysis is different from normal sensory analysis in that its result can be obtained by one or more sniffers. Recently, a novel, fully computerized GC-O system was used, where eight synchronized sniffers detected volatile compounds obtained from a single chromatographic separation and the software developed was applied to analyze data (Berdague et al., 2007).

5.1.2 Factors Affecting GC-O Analysis

Factors that are considered to affect the value of GC-O analysis are the sample character, GC conditions, design and operation of the sniffing port, sniffer condi-

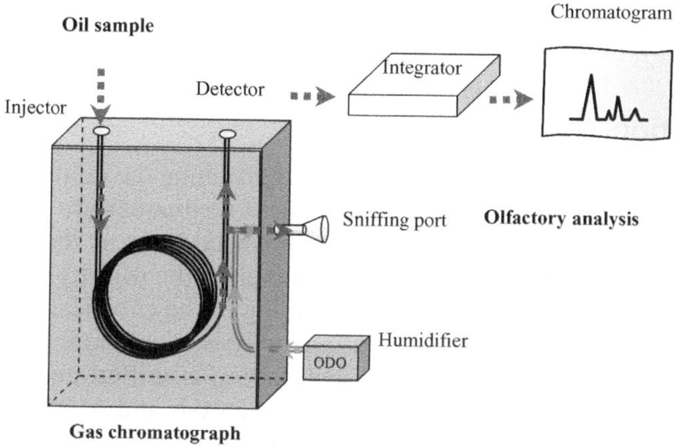

Figure 5.1. Schematic procedure of gas chromatography–olfactometry analysis.

tions, including position when sniffing, duration of accessing the effluents (usually less than 30 min), and sniffer age and sex. The sniffer should be trained to manage sniffer breath (around 20 breaths/min), and the experimental design should control the potential for human assessor bias. Considerable emphasis is placed on the requirement for multidimensional GC analysis, and on best practice and training human assessors (Delahunty et al., 2006). Though GC-O can be carried out by one sniffer, a group of assessors is considered a prerequisite for reliable gas chromatography–olfactometry analysis (van Ruth and O'Connor, 2001). GC-O is different from the other sensory analyses in that it is affected by the breathing process due to the unpredictable elution of compounds from the GC column. A tendency for higher odor detection frequency by fast-breathing subjects was observed in the three experiments. The experiments carried out by (Hanaoka et al., 2001) suggested that there was possibly an influence of individual breathing on the tendency of rating odor intensity, that a subject who was asked to breath faster rated odors more intensively.

5.1.3 GC-Olfactometry Techniques

Gas chromatography–olfactometry was, at the beginning, simply a direct-column sniffing method of qualification. Applications of the GC-O techniques were first developed for quantitation around 1976 as dilution analysis in parallel by two groups: in America, by Terry Acree et al., called *Combined Hedonic Aroma Response Measurements (CHARM)* (Acree, 1997), and in Germany, by Grosch et al., called *Aroma Extract Dilution Analysis (AEDA)* (Grosch, 1994). The other techniques were *time-intensity (OSME)* (Miranda-Lopez et al., 1992), *detection frequency* (van Ruth and Roozena, 1994), and *posterior-intensity* (van Ruth and O'Connor, 2001). The *dilution-to-threshold* method measures the potency of odor-active compounds by using a series of extract dilutions, whereas detection frequency and time-intensity methods measure odor-active compound intensity in a single concentrated extract (Delahunty et al., 2006).

5.1.4 Dilution Techniques

The incremental dilution techniques aim at determining the relative odor potency of compounds present in an odor extract. These techniques are the most simplified way of estimating the potential role of an odorant in the flavor mixture without pre-isolation or synthesis. The method gives the priority order for chemical identification and adds to the understanding of the chemical origins of olfactory differences (Grosch, 2001). In dilution analysis, a sample is diluted stepwise, usually two-, three-, or fivefold, and each dilution is sniffed until no significant odor is detected. Dilution techniques (CharmAnalysis and AEDA) are based on the principle of *odor detection threshold*. Therefore, the dilution value is the number of dilutions a sample must undergo to reach a subject's threshold. The primary difference between the two methods is that CharmAnalysis measures the dilution value over the entire elution time of odorant, whereas AEDA determines the maximum dilution value detected (Acree, 1993). In another way, in CharmAnalysis the duration of perception is taken into account together with the final dilution (or dilution value) in which a compound is detected. This dilution value is analogous to the dilution factor (FD-value) in AEDA. In fact, the dilution value at the peak maximum in a Charm chromatogram is identical to the FD factor calculated when the data are plotted on an AEDA basis (Grosch, 1994)). Dilution methods are widely used for screening of aroma-active compounds in GC-olfactory analysis to find out the odor-impact components that play important roles in a certain flavor mixture (Hwan Kim et al., 2003; van Ruth and O'Connor, 2001).

Aroma Extract Dilution Analysis (AEDA). In AEDA, the flavor dilution factor (FD-factor) is simply the last dilution at which an odor-active compound is detected. Flavor dilution factor is defined as the highest dilution at which an odorant could be recognized. The outline of procedure for AEDA is shown in Figure 5.2. This example shows the basis of N-fold stepwise dilution. FD-factor is n^i and sometimes expressed as the following:

$$\text{FD-factor} = \log N^n \quad (n\text{: number of dilution repetitions})$$

The results can also be illustrated as a bar graph and the height of each bar is the FD factor. AEDA data are also presented as the logarithm of the flavor dilution factor versus the retention index/retention time or by listing the FD-factors. The method has been used to determine the potent odor-active compounds in many different food products and citrus essential oils. Recently, a new concept of AEDA using static headspace instead of extracts has been reported. Dilution steps were made by injecting decreasing headspace volumes to evaluate the contribution of a compound to the whole composition (van Ruth, 2001). A typical gas chromatogram and aromagram from AEDA for *C. aurantifolia* Persa (lime) is shown in Figure 5.3 (Lan Phi et al., 2006). Of the 92 compounds identified in the lime oil from Vietnam, limonene was the major component (73.5%), followed by geranial (8.4%), neral (4.9%), myrcene (2.1%), and β-bisabolene (1.6%). Eight compounds—limonene, geranial, neral, myrcene, geranyl acrtate, α-pinene,

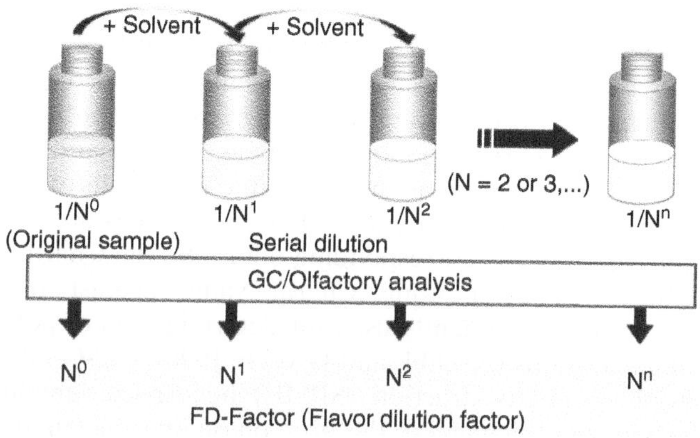

Figure 5.2. Aroma extraction dilution analysis (AEDA) technique.

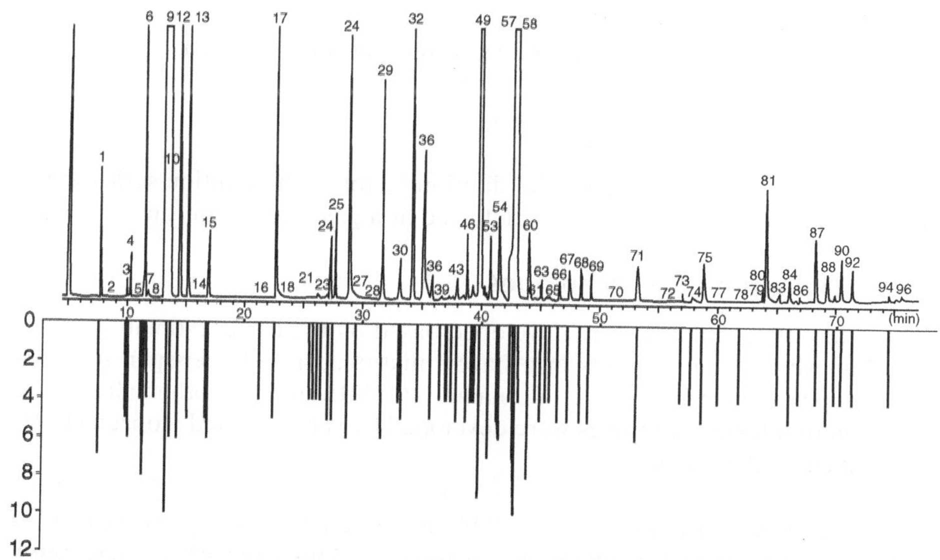

Figure 5.3. A gas chromatogram and an aromagram (FD value vs. retention time) resulting from AEDA of the volatile components of *C. aurantifolia* Persa (lime) peel oil. In the flavor dilution (FD) aromagram (cf. Figure 5.1), the logarithm with base 3 of the FD factors obtained for each odorant were plotted against their retention times (Rt).

α-terpineol, and β-bisabolene—were evaluated as the odor-active compounds, showing high FD-factors (FD-factor >3^6). From the GC-sniffing results, several compounds such as neryl acetate, β-bisabolene, germacrene D, and others were suggested as contributors to the characteristic aroma of this lime.

CharmAnalysis. Acree et al. (1984) developed a dilution analysis technique called *CharmAnalysis* based on the sniffing of decreasing serial dilutions of volatiles. In order to avoid bias introduced by knowledge of the samples, the dilutions are presented in a randomized manner (Acree et al., 1984). The assessor points out the beginning and end of each particular odor perception (duration of the smell) with a sensorial descriptor. Times of individual sniffing are combined and graphed to yield a chromatogram with peaks and quantified peak areas (Charm values), which are used to quantify potency. The results of CharmAnalysis are usually illustrated by an *aromagram*, where peak areas are proportional to the odor concentration of the corresponding odorants. The CharmAnalysis data are usually illustrated by plotting Charm value against retention time. CharmAnalysis has been frequently used for determination of potency of odor-active compounds in foods (Rychlik and Grosch, 1996). GC-O dilution analysis with the solid-phase microextraction (SPME) headspace sampling has been achieved by varying the thickness of the fiber phase and the length of exposure, and also by splitting of the injected sample into different ratios in the GC injection port. The calibration of nominal split ratios of the hardware to achieve the actual dilutions desired was successfully applied to the CharmAnalysis of brewed coffee (Deibler et al., 2004).

Charm value is calculated according to the following formula:

$$C = d^{n-1}$$

where C is the Charm value, d is the dilution factor of the dilution series, and n is the number of times an odor was detected at a given retention time.

5.1.5 Time-Intensity Techniques

Time-intensity techniques were developed based on the direct estimation of the odor intensity of the odorants in a flavor mixture. These finger-span methods were proposed by McDaniel et al., namely OSME, and the other alternative detection frequency techniques were developed by van Ruth and Roozen (1994) and Pollien et al. (1999).

OSME. OSME (McDaniel et al., 1990) is a time-intensity approach to GC-O that uses a cross-modal matching device to continuously record the perception of odorant intensity perceived at the sniffing port. The panelist moves the cursor of a variable resistor as a function of the intensity of perception, thus providing the odor peak. The verbal description of the odor peaks are also recorded at the same time. Only a few applications have been published. A panel-training procedure is necessary before using the time-intensity method. The odor-active volatile composition of the extracts of blue cheese has been carried out by eight trained assessors (Hulin-Bertaud et al., 2001). To improve the reliability of aromagrams, two research groups proposed to calculate peak detection frequencies from the odors perceived by assessors.

Detection Frequency Technique. Detection frequency is a GC-O technique used to estimate the odor intensity based on recording detected odors from a number of sniffers. The detection frequency method calculates the peak detection frequencies from the odors perceived to improve the reliability of aromagrams that show the repeatable and reproducible abilities. To compare detection frequencies, both peak height and peak area are used. When the peak height is used, it is called *nasal impact frequency (NIF)* and *surface of nasal impact frequency (SNIF)* regarding the use of peak area.

A panel of eight assessors evaluate six volatile flavor compounds at various concentration levels using the detection frequency method and the perceived intensity method (van Ruth, 2004). The detection frequency method was more accurate in terms of repeatability and the range of sensitivity was similar for both methods (van Ruth, 2004).

The detection frequency method was evaluated for attribution of odor potency to eight volatile compounds at seven concentration levels. Detection frequency data were also highly correlated with sensory odor intensities (van Ruth and O'Connor, 2001). An aroma compound was quantitated for the first time by GC-olfactometry (GC-O) on the basis of the detection frequency of odorants by a panel of 8–12 sniffers. The results concluded that GC-O can compete with the most sensitive and selective techniques for determination of extremely intense odorants, because little sample preparation is required and there is no need for the synthesis of labeled compounds (Pollien et al., 1999).

Posterior-Intensity Technique. Two gas chromatography–olfactometry methods were evaluated in terms of repeatability, range of sensitivity, and discriminating properties (van Ruth, 2004). The intensity method was more accurate with regard to discrimination between concentration levels (van Ruth, 2004).

The posterior-intensity method was evaluated for attribution of odor potency to eight volatile compounds at seven concentration levels in addition to the sensory odor intensity of the compounds at eight concentration levels. It was suggested that posterior intensities correlated reasonably well with sensory odor intensities (van Ruth and O'Connor, 2001).

5.1.6 Omission Test

The omission test (Grosch, 2001), based on the reconstruction of an aroma model, is often carried out according to the data resulting from GC-sniffing and its techniques. The model sample of a certain citrus flavor is made up of the authentic chemicals and dilution solvent. The solvents used in the experiments studied were water (Song et al., 2000a), methanol, ethanol, and so on. The reconstruction of the aroma-impact compounds in the concentrations naturally occurring in the peel oil elicits the overall aroma of the peel oil itself and proves the identification results.

The sensory panelists are employed to evaluate the aroma model of a mixture of odorants judged from GC-O data. The closest match of a fresh citrus aroma and its aroma model was assigned according to a score of 0–9 points. The least close gets 0 points, and the highest score is 9 for the best match to fresh fruit aroma.

Limonene and linalool were sometimes considered as dilution solvents due to their abundance in citrus essential oils and limonene was used as a background in the aroma model of some citrus essential oils (Song et al., 2000a).

5.2 FLAVOR AND ODOR/AROMA IMPACT COMPOUNDS IN CITRUS ESSENTIAL OILS

Citrus oils are the oils extracted directly (by hand or mechanically) by pressing the fruit peel or by concentrating/centrifuging the fruit juice. The odor-impact components can be found in all chemical classes of citrus essential oils. The key compounds of citrus oils, including oils such as orange, mandarin/tangerine, grapefruit/pummelo, lime, lemon, yuzu, and hybrids, will be presented.

5.2.1 Sweet Orange (*C. sinensis* L. Osbeck)

The main orange varieties have been investigated, including Hamlin, Valencia, Pera, Navelina, Moro, Tarocco, and Washington Navel, both as juices and essential oils, at different mature stages. More than 300 volatile compounds have been detected by GC and GC-MS; however, only a small number of compounds really contributed to orange aroma characterized by GC-O. Although the terpene hydrocarbons make up about 96% of the orange oil composition, the aroma-active components of orange have been found to be major in oxygenated groups, of which aldehydes and esters are the primary volatile components contributing to fresh orange flavor. The odor-active aldehydes include saturated and unsaturated aliphatic aldehydes, terpene aldehydes, and phenolic aldehydes. They produced the most aroma activity although present in small amounts. Aldehydes such as citronellal, neral, geranial, and β-sinensal contributed to the citrusy, floral, fatty, and green aroma notes. The terpenic and the saturated aliphatic aldehydes usually impart fruity (citrus-like) and green notes. Neral and geranial, the two isomeric monoterpene aldehydes, are typical constituents of orange peel oil and are believed to be important contributors to orange flavor (Ahmed et al., 1978a). Other minor terpene aldehydes of peel oil include sinensal and citronellal. Sinensal is a sesquiterpene aldehyde that occurs in orange peel oil in two isomeric forms as a 2:1 ratio of α-sinensal to β-sinensal and both of them have very similar aromas (Shaw, 1991). The three homologous straight-chain aldehydes, octanal, nonanal, and decanal, have been implicated as important contributors to orange flavor (Shaw, 1991). Octanal and decanal are generally considered important contributors to orange flavor. Their contents are the standard of identity for orange peel oil. However, decanal at the level of 0.72 ppm made a negative contribution to orange juice flavor (Ahmed et al., 1978a). Researchers indicated that acetaldehyde, hexanal, octanal, decanal, dodecanal, (*R*)-limonene (Ahmed et al., 1978a), and linalool were important contributors to orange flavor (Shaw, 1991) based on the ratio of concentration to odor threshold (odor unit). Sensory evaluation of model orange juices revealed the highest flavor scores for a mixture of acetaldehyde, citral, ethyl butanoate, d-limonene, and octanal that can provide an acceptable orange flavor (Ahmed et al., 1978b). (*Z*)-Hex-3-enal is an important contributor to the green, grassy top-note of freshly prepared orange juices (Hinterholzer and Schieberle, 1998).

The three esters, ethyl acetate, methyl butyrate, and ethyl butyrate, are known to contribute to the top-note of citrus flavor. Ethyl butanoate, ethyl propionate, and ethyl 2-methylbutanoate were also important to orange flavor (Shaw, 1991). Two unsaturated alcohols, *cis*-3-hexenol and *trans*-2-hexenol, are important contributors to the green, leafy top-note in fresh orange and other fruit flavors. Ahmed et al. (1978a) found limonene to be an important contributor to orange flavor when added at a level of 190 ppm (0.019%) to processed juice.

GC-Olfactometry and AEDA analysis results of the volatiles extracted from the fresh juice of Valencia late oranges revealed the six most odor-active compounds with fruity (ethyl 2-methylpropionate, ethyl butanoate and (*S*)-ethyl 2-methylbutanoate), green and leaf-like (*Z*)-hex-3-enal), sweet and spicy (3a, 4, 5, 7a-tetrahydro-3,6-dimethyl-2(3*H*)-benzofuranone), and metallic (4,5-epoxy-(*E*)-dec-2-enal) odor notes. Among 18 odor-active compounds identified, 3a,4,5,7a-tetrahydro-3,6-dimethyl-2(3*H*)-benzofuranone, oct-1-en-3-one, methional, 4,5-epoxy-(*E*)-dec-2-enal, and 4-hydroxy-2,5-dimethyl-3(2*H*)-furanone are considerable contributors to the orange flavor with high FD factors (Hinterholzer and Schieberle, 1998).

Using stable isotope dilution assays, it was shown that the fruity-smelling esters, ethyl 2-methylpropanoate, ethyl butanoate, (*S*)-ethyl 2-methylbutanoate, and wine lactone, the grassy-smelling (*Z*)-hex-3-enal, and the citrus-like decanal were the most potent odorants due to their high OAVs in both Valencia late and Navel hand-squeezed orange juices (Buettner and Schieberle, 2001).

In fresh orange juice, seven odor-active esters have been reported, including ethyl esters. Ethyl butanoate contributes the most to orange juice and is the single most important ester. Ethyl butanoate has been found in late Hamlin, late pineapple, mid- and late-Valencia, Pera, Navelina, Moro, Tarocco, and Washington Navel juices (Arena et al., 2006; Buettner and Schieberle, 2001; Rega et al., 2003). Ethyl butanoate concentration has been used as one of the key measures of desirable flavor in orange products (Perez-Cacho and Rouseff, 2008).

Identification of aroma-active compounds in orange essence oil using gas chromatography–olfactometry and time-intensity methods revealed octanal, decanal, citronellal, and β-sinensal, and linalool as the key aroma-impact compounds. A cyclic ester, wine lactone, was the key aroma-impact compound of orange essence oil, imparting a strong herbal and spicy note at trace amounts (Högnadóttir and Rouseff, 2003).

CharmAnalysis of Valencia and Pera sweet orange oils exposed the six most odor-active compounds, octanal, nonanal, decanal, unknown licorice compound, linalool, and β-sinensal, acounting for 90% of the total Charm. β-Sinensal, the sesquiterpene aldehyde, with a Charm value of 14% makes a significant contribution to the flavor of orange oil. The straight-chain aldehydes (C_8–C_{14}), β-sinensal, and linalool, were judged to be key to the future flavor formulations and improved quality-control monitoring of the oil (Gaffney et al., 1996). An unknown compound of licorice odor, which co-eluted with limonene, was determined to be the most odor-active compound in the Pera oil (Gaffney et al., 1996). The primary odor-active volatiles of Florida Valencia and Brazilian Pera orange oils reported by Gaffney et al. (1996) by % Charm values are shown in Table 5.1.

Application of the cross-matching test and correspondence analysis based on a nonverbal method and reflex human decision-making demonstrated linalool (refreshing floral-woody) and nonanal (fatty-floral) as the potent character-impact compounds of orange oil. Based on the limited odor unit values, linalool, limonene (fresh, light, and sweet citrusy), octanal (harsh-fatty), nonanal (powerful and diffusive fatty-floral, waxy), decanal (orange-like aroma), dodecanal (sweet, waxy-herbaceous and floral), and myrcene (sweet, balsamic-resinous), were also selected as character-impact compounds of Valencia orange oil (Chida et al., 2006).

GC-Olfactometry and four-scale rating intensity were used to determine the aroma-active compounds of fruit juice and peel oil of Jinchen sweet orange. There are 22 components that appear to be the major contributors to the peel oil aroma. Linalool, α-pinene, and decanal presented the highest aroma intensity in this orange peel oil (Qiao et al., 2008).

TABLE 5.1. Charm values of Valencia and Pera orange oils adapted from Gaffney et al. (1996)

Compound	Attribute	Valencia Orange Oil (%)	Pera Orange Oil (%)
Octanal	citrus/aldehydic	45.0	35.0
Linalool	fruity	39.7	12.8
Nonanal	fattyfloral	4.2	4.2
Decanal	sweet/citrus/orange	5.5	4.0
Undecanal	citrus/peely/orange	6.4	3.5
β-Sinensal	fishy/herbal	14.0	8.2

Valencene, the major sesquiterpene in orange peel oil, and its concentration has been traditionally used as an indicator of the commercial orange oil value. However, using multidimensional GC analysis coupled with mass spectrometry and olfactometry, Elston et al. (2005) reported that valencene possessed no aroma activity at the levels present in orange oils (54–68 μg/g). The level of valencene in orange oils may positively correlate with the aroma quality of the oil due to maturity effects (Elston et al., 2005).

5.2.2 Sour Orange (*C. aurantium* L.)

The characteristic flavor components of daidai (*Citrus aurantium* L. var. *cyathifera* Y. Tanaka), a sour Japanese citrus, were examined by GC-O and AEDA. Geranial, octyl acetate, geraniol, octanal, cedrol, *cis*-limonene oxide, *trans*-2-decenal, linalyl acetate, and β-elemol were identified as characteristic flavor components of daidai. Linalyl acetate and β-elemol had the highest flavor dilution factors. Geraniol, octanal, linalyl acetate, and *cis*-limonene oxide were reported as the active components of the daidai peel oil as proven by GC-sniffing and the omission test (Song et al., 2000a).

5.2.3 Grapefruit (*C. paradisi*)

Grapefruit Juice. It was first reported that the characteristic flavor of grapefruit juice is nootkatone and its derivatives (Demole and Enggist, 1983) and 1-*p*-menthen-8-thiol (Demole et al., 1982). By calculation of the odor activity values of the odorants (ratio of their concentrations in juice to their odor thresholds in water), it was shown that the fruity esters, ethyl 2-methylpropanoate, ethyl butanoate, and (*S*)-ethyl 2-methyl-butanoate, and the fruity and sweet wine lactone were among the most potent odorants of fresh grapefruit juice, as well as the grassy-smelling (*Z*)-hex-3-enal, and *trans*-4,5-epoxy-(*E*)-dec-2-enal with metallic odor. The typical sulfurous, grapefruit-like odor quality was mainly due to the catty, blackcurrant-like 4-mercapto-4-methylpentan-2-one and the grapefruit-like-smelling 1-*p*-menthene-8-thiol (Buettner and Schieberle, 2001). These findings were confirmed by reconstitution experiments to simulate the aroma of fresh grapefruit juice.

The gas chromatographic separation of the 1-*p*-menthene-8-thiol enantiomers has been achieved using (2,3-*di*-*O*-methyl-6-*O*-TBDMS)-β-cyclodextrin as the chiral stationary phase in enantioselective gas chromatography. The sensory evaluation of the pure enantiomers has been realized by enantioselective gas chromatography–olfactometry. (*R*)-1-*p*-Menthene-8-thiol was found to be of formative influence on the natural odor of grapefruit, whereas the odor of the (*S*)-enantiomer was weak and nonspecific (Lehmann et al., 1995).

An ion-trap mass spectrometer chemical sensor has been utilized to differentiate between grapefruit juices that differ only in the concentration of a single component. Grapefruit juice was fortified with 40 to 2000 ppm vanillin, a low-level, naturally occurring compound in citrus juices. Principal component analysis and discriminative analysis of mass spectral data (*m/z* 50–200) provided clear separation of the grapefruit juice samples. Vanillin was observed in the juice headspace at the 40 ppm level, with identification possible at the 100 ppm level using either MS or MS/MS (Goodner and Rouseff, 2001).

By application of AEDA on an extract prepared from fresh grapefruit juice, 37 odor-active compounds were detected in the flavor dilution (FD) factor range of 256 and subsequently identified. Among them, the highest odor activities (FD-factors) were determined for ethyl butanoate, *p*-1-menthene-8-thiol, (*Z*)-3-hexenal, 4,5-epoxy-(*E*)-2-decenal, 4-mercapto-4-methylpentane-2-one, 1-heptene-3-one, and wine lactone (Buettner and Schieberle, 1999). The data confirmed results of the literature on the significant contribution of 1-*p*-menthene-8-thiol in grapefruit aroma.

Peel Oil. Thirty-eight aroma-active compounds were detected in commercial cold-pressed grapefruit oil using a time-intensity GC-olfactometry procedure. Compounds with the greatest aroma intensities include: 1,8-cineole, octanal, dodecanal, *trans*-4,5-epoxy-(*E*)-2-decenal, β-sinensal, and nootkatone. The aroma activities of sulfur compounds such as 4-mercapto-4-methyl-2-pentanol and methional were surprisingly low. Over 200 volatiles have been reported in grapefruit oil, but only 38 have significant aroma activity and 22 of these can be considered major aroma-impact compounds (Lin and Rouseff, 2001). The terpene thiol, 1-*p*-menthene-8-thiol, has been shown to impart strong grapefruit-like characteristics (Arthur and Reeve, 2004). Nootkatone and 1-*p*-menthen-8-thiol would be the characteristic compounds of grapefruit aroma.

5.2.4 Mandarin (*C. reticulata*)

Satsuma Mandarin. The mandarin is assumed to have originated in Southeast Asia (Kale and Adsule, 1995). Satsuma mandarin (*Citrus unshiu* Marcov.) was originally developed in Japan. Three different Korean Satsuma mandarin cultivars, Miyamoto, Aoshima, and Miyagawa-wase, exhibited a similar aroma character with herbaceous, sweet, green, and sour notes characterized by GC-O (Choi, 2004). Among 51 volatiles characterized, linalool (citrus-like), *trans*-linalool furanoxide (sweet) and *cis*-linalool pyranoxide (sweet), and *l*-carvone (floral and herbaceous) contributed to the pleasant aroma of Miyamoto and Miyagawa-wase mandarins, respectively (Choi, 2004). Thymol and methyl N-methyl anthranilate have been reported as major aroma compounds in mandarin oil (Wilson and Shaw, 1981) but have not been fully proven.

Clementine. Clementine (*Citrus reticulata* Blanco cv. *Clementine*) oil has large amounts of decanal, a-sinensal and linalool that are major aroma impact compounds. They contributed orangy, lavender-like and fishy, metallic odor notes, respectively, to the flavor of Spanish clementine oil (Chisholm et al., 2003a). Almost 50 odorants were identified in Spanish clementine oil by using GC-O, and most of them were composed of unsaturated aldehydes with high odor spectrum values (OSV). α- and β-Sinensal, *trans*-4,5-epoxy-(*E*)-2-decanal, (*E*,*Z*)-2,6-

dodecadienal, and linalool dominated clementine oil aroma (Chisholm et al., 2003a). Aldehydes contributed most to clementine aroma. Limonene (82–87.5%) with high odor threshold (~0.2mg/l) and minty, citrusy notes also contributed to the overall aroma of Spanish clementine oil.

Instrumental and sensory analysis (AEDA) revealed linalool, (*E,E*)-deca-2,4-dienal, wine lactone, a-pinene, myrcene and octanal as the most important components in Spanish clementine oil investigated by Buettner et al., 2003. The clementine aroma was dominated by fatty, metallic and green coriander-like resulted from (*E*)-alk-2-enals. Among them, (*E*)-dodec-2-enal and (*E*)-tridec-2-enal were suggested to contribute to the aroma of clementine peel oil.

Pontianak. The peel of Pontianak orange (*Citrus nobilis* var. Lour. *microcarpa* Hassk.) possesses a characteristic sulphurous and resinous aroma (Fischer et al., 2008) and the green, fatty, fresh, peely, floral, and tarry attributes (Dharmawan et al., 2009). Pontianak oil extracted by a solvent extraction/vacuum distillation process and investigated by GC-O and AEDA revealed 26 out of 32 odor-active compounds detected in the FD-factor range of 4–2048. (*R*)/(*S*)-Linalool, myrcene, (*R*)-limonene, and 1,8-cineole were characterized as the most potent odorants, followed by octanal, (*E,E*)-2,4-decadienal, nerol, (*E*)-2-dodecenal, geraniol, and (*E,E*)-2,4-nonadienal due to their high FD-factors (Fischer et al., 2008). 1-Phenylethanethiol, occurring as a mixture of the (*R*) (76%) and the (*S*)-enantiomer (24%), exhibited an intense sulphurous, resinous smell at the very low odor threshold of 0.005 ng/L in air, and was found to be responsible for the odor impression detected in the extract. Application of static headspace aroma dilution analysis (SHA) revealed the green, grassy notes of hexanal and (*Z*)-3-hexenal as further important odorants in the headspace of Pontianak peel oil (Fischer et al., 2008). Furthermore, omission experiments showed that the unique odor quality of the peel is significantly influenced by the resinous, sulphurous odor notes of 1-phenylethanethiol, although its concentration was only 38 ng/g peel (Fischer and Schieberle, 2009).

Another study of Pontianak orange peel oil carried out by using GC-O, AEDA, and omission tests confirmed (*Z*)-5-dodecenal and 1-phenylethyl mercaptan as key-aroma compounds of Pontianak orange oil (Dharmawan et al., 2009). Forty-one compounds were found to be aroma active, which were mainly dominated by saturated and unsaturated aldehydes. The FD-factor was within the range in agreement with Fischer et al. (2008), and compounds having the highest FD-factor were α-pinene, β-pinene, linalool, and 2-methoxy-3-(2-methylpropyl) pyrazine. On the basis of GC-O results, OAV, and relative flavor activity (RFA), an aroma model was reported as closest to Pontianak original oil aroma (Dharmawan et al., 2009).

5.2.5 Lime (*C. aurantifolia*)

Chisholm et al. (2003b) evaluated the most intense aroma volatiles of extracted and distilled oils from the peels of key lime (*Citrus aurantifolia* Swingle) by using GC-O (Charm analysis) and gas chromatography–mass spectrometry (GC-MS).

More than 50 and 60 odor-active volatiles were detected in the extracted oil, respectively. The characteristic lime-like odor was described as fragrant, fresh and citrusy. Aldehydes, especially geranial, neral, and linalool were found to dominate the lime oil aroma, which contributed for the fresh, floral, citrus-like characters. The distilled oil contained alcohols, ethers and sesquiterpenes, which imparted woody, musty, spicy, and balsamic notes to its aroma. Germacrene B and caryophylene oxide were identified as the odor active compounds in key lime oil. They contributed woody/spicy and the sawdust-like odor notes, respectively, to the extracted oil (Chisholm et al., 2003b). The cold-pressed lime oil of *C. aurantifolia* Persa was subjected to GC-O (AEDA) analysis (Lan Phi et al., 2006a). Limonene, geranial, neral, myrcene, geranyl acetate, a-pinene, a-terpineol and b-bisabolene were the most odor-active compounds in this lime oil. Germacrene B with high FD factor (3^5) was evaluated as having lime-like odor from GC-sniffing. Neryl acetate, b-bisabolene, *l*-carvone, geranyl acetate, a- and b-citronellol, cumin aldehyde, perilladehyde, nerol, tridecanal, geraniol and dodecyl acetate also contributed to the characteristic aroma of lime. It was suggested that, b-bisabolene and geranyl acetate were the key aroma compounds of *C. aurantifolia* Persa cold-pressed oil.

5.2.6 Lemon (*Citrus limon*)

Schieberle and Grosch (1988) reported that important volatile flavor compounds of fresh lemon oil were myrcene, limonene, g-terpinene, octanal, nonanal, linalool, citronellal, (E)-2-nonenal, decanal, neral and geranial. On the basis of their high FD factor and identification data, neral and geranial together with linalool were the most potent aroma compounds of fresh Italian lemon oil. In contrast, carvone, *p*-methylacetophenone, *p*-cresol, and *p*-cymene were indicators for the deterioration of lemon oil flavor, showing high FD factors after storage. (Schieberle and Grosch, 1989). The application of the cross-matching by sensory test and correspondence analysis of lemon oil purchased from the USA found that citrals (neral and geranial) are the potent character-impact compounds on the basis of their limited odor unit values, with a high matching frequency of 0.89 (Chida et al., 2006). Neral and geranial are two isomeric monoterpene aldehydes, generally in the ratio of 2:3, responsible for the unique character of lemon oil.

5.2.7 Ichang-Papeda (*C. ichangensis*)

Yuzu. Yuzu (*Citrus junos* Sieb. ex Tanaka) is classified as a native mutant belonging to the species Papeda according to the taxonomy by Swingle. To clarify the odor-active compounds that differentiate yuzu from other citrus fruits, sensory evaluations were conducted on yuzu peel oil by using GC-O analysis. Song et al. (2000b) reported that the terpenes were the major components of yuzu peel oil, but they contributed little to the characteristic flavor of yuzu. Methyltrisulfide, borneol, *n*-octanol, *trans*-undec-2-enal, (+)-*p*-mentha-1-en-9-ol, eugenol, and carvacrol were found to be strongly involved in the characteristic flavor of yuzu, together with 6-methyl-5-hepten-2-ol and methyltrisulfide having the highest FD-factor.

During GC-O analysis of yuzu peel oil, the oxygenated part emerged to be the characteristic aroma group of fresh yuzu fruit. Miyazawa et al. (2009) have examined the oxygenated part of yuzu peel oil by aroma extract dilution analysis (AEDA) and reported seven odorants as odor-active volatiles in the highest flavor dilution (FD) factors of 128 and 32: oct-1-en-3-one, (*E*)-non-4-enal, (*E*)-dec-4-enal, 4-methyl-4-mercaptopentan-2-one, (*E*)-non-6-enal, (6*Z*,8*E*)-undeca-6,8,10-trien-3-one (Yuzunone), and (6*Z*,8*E*)-undeca-6,8,10-trien-4-ol (Yuzuol). Among the most odor-active volatiles in yuzu, (*E*)-non-6-enal and Yuzunone were identified for the first time solely in yuzu peel oil and not in the peel of other citrus species, and Yuzuol was identified for the first time in nature. Sensory evaluation of yuzu aroma reconstitutions revealed that the newly identified compound, Yuzunone, contributes greatly to the distinct yuzu aroma (Miyazawa et al., 2009). Applying GC-O and AEDA on the hexane extract concentrate of yuzu oil revealed *trans*-4,5-epoxy-(*E*,*Z*)-2,7-decadienal as one of 28 potent aroma compounds characterized (Miyazato et al., 2008).

From the aspect of a different viewpoint, Lan Phi and Sawamura (2008) demonstrated the yuzu characteristic flavor as a verbal profile through GC-sniffing. Odor notes of 67 recognized compounds were described and totaled. The frequency of sensory note occurrence is suggested to present a food aroma profile. The total frequency of each descriptive note is considered to constitute a common profile for the characteristic aroma of yuzu. The frequent descriptive notes as judged were as follows: grassy (which occurred 230 times), herbal (219 times), floral (212 times), sweet (175 times), citrusy (92 times), and fatty (75 times). These terms represent a sense of yuzu aroma, and may play roles in the quality of yuzu aroma.

Sudachi. Application of the cross-matching test and correspondence analysis in the characterization of sudachi (*C. sudachi*) aroma revealed α- and β-pinene, α-sinensal, and myrcene as important components of this citrus oil (Chida et al., 2006).

5.2.8 *Citrus* Hybrids

Hallabong. An artificial hybrid, "Shiranui" (*C. unshiu* Marcov. × *C. sinensis* Osbeck × *C. reticulata* Blanco), was first developed in Nagasaki, Japan. The common Japanese name is *Dekopon*. Recently, it has become popular in Korea, called *Hallabong*. Hallabong oil has a characteristic sweet flavor much like sweet orange and ponkan. Instrumental and sensory analysis results from GC-sniffing and AEDA of the cold-pressed oil and its oxygenated fraction revealed citronellal (citrus peel-like), *cis*-β-farnesene (green, citrus-like), and citronellyl acetate (citrus-like, oily) as the character-impact odorants of Hallabong peel oil. Among them, citronellal gave the strongest character of Hallabong aroma (Choi, 2003).

Hyuganatsu. Choi et al. (2001) have investigated the volatile components of Hyuganatsu (*Citrus tamurana* Hort. ex Tanaka) cold-pressed peel oil by chemical and sensory analyses. Monoterpene hydrocarbons were predominant in Hyuganatsu peel oil, however, the characteristic flavor was present in the oxygenated fraction. Ten odor compounds having hyuganatsu-like aroma were limonene, linalool, octanol, neral, neryl acetate, tridecanal, *trans*-carveol, *cis*-nerolidol, *trans,trans*-farnesyl acetate, and *trans,trans*-farnesol. Linalool and octanol were the most odor-active or key compounds of Hyuganatsu aroma (Choi et al., 2001).

Sanbokan. Sanbokan (*Citrus sulcata* Hort. ex Takahashi) is a Japanese citrus. Results from AEDA of the oxygenated fraction revealed that linalool (4^8), octanal (4^7), 4,5-epoxy-(2*E*)-decenal (4^7), (4*Z*)-decenal (4^6), and methyl epijasmonate (4^6) had high FD-factors in the peel oil extract (Tomiyama et al., 2008).

5.2.9 Kumquat

The aroma profile of kumquat (*Fortunella japonica* Swingle) cold-pressed peel oil was characterized by fruity, sweet and citrusy top notes, middle green and woody notes, and an oily undertone (Choi, 2005). Flavor dilution (FD) factors and relative flavor activities (RFA) of volatile constituents were evaluated by aroma extract dilution analysis with GC-O. Choi (2005) reported that a-pinene, sabinene, myrcene, limonene, b-elemene and terpinen-4-ol showed the highest FD values of 3^7. Camphene, terpinen-4-ol, citronellyl formate, and citronellyl acetate are regarded as important aroma compounds of kumquat oil. Among them, citronellyl acetate was the characteristic odor component of kumquat cold-pressed peel oil. (Choi, 2005).

5.2.10 Aroma Models of Some Citrus Essential Oils

Daidai. The full aroma model of daidai (*Citrus aurantium* L. var. *cyathifera* Y. Tanaka) is composed of nine odorants (geranial, octyl acetate, geraniol, octanal, cedrol, *trans*-2-decenal, *cis*-limonene oxide, linalyl acetate, and β-elemol) with a score of 6.4, as reported by Song et al. (2000a).

Hyuganatsu. Linalool and octanol were considered the key aroma compounds of hyuganatsu oil. The diluted solutions of linalool and octanol of 2 ppm gave a fresh-and-fruity aroma note similar to Hyuganatsu flavor (Choi et al., 2001).

Kabosu. *C. sphaerocarpa* Tanaka (kabosu) is one of the most popular sour citrus fruits in Japan. Minh Tu et al. (2002) reported the aqueous solutions of (R)-(+)-citronellal of 0.25% (by smelling trip) or of 0.016% (by headspace-sniff in a 30-ml vial), gave an odor similar to that of kabosu aroma.

Bergamot. *C. bergamia* Risso (bergamot) is said to be a variety of sour/bitter orange. This fruit is mainly cultivated in Italy and possesses a fresh and attractive aroma. An aroma model of bergamot was introduced by Sawamura et al. (2006). Of a 2-ml aroma model mixture, the compositions (mg) of 10 authentic compounds are as follow: limonene (2.00), linalyl acetate (1.50), linalool (0.50), g-terpinene (0.35), b-pinene (0.30), citral (0.30), geraniol (0.10), limonene oxide (0.03), (Z)-b-ocimene (0.01) and decanal (0.01). The scoring test result of this aroma model to the original bergamot oil was 7.1 out of the 9-score scale.

5.3 FUNCTIONAL GROUPS RELATED TO CITRUS FLAVOR ACTIVITY

5.3.1 Aliphatic Hydrocarbons

Among six aliphatic hydrocarbons characterized from 10 citrus varieties, tetradecane showed the highest aroma activity. This component is the characteristic component of Ki-mikan (*Citrus flaviculpus* Hort. ex Tanaka) cold-pressed oil (Choi et al., 2002).

5.3.2 Monoterpenes

AEDA revealed three odorants with higher FD factors in 10 samples: limonene, myrcene, and α-pinene. Other compounds with high FD-factor values were β-pinene, camphene, and terpinolene. Myrcene showed the highest FD-factor (3^{10}) in kiyookadaidai (*Citrus sp.*) oil. The concentration of this component in kiyookadaidai was also found to be rather high (62.4%) compared to that of limonene (16.8%). Myrcene was noted as a kiyookadaidai-like and mochiyu-like aroma in kiyookadaidai (Tu et al., 2003a) and mochiyu (*Citrus inflata* Hort. ex Tanaka) (Tu et al., 2003b) peel oils, respectively. The concentration of limonene is normally predominant in citrus essential oils. Its FD-factor was also high in most citrus oils. However, limonene was not indicated as an impact component in any of these samples. Limonene in Hyuganatsu oil, though, not only had Hyuganatsu-like odor but also had a high FD-factor value of 3^7. It is obvious that the higher concentration often shows higher FD factors and they do not always contribute to the overall aroma of a certain flavor mixture. Among monoterpene compounds, two isomeric compounds, (*Z*)- and (*E*)-ocimene, were characterized as the aroma-characteristic components of kiyookadaidai and mochiyu oils, accordingly.

5.3.3 Sesquiterpenes

Thirty compounds have been identified and quantified. Only 18 compounds among them were characterized as odor-active components as revealed from GC-O and AEDA results. Sesquiterpenes were present at low concentration in citrus oils. Tu et al. (2003b) reported only 0.5% of sesquiterpenes among 98.1% hydrocarbons found in mochiyu oil. In natsudaidai oil, the concentration of sesquiterpenes was 0.58% while that of monoterpenes was 91.19% of the total volatile fraction. Some sesquiterpenes, however, were reported as important components in citrus oils. α-Bergamotene is, for example, the characteristic component of kiyookadaidai. δ-Elemene and β-elemene are two major sesquiterpenes among the essential oils studied. They were not only shown as aroma-active components (FD > 3^4) but also as the odor-characteristic components of mochiyu, natsudaidai, and Japanese yuzu aroma. Among other sesquiterpenes, β-caryophyllene, β-elemene, *trans*-β-farnesene, and germacrene D were predominant. They had rather high FD factors. However, these studies suggested that they did not contribute to the organoleptic profiles of aroma for these oils. In another case, α-humulene occurred at very low concentration in Hyuganatsu (0.02%), yuzu (0.02%) and Tosa-buntan (0.01%), and was not detected in kabosu (Tu et al., 2002) oil by GC-MS. This compound, however, showed very high FD factors, that is, 2^{12} in yuzu and 3^7 in the other three samples from the sniffing test. Therefore, it is suggested that α-humulene is an aroma contributor of citrus flavor. The results also list a trace amount of components that were not detected by conventional methods such as GC and GC-MS, but were identified and characterized by GC-O and its combining technique. GC-O also has been a useful tool for identifying a trace amount of unknown aroma compounds on the basis of their odor characters.

5.3.4 Aldehydes

The minor group to consider in citrus oils is aldehydes. These have been identified as important components contributing to the citrus aroma. Although present at very low concentration, 18 aldehydes were identified as the aroma-active components. Aliphatic aldehydes seem to be predominant in these identified compounds. Among a series of saturated aliphatic aldehydes, octanal and tridecanal are the most important. Octanal shows the characteristic odor of daidai and yuzu oils. This compound was also suggested as an aroma-impact component of daidai aroma (Song et al., 2000a). Tridecanal was the aroma-characteristic compound of Hyuganatsu oil, presenting Hyuganatsu-like aroma. Three unsaturated aliphatic aldehydes, (*E*)-2-decenal, (*E*)-2-undecenal, and 2-dodecenal, play a vital role in some citrus oils. Buettner et al. (2003) reported that the long-chain (*E*)-alk-2-enals, exhibiting the characteristic odor quality of green coriander, contributed to the aroma of clementine oil. (*E*)-2-Decenal and (*E*)-2-undecenal were identified as characteristic flavor components of daidai and yuzu cold-pressed oils, respectively. As mentioned before, 2-dodecenal was the key aroma compound of Tosa-buntan (*Citrus grandis* Osbeck froma *Tosa-buntan*) essential oil (Sawamura et al., 2001). The authors proved this result by showing the presence of a pleasant and refreshing aroma similar to Tosa-buntan flavor even at a low concentration (2 ppm) of 2-dodecenal.

5.3.5 Alcohols

Forty-one alcohols have been identified and characterized by using GC-O and AEDA. The most common alcohols were linalool, octanol, α-terpineol, nerol, and geraniol. Linalool is the odor-active compound, with higher flavor dilution factors ranging from 3^6 to 3^8 in most citrus oils, and of 2^{15} in yuzu oil. This alcohol is a main odor-characteristic compound of Hyuganatsu and Ki-mikan oil. Octanol was found to be strongly involved in the characteristic flavor of yuzu and also the key or impact compound of Hyuganatsu and natsudaidai cold-pressed oils. This compound presented Hyuganatsu-like and natsudaidai-like notes with rather high flavor dilution values of 3^8 and 3^5, accordingly. α-Terpineol together with linalool summed up the concentration of alcohols found in citrus oils. In Vietnamese lime oil, α-terpineol had rather high odor intensity (FD-factor of 3^7). This component was characterized as an impact compound of ki-mikan peel oil. The alcohol group, in particular, plays a significant role in yuzu cold-pressed oil aroma. Eighteen compounds have been aroma-active components in yuzu oil, showing flavor dilution factors from 2^{12} to 2^{18}. Nine compounds of them showed a yuzu-like odor note. 6-Methyl-5-hepten-2-ol at a trace amount did show yuzu-like odor by sensory analysis as well as the highest FD factor (2^{18}). This compound would be a strong contributor of the yuzu aroma model. Methyltrisulfide is considered to be a significantly important component in yuzu oil as well. Song et al. (2000a) reported that 1 ppb of methyltrisufide showed a yuzu-like aroma. Two monoterpene alcohols, nerol and geraniol, represented the characteristic aroma of *C. aurantifolia* Persa (lime) oil (Lan Phi et al., 2006). Nerol and geraniol also had the characteristic odor of mochiyu and daidai oils, respectively. Geraniol is particularly the aroma-active component of daidai oil.

5.3.6 Esters

Minor group components such as esters have contributed to the specification of citrus oil aroma. Octyl acetate, linalyl acetate, neryl, and geranyl acetate are four major esters found in these oil samples. Octyl acetate and linalyl acetate were associated with the aroma character note of kabosu and daidai flavor. These compounds showed high flavor dilution factors of 2^{12} and 2^{15}, accordingly, in yuzu peel oil. Geranyl acetate had a lime-like odor in Vietnamese lime oil (Lan Phi et al., 2006a), while neryl acetate showed both lime-like and Hyuganatsu-like odor notes in both varieties. These two compounds are also rather active in other citrus oils as given in their FD-factor values. *trans,trans*-Farnesyl acetate is also a contributor of Hyuganatsu oil since it presents Hyuganatsu-like odor with high a FD factor of 3^7.

5.3.7 Ketones and Acids

The most common ketone, carvone, occurs naturally in many kinds of essential oils, being the major ketone constituent of some citrus oils such as Hyuganatsu, daidai, Vietnamese lime, and yuzu. Cavone was reported for the first time as an important contributor to clementine peel aroma. This compound shows a lime-like odor note from GC-sniffing of *C. aurantifolia* Persa (lime) cold-pressed oil (Lan Phi, 2006a). Nootkatone, a character-impact component of grapefruit and pummelo, is also present as an odor-active component in Tosa-buntan (FD-factor of 3^7) (Sawamura et al., 2001) and natsudaidai (3^5) (Lan Phi, 2006b) peel oils. α-Thujone, a trace amount of component in both Hyuganatsu and Ki-mikan oils, had rather high FD factors of 3^6 and 3^5, respectively. Only three acids were found to be odor-active compounds in Tosa-buntan and Ki-mikan oils.

5.3.8 Oxides and Epoxides

A minor group in citrus oil, oxides and epoxides, plays a significant role in contributing to the citrus aroma. (*Z*)- and (*E*)-Limonene oxides and (*Z*)- and (*E*)-linalool oxides are representatives. Song et al. (2000a) reported that (*Z*)-limonene oxide was an aroma-active component of daidai oil, whereas (*Z*)- and (*E*)-linalool oxides (furanoid form) were the characteristic components of mochiyu oil, showing mochiyu-like odor at a high FD factor of 3^7. Two epoxides, *trans*-caryophyllene epoxides and myrcene epoxide, also had high odor activity in yuzu essential oil.

5.3.9 Sulfur-Containing Compounds

Sulfur-containing compounds such as diallyl disulfide and diallyl trisulfide are the major components in garlic aroma. These components are described as having strong garlic and very ripe cheese odors as reviewed by Curionia and Bosset (2002). The only sulfur-containing compound that was identified and characterized in yuzu oil is methyltrisulfide. This compound plays an important role in yuzu aroma as reported by Song et al. (2000b). Tajima (Tajima et al., 1990) reported for the first time that dimethyl trisulfide was the important component in yuzu oil. A trace amount of methyltrisulfide had the highest FD factor of 2^{18} among the other odor-active components found in yuzu oil. Moreover, due to its low odor threshold, methyltrisulfide presented a yuzu-like aroma at a very low concentration of 1 ppb as described by Song et al. (2000b).

Another sulfur-containing group is terpene thiols, which has a major organoleptic impact on citrus aroma. The representative compound is 1-*p*-menthene-8-thiol, having a very low aroma threshold, and imparting a strong grapefruit-like odor (Goeke, 2002).

5.4 PROSPECTS FOR GC-O

A limitation of conventional GC-O is that it is performed using a single column where co-elution of peaks is likely to occur, making identification of the compound responsible for a perceived odor difficult or uncertain. There is also the possibility of making an incorrect identification if a trace odorant is masked by a large odorless compound or even a large odor compound like limonene. Alternatively, co-elution of more than one odor-active compound during GC-O analysis may result in a mixed-odor perception, known as an *odor cluster*.

To resolve those co-elution problems, researchers have used comprehensive two-dimensional gas chromatography (GC × GC) (Eyres et al., 2007) and two-dimensional gas chromatography–olfactometry (GC × GC-O) (d'Acampora et al., 2007) in identifying character-impact odorants.

5.5 CLOSING REMARKS

Knowledge of volatile composition alone is not enough to completely understand the overall citrus aroma due to complex interactions of odorants. Applications of GC-O and combined techniques (mostly dilution techniques) allow us to characterize key aroma compounds and screen individuals for differences in citrus flavors. The characteristic volatile profile of citrus oil seems to be associated with a much higher proportion of oxygenated compounds such as alcohols, aldehydes, and esters.

Most of the odor-active compounds are found in the minor prevalent chemical functional groups of aldehydes, esters, alcohols, and ketones. Studies on citrus oils and juices have subsequently demonstrated that only a small fraction of the total volatiles actually contribute to their odor/aroma. The odor-active volatiles responsible for citrus odor are typically present at low concentrations. In some kinds of citrus fruits, the character-impact compounds are recognized, for example, 1-*p*-methene-8-thiol in grapefruit oil and citral (neral and geranial) in lemon oil. In other cases, no single compound is considered a character-impact component; the aroma/odor of that oil is a mixture of several or dozens of aroma-active volatiles present at low concentrations, such as in orange oil. It is suggested that the evaluation and grouping of the odor-impact components and their odor activities are valuable in flavor systems that can be used in flavor formulations and quality control.

REFERENCES

Acree, T.E. (1993). Bioassay for flavor. In: Acree, T.E., Teranishi, R. (eds.), *Flavor science: Sensible principles and techniques*. Washington DC: American Chemical Society, pp. 1–20.

Acree, T.E. (1997). GC/Olfactometry: GC with a sense of smell: A report. *Analytical Chemistry News & Features*, 170A–175A.

Acree, T.E., Barnard, J., Cummingham, D. (1984). A procedure for the sensory analysis of gas chromatographic effluents. *Food Chemistry* **14**: 273–286.

Ahmed, E.M., Dennison, R.A., Dougherty, R.H., Shaw, P.E. (1978a). Flavor and odor thresholds in water of selected orange juice components. *Journal of Agricultural and Food Chemistry* **26**: 187–191.

Ahmed, E.M., Dennison, R.A., Shaw, P.E. (1978b). Effect of selected oil and essence volatile components on flavor quality of pumpout orange juice. *Journal of Agricultural and Food Chemistry* **26**: 368–372.

Arena, E., Guarrera, N., Campisi, S., Nicolosi, A.C. (2006). Comparison of odour active compounds detected by gas chromatography-olfactometry between hand-squeezed juices from different orange varieties. *Food Chemistry* **98**: 59–63.

Arthur, D., Reeve, D. (2004). Grapefruit: The "forbidden" fruit. *Perfumer & Flavorist* **29**: 26–28.

Berdague, J.L., Tournayre, P., Cambou, S. (2007). Novel multi-gas chromatography–olfactometry device and software for the identification of odour-active compounds. *Journal of Chromatography A* **1146**: 85–92.

Blank, I., Grosch, W. (1991). Evaluation of potent odorants in dill seed and dill herb (*Anethum graveolens* L.) by Aroma Extract Dilution Analysis. *Journal of Food Science* **56**: 63–67.

Buchbauer, G., Jirovetz, L., Nikiforov, A. (1996). Comparative investigation of essential clover flower oils from Austria using gas chromatography–flame ionization detection, gas chromatography–mass spectrometry, and gas chromatography–olfactometry. *Journal of Agricultural and Food Chemistry* **44**: 1827–1828.

Buettner, A., Mestres, M., Fischer, A., Guasch, J., Schieberle, P. (2003). Evaluation of the most odour-active compounds in the peel oil of clementines (*Citrus reticulata* Blanco cv. *clementine*). *European Food Research and Technology* **216**: 11–14.

Buettner, A., Schieberle, P. (1999). Characterization of the most odor-active volatiles in fresh, hand-squeezed juice of grapefruit (*Citrus paradisi* Macfadyen). *Journal of Agricultural and Food Chemistry* **47**: 5189–5193.

Buettner, A., Schieberle, P. (2001). Evaluation of aroma differences between hand-squeezed juices from Valencia late and Navel oranges by quantitation of key odorants and flavor reconstitution experiments. *Journal of Agricultural and Food Chemistry* **49**: 2387–2394.

Chida, M., Yamashita, K., Izumiya, Y., Watanabe, K., Tamura, H. (2006). Aroma impact compounds in three citrus oils: Cross-matching test and correspondence analysis approach. *Journal of Food Science* **71**: S54–S58.

Chisholm, M.G., Jell, J.A., Cass, D.M. (2003a). Characterization of the major odorants found in the peel oil of *Citrus reticulata* Blanco cv. *Clementine* using gas chromatography–olfactometry. *Flavour and Fragrance Journal* **18**: 275–281.

Chisholm, M.G., Wilson, M.A., Gaskey, G.M. (2003b). Characterization of aroma volatiles in key lime essential oils (*Citrus aurantifolia* Swingle). *Flavour and Fragrance Journal* **18**: 106–115.

Choi, H.-S. (2003). Character impact odorants of *Citrus* Hallabong [(*C. unshiu* Marcov. × *C. sinensis* Osbeck) × *C. reticulata* Blanco] cold-pressed peel oil. *Journal of Agricultural and Food Chemistry* **51**: 2687–2692.

Choi, H.-S. (2004). Volatile constituents of satsuma mandarins growing in Korea. *Flavour and Fragrance Journal* **19**: 406–412.

Choi, H.-S. (2005). Characteristic odor components of Kumquat (*Fortunella japonica* Swingle) peel oil. *Journal of Agricultural and Food Chemistry* **53**: 1642–1647.

Choi, H.-S., Kondo, Y., Sawamura, M. (2001). Characterization of the odor-active volatiles in citrus Hyuganatsu (*Citrus tamurana* Hort. ex Tanaka). *Journal of Agricultural and Food Chemistry* **49**: 2404–2408.

Choi, H.-S., Sawamura, M., Kondo, Y. (2002). Characterization of the key aroma compounds of *Citrus flaviculpus* Hort. ex Tanaka by aroma extraction dilution analysis. *Journal of Food Science* **67**: 1713–1718.

Christensen, K.R., Reineccius, G.A. (1995). Aroma extract dilution analysis of aged Cheddar cheese. *Journal of Food Science* **60**: 218–220.

Counet, C., Callemien, D., Ouwerx, C., Collin, S. (2002). Use of gas chromatography–olfactometry to identify key odorant compounds in dark chocolate. Comparison of samples before and after conching. *Journal of Agricultural and Food Chemistry* **50**: 2385–2391.

Curionia, P.M.G., Bosset, J.O. (2002). Key odorants in various cheese types as determined by gas chromatography–olfactometry. *International Dairy Journal* **12**: 959–984.

d'Acampora, Z.B., Casilli, A., Dugo, P., Dugo, G., Mondello, L. (2007). Odour fingerprint acquisition by means of comprehensive two-dimensional gas chromatography–olfactometry and comprehensive two-dimensional gas chromatography–mass spectrometry. *Journal of Chromatography A* **1141**: 279–286.

d'Acampora, Z.B., Dugo, P., Dugo, G., Mondello, L. (2008). Gas chromatography–olfactometry in food flavour analysis. *Journal of Chromatography A* **1186**: 123–143.

Deibler, K.D., Llesca, F.M., Lavin, E.H., Acree, T.E. (2004). Calibration of gas chromatography inlet splitting for gas chromatography–olfactometry dilution analysis. *Flavour and Fragrance Journal* **19**: 518–521.

Delahunty, C.M., Eyres, G., Dufour, J.-P. (2006). Gas chromatography–olfactometry. *Journal of Separation Science* **29**: 2107–2125.

Demole, E., Enggist, P., Ohloff, G. (1982). 1-*p*-Menthen-8-thiol: A powerful flavor impact constituent of grapefruit juice (*Citrus paradisi* Macfadyen). *Helvetica Chimica Acta* **65**: 1785–1794.

Demole, E., Enggist, P. (1983). Further investigation of grapefruit juice flavor components (*Citrus paradisi* Macfadyen). Valencene- and eudesmane-type sesquiterpene ketones. *Helvetica Chimica Acta* **66**: 1381–1391.

Dharmawan, J., Kasapis, S., Sriramula, P., Lear, M.J., Curran, P. (2009). Evaluation of aroma-active compounds in Pontianak orange peel oil (*Citrus nobilis* Lour. var. *microcarpa* Hassk.) by gas chromatography–olfactometry, aroma reconstitution, and omission test. *Journal of Agricultural and Food Chemistry* **57**: 239–244.

Elston, A., Lin, J., Rouseff, R. (2005). Determination of the role of valencene in orange oil as a direct contributor to aroma quality. *Flavour and Fragrance Journal* **20**: 381–386.

Eyres, G., Marriott, P.J., Dufour, J.-P. (2007). The combination of gas chromatography–olfactometry and multidimensional gas chromatography for the characterisation of essential oils. *Journal of Chromatography A* **1150**: 70–77.

Fischer, A., Grab, W., Schieberle, P. (2008). Characterisation of the most odour-active compounds in a peel oil extract from Pontianak oranges (*Citrus nobilis* var. Lour. *microcarpa* Hassk.). *European Food Research and Technology* **227**: 735–744.

Fischer, A., Schieberle, P. (2009). Characterisation of the key aroma compounds in the peel oil of Pontianak oranges (*Citrus nobilis* Lour. var. *microcarpa* Hassk.) by aroma reconstitution experiments. *European Food Research and Technology* **229**: 319–328.

Fuller, G.H., Steltenkamp, R., Tisserand, G.A. (1964). The gas chromatography with human sensor: Perfumer model. *Annals of the New York Academy of Sciences* **116**: 711–724.

Gaffney, B.M., Havekotte, M., Jacobs, B., Costa, L. (1996). CharmAnalysis of two *Citrus sinensis* peel oil volatiles. *Perfumer & Flavorist* **21**: 1–5.

Goeke, A. (2002). Sulfur-containing odorants in fragrance chemistry. *Sulfur Reports* **23**: 243–278.

Goodner, K.L., Rouseff, R.L. (2001). Using an Ion-trap MS sensor to differentiate and identify individual components in grapefruit juice headspace volatiles. *Journal of Agricultural and Food Chemistry* **49**: 250–253.

Grosch, W. (1994). Determination of potent odourants in foods by Aroma Extract Dilution Analysis (AEDA) and calculation of Odour Activity Values (OAVs). *Flavour and Fragrance Journal* **9**: 147–158.

Grosch, W. (2001). Evaluation of the key odorants of foods by dilution experiments, aroma models and omission. *Chem Sense* **26**: 533–545.

Gurbuz, O., Rouseff, J.M., Rouseff, R.L. (2006). Comparison of aroma volatiles in commercial merlot and cabernet sauvignon wines using gas chromatography–olfactometry and gas chromatography–mass spectrometry. *Journal of Agricultural and Food Chemistry* **54**: 3990–3996.

Guth, H. (1997). Identification of character impact odorants of different white wine varieties. *Journal of Agricultural and Food Chemistry* **45**: 3022–3026.

Hanaoka, K., Vallet, N., Giampaoli, P., Heyd, B., MacLeod, P. (2001). Possible influence of breathing on detection frequency and intensity rating in gas chromatography–olfactometry. *Food Chemistry* **72**: 97–103.

Hinterholzer, A., Schieberle, P. (1998). Identification of the most odour-active volatiles in fresh, hand-extracted juice of Valencia late oranges by odour dilution techniques. *Flavour and Fragrance Journal* **13**: 49–55.

Högnadóttir, A., Rouseff, R.L. (2003). Identification of aroma active compounds in orange essence oil using gas chromatography–olfactometry and gas chromatography–mass spectrometry. *Journal of Chromatography A* **998**: 201–211.

Hulin-Bertaud, S., O'Riordan, P.J., Delahunty, C.M. (2001). Gas chromatography/olfactometry panel training: A time-intensity approach for odor evaluation. In: Spanier, A.M., Shahidi, F., Parliment, T.H., Mussinan, C., Ho, C.-T., Contis, E.T. (eds.), *Food flavors and chemistry: Advances of the new millennium*. Cambridge, UK: Royal Society of Chemistry, pp. 394–403.

Hwan Kim, T., Mi Lee, S., Kim, Y.-S., Heon Kim, K., Oh, S., Lee, H.J. (2003). Aroma dilution method using GC injector split ratio for volatile compounds extracted by headspace solid phase microextraction. *Food Chemistry* **83**: 151–158.

Kale, P.N., Adsule, P.G. (1995). Citrus. In: Salunkhe, D.K., Kadam, S.S. (eds.), *Handbook of fruit science and technology: Production, composition, storage, and processing*. New York: Marcel Dekker, pp. 39–66.

Kamath, A., Asha, M.R., Ravi, R., Narasimhan, S., Rajalakshmi, D. (2001). Comparative study of odour and GC-olfactometric profiles of selected essential oils. *Flavour and Fragrance Journal* **16**: 401–407.

Lan Phi, N.T., Minh Tu, N.T., Nishiyama, C., Sawamura, M. (2006a). Characterisation of the odour volatiles in *Citrus aurantifolia* Persa lime oil from Vietnam. In: Bredie, W.L.P., Petersen, M.A. (eds.), *Flavour science: Recent advances and trends*. Amsterdam: Elsevier, pp. 193–196.

Lan Phi, N.T., Nishiyama, C., Choi, H.S., Sawamura, M. (2006b). Evaluation of characteristic aroma compounds of *Citrus natsudaidai* Hayata (Natsudaidai) cold-pressed peel oil. *Bioscience, Biotechnology, and Biochemistry* **70**: 1832–1838.

Lan Phi, N.T., Sawamura, M. (2008). Characteristic aroma composition profile of mature stage *Citrus junos* (Yuzu) peel oil from different origins. *Food Science and Technology Research* **14**: 359–366.

Lan-Phi, N.T., Shimamura, T., Ukeda, H., Sawamura, M. (2009). Chemical and aroma profiles of yuzu (*Citrus junos*) peel oils of different cultivars. *Food Chemistry* **115**: 1042–1047.

Le Guen, S., Prost, C., Demaimay, M. (2000). Critical comparison of three olfactometric methods for the identification of the most potent odorants in cooked mussels (*Mytilus edulis*). *Journal of Agricultural and Food Chemistry* **48**: 1307–1314.

Lehmann, D., Dietrich, A., Hener, U., Mosandl, A. (1995). Stereoisomeric flavour compounds. Vol. LXX: 1-*p*-menthene-8-thiol: Separation and sensory evaluation of the enantiomers by enantioselective gas chromatography–olfactometry. *Phytochemical Analysis* **6**: 255–257.

Lin, J., Rouseff, R.L. (2001). Characterization of aroma-impact compounds in cold-pressed grapefruit oil using time-intensity GC-olfactometry and GC-MS. *Flavour and Fragrance Journal* **16**: 457–463.

Marin, A.B., Acree, T.E., Hotchkiss, J.H., Nagy, S. (1992). Gas chromatography–olfactometry of orange juice to assess the effects of plastic polymers on aroma character. *Journal of Agricultural and Food Chemistry* **40**: 650–654.

McDaniel, M.R., Miranda-Lopez, R., Watson, B.T., Micheals, N.J., Libbey, L.M. (1990). Pinot noir aroma: A sensory/gas chromatographic approach. In: Charalambous, G. (ed.), *Flavors and off-flavors '89: Proceedings of the 6th International Flavor Conference, Rethymnon, Crete, Greece, 5–7 July 1989*. New York: Elsevier Science, pp. 23–36.

Miranda-Lopez, R., Libbey, L.M., Watson, B.T., McDaniel, M.R. (1992). Odor analysis of pinot noir wines from grapes of different maturities by a gas chromatography–olfactometry technique (Osme). *Journal of Food Science* **57**: 985–993.

Miyazato, H., Hashimoto, S., Hayashi, S. (2008). Investigation on potent aroma compound in Yuzu (*Citrus junos* Tanaka) (II). *Proceedings of Symposium on Chemistry of Terpenes, Essential Oils and Aromatics*, Gunma, Japan, pp. 69–71.

Miyazawa, N., Tomita, N., Kurobayashi, Y., Nakanishi, A., Ohkubo, Y., Maeda, T., Fujita, A. (2009). Novel character impact compounds in yuzu (*Citrus junos* Sieb. ex Tanaka) peel oil. *Journal of Agricultural and Food Chemistry* **57**: 1990–1996.

Ott, A., Fay, L.B., Chaintreau, A. (1997). Determination and origin of the aroma impact compounds of yogurt flavor. *Journal of Agricultural and Food Chemistry* **45**: 850–858.

Perez-Cacho, P.R., Rouseff, R.L. (2008). Fresh squeezed orange juice odor: A review. *Critical Reviews in Food Science and Nutrition* **48**: 681–695.

Poisson, L., Schieberle, P. (2008). Characterization of the most odor-active compounds in an American Bourbon Whisky by application of the Aroma Extract Dilution Analysis. *Journal of Agricultural and Food Chemistry* **56**: 5813–5819.

Pollien, P., Fay, L.B., Baumgartner, M., Chaintreau, A. (1999). First attempt of odorant quantitation using gas chromatography–olfactometry. *Anal Chem* **71**: 5391–5397.

Qiao, Y., Xie, B.J., Zhang, Y., Zhang, Y., Fan, G., Yao, X.L., Pan, S.Y. (2008). Characterization of aroma active compounds in fruit juice and peel oil of Jinchen sweet orange fruit (*Citrus sinensis* (L.) Osbeck) by GC-MS and GC-O. *Molecules* **13**: 1333–1344.

Rega, B., Fournier, N., Guichard, E. (2003). Solid phase microextraction (SPME) of orange juice flavor: Odor representativeness by direct gas chromatography olfactometry (D-GC-O). *Journal of Agricultural and Food Chemistry* **51**: 7092–7099.

Rychlik, M., Grosch, W. (1996). Identification and quantification of potent odorants formed by toasting of wheat bread. *Lebensm-Wiss u-Technol* **29**: 515–525.

Sawamura, M., Onishi, Y., Ikemoto, J., Minh Tu, N.T., Lan Phi, N.T. (2006). Characteristic odour components of bergamot (*Citrus bergamia* Risso) essential oil. *Flavour and Fragrance Journal* **21**: 609–615.

Sawamura, M., Song, H.-S., Choi, H.-S., Sagawa, K., Ukeda, H. (2001). Characteristic aroma components of Tosa-buntan (*Citrus grandis* Osbeck forma *Tosa*) fruit. *Food Science and Technology Research* **7**: 45–49.

Schieberle, P., Grosch, W. (1988). Identification of potent flavor compounds formed in an aqueous lemon oil/citric acid emulsion. *Journal of Agricultural and Food Chemistry* **36**: 797–800.

Schieberle, P., Grosch, W. (1989). Potent odorants resulting from the peroxidation of lemon oil. *Z Lebensm Unters Forsch* **189**: 26–31.

Schnermann, P., Schieberle, P. (1997). Evaluation of key odorants in milk chocolate and cocoa mass by aroma extract dilution analyses. *Journal of Agricultural and Food Chemistry* **45**: 867–872.

Semmelroch, P., Grosch, W. (1996). Studies on character impact odorants of coffee brews. *Journal of Agricultural and Food Chemistry* **44**: 537–543.

Shaw, P.E. (1991). Fruits II. In: Maarse, H. (ed.), *Volatile compounds in foods and beverages*, New York: Marcel Dekker Inc., pp. 305–328.

Song, H.S., Sawamura, M., Ito, T., Ido, A., Ukeda, H. (2000a). Quantitative determination and characteristic flavour of daidai (*Citrus aurantium* L. var. *cyathifera* Y. Tanaka) peel oil. *Flavour and Fragrance Journal* **15**: 323–328.

Song, H.S., Sawamura, M., Ito, T., Kawashimo, K., Ukeda, H. (2000b). Quantitative determination and characteristic flavour of *Citrus junos* (yuzu) peel oil. *Flavour and Fragrance Journal* **15**: 245–250.

Tajima, K., Tanaka, S., Yamaguchi, T., Fujita, M. (1990). Analysis of green and yellow yuzu peel oils (*Citrus junos* Tanaka). Novel aldehyde components with remarkably low odor thresholds. *Journal of Agricultural and Food Chemistry* **38**: 1544–1548.

Tomiyama, K., Kasuga, H., Nozaki, O., Ogasawara, H., Kawakami, Y. (2008). Volatile components of Sanbokan (*C. sultaca* Hort. ex Takahashi). *Proceedings of Symposium on the Chemistry of Terpenes, Essential Oils and Aromatics*, Gunma, Japan, pp. 75–77.

Tu, N.T.M., Onishi, Y., Choi, H.-S., Kondo, Y., Bassore, S.M., Ukeda, H., Sawamura, M. (2002). Characteristic odor components of *Citrus sphaerocarpa* Tanaka (Kabosu) cold-pressed peel oil. *Journal of Agricultural and Food Chemistry* **50**: 2908–2913.

Tu, N.T.M., Onishi, Y., Choi, H.S., Kondo, Y., Ukeda, H., Sawamura, M. (2003a). Characteristic odour components of *Citrus sp* (Kiyookadaidai) cold-pressed peel oil. *Flavour and Fragrance Journal* **18**: 515–520.

Tu, N.T.M., Onishi, Y., Son, U.S., Ogawa, E., Ukeda, H., Sawamura, M. (2003b). Characteristic odour components of *Citrus inflata* Hort. ex Tanaka (Mochiyu) cold-pressed peel oil. *Flavour and Fragrance Journal* **18**: 454–459.

van Ruth, S.M. (2001). Methods for gas chromatography–olfactometry: A review. *Biomolecular Engineering* **17**: 121–128.

van Ruth, S.M. (2004). Evaluation of two gas chromatography–olfactometry methods: The detection frequency and perceived intensity method. *Journal of Chromatography A* **1054**: 33–37.

van Ruth, S.M., O'Connor, C.H. (2001). Evaluation of three gas chromatography–olfactometry methods: Comparison of odour intensity–concentration relationships of eight volatile compounds with sensory headspace data. *Food Chemistry* **74**: 341–347.

van Ruth, S.M., Roozen, J.P. (1994). Gas chromatography/sniffing port analysis and sensory evaluation of commercially dried bell peppers (*Capsicum annuum*) after rehydration. *Food Chemistry* **51**: 165–170.

Wilson, C.W., Shaw, P.E. (1981). Importance of thymol, methyl *N*-methylanthranilate, and monoterpene hydrocarbons to the aroma and flavor of mandarin cold-pressed oils. *Journal of Agricultural and Food Chemistry* **29**: 494–496.

6

FUNCTIONAL PROPERTIES

Hyang-Sook Choi

Kyungin Women's College
Inchon, Korea

Aromatic plants and their preparations belong to the oldest known health-care products that have been used by human beings all over the world. Plants contain pharmacologically and physiologically active compounds. *Nutraceuticals*, often referred to as *phytochemicals* or functional foods, are natural bioactive chemical compounds that provide demonstrated physiological benefits or reduce the risk of chronic diseases, above their basic nutritional function. The beneficial role of many nutraceuticals and functional foods may relate to their protective effects against degenerative diseases, such as cancer and cardiovascular diseases. Typically the active ingredients in the food are believed to help the body combat metabolic processes that lead to degenerative conditions. In this way, supplementing the diet with beneficial phytonutrients may reduce the risk of degenerative diseases during aging.

Several groups of plant phytochemicals, including carotenoids, tocopherols, and polyphenols, are extremely effective antioxidants; these antioxidants are found at various levels in fruits, vegetables, and nonfood plants. Thus, "nutraceuticals" and "functional foods" refer to fresh or processed fruits or vegetables that are particularly high in antioxidants. Phenolics of plant origin have been

Citrus Essential Oils: Flavor and Fragrance, Edited by Masayoshi Sawamura

found to act as free radical scavengers and inhibitors of cholesterol oxidation and DNA breakage, thus serving as potential cancer-preventing agents.

Antioxidants are substances that can delay onset, or slow the rate, of oxidation. Literally hundreds of compounds, both natural and synthesized, have been reported to possess antioxidant properties. Their use in foods, however, is limited by certain obvious requirements not the least of which is adequate proof of safety. The main lipid-soluble antioxidants currently used in food are monohydric or polyhydric phenols with various ring structures. The effectiveness of an antioxidant is related to many factors, including activation energy, rate constants, oxidation-reduction potential, ease of antioxidant loss or destruction, and solubility properties.

Oxidation occurs when electrons are removed from an atom or group of atoms. Simultaneously, there is a corresponding reduction reaction that involves the addition of electrons to a different atom or group of atoms. Oxidation reactions may or may not involve the addition of oxygen atoms or the removal of hydrogen atoms from the substance being oxidized. Oxidation-reduction reactions are common in biological systems, and also are common in foods. Although some oxidation reactions are beneficial in foods, others can lead to detrimental effects, including degradation of vitamins, pigments, and lipids, with loss of nutritional value and development of off flavors. Control of undesirable oxidation reactions in foods is usually achieved by employing processing that excludes oxygen or involves the addition of appropriate chemical agents. More recently, the term "food antioxidants" often has been applied to those compounds that interrupt the free-radical chain reaction involved in lipid oxidation and those that scavenge singlet oxygen; however, the term should not be used in such a narrow sense. Many naturally occurring substances possess antioxidant capabilities, and the tocopherols are noted examples that are widely employed. Recently, extractives of aromatic plants, including spices, have been successfully commercially exploited as natural antioxidants (Lindsay, 1996).

Microbial activity is one of the primary modes of deterioration of many foods and is often responsible for food quality reduction, spoilage, and economic loss. The approaches to regulating microbial deterioration of foods are the direct addition of antimicrobials and the use of antimicrobials in food-contact surfaces such as packaging materials. Despite the widespread use and effectiveness of chemical interventions, researchers are continually investigating the use of other novel antimicrobial agents such as natural plants.

Essential oils are rich sources of biologically active compounds. Recently there has been a profound interest in the functional properties, including antimicrobial effects of extracts from aromatic plants, particularity essential oils (Morris et al., 1979). Many oils and extracts from different plants have been investigated for their antimicrobial properties against a series of bacteria and yeasts (Saller et al., 1995; Zhu et al., 2005). Essential oils have been found to be antibacterial, antifungal, and therapeutic in cancer treatment (Crowell, 1997). Some oils have been shown to have applications in food preservation, while others have pharmacological properties such as antiseptic, and expectorant, and some are used in aromatherapy (Arldoğan et al., 2002). The use of natural antimicrobial compounds seems to be important not only in the preservation of food but also in the control of human and plant diseases of microbial origin.

As mentioned earlier, aromatic plants, including fruits and vegetables, possess many physiological activities. However, functional properties of citrus essential oils have not been studied to date. Therefore, we will introduce the antioxidative, anticarcinogenic, and antimicrobial activities of citrus essential oils.

6.1 ANTIOXIDATIVE ACTIVITY

Hyang-Sook Choi

Fruits and vegetables are a rich source of phytochemicals that may promote good health. They include thousands of compounds, pigments, and natural antioxidants, many of which have been associated with protection from heart disease, hypertension, cancer, and many chronic diseases. Singly and together, these compounds help plants resist the attacks of bacteria and fungi, the ravages of free radicals, and high levels of ultraviolet light from the sun. When we eat these plants, the phytochemicals end up in our tissues and provide many of the same protections (Tsushida et al., 1994, Baratta et al., 1998, Dorman et al., 2000, Teow et al., 2007).

Some phytochemicals show antioxidant activity. Natural antioxidants found in dietary plants may play an important role in the prevention of cardio- and cerebrovascular diseases, carcinogenesis, and various chronic diseases. Plants provide food antioxidants like vitamin C, vitamin E, and carotenes. Polyphenol compounds and phytoestrogens also have been recognized as having the potential to reduce disease risk. Antioxidants are often used to delay autoxidations in food lipids, a process responsible for off-flavors and formation of constituents that might pose a potential health risk. According to the mode of action, antioxidants may be classified as free radical terminators, and chelators of metal ion (Khanum et al., 1999).

Antioxidant compounds in food play an important role as health-protecting factors. Some phytochemicals neutralize free radicals. Free radicals are continually produced in our cells and over time can result in damage both to DNA and important cell structures. Eventually, this damage can promote both cancer and cell aging. Many different plant chemicals are able to neutralize or reduce concentrations of free radicals, thus protecting us against the development of both cancer and heart disease (Cao et al., 1996, Bandoniene and Murkovic, 2002).

The relative effectiveness of antioxidants is dependent on the action type of antioxidants (free radical inhibitor, peroxide decomposer, metal inactivator, or oxygen scavenger), test system, emulsion system, concentration, oxidation time, method used, and growth stage of plant samples (Yagi, 1970). The various methods used to measure antioxidant activity of food products can give varying results depending on the specific free radical being used as a reactant. Several studies have reported correlations among the antioxidative activities measured by different methods, as well as the correlations between those methods and phytochemical concentrations in various food commodities (Awika et al., 2003). Therefore, it is necessary to combine the results of antioxidative activities of a sample in order to establish a credible result that can be readily adapted in human health. Now we introduce the antioxidative activities of citrus essential oils by (1) the HPLC-DPPH screening method for determining radical-scavenging activity, (2) the assay of proxide value with the thiocyanate method, and (3) tocopherol analysis.

6.1.1 Radical-Scavenging Activities of Citrus Peel Essential Oils and Their Components

Free radicals are generated in the human body through aerobic respiration and exist in different forms. Reactive oxygen species such as superoxide anion, hydroxyl radical, hydrogen peroxide, peroxyl radical, and singlet oxygen are known to cause oxidative damage, contributing to the development of chronic diseases such as cancer, cerebrovascular disease, and heart disease. The prevention and removal of reactive oxygen species is achieved through enzymatic and nonenzymatic reactions. Living cells have biological defense mechanisms composed of enzymatic antioxidant systems that remove free radical species. Nonenzymatic reactions can also effectively scavenge free radicals. Thus, the efficiency of antioxidant defense relies on a variety of nonenzymatic antioxidants such as vitamins C and E, and many phytochemicals that possess the scavenging activity of oxidants and free radicals, which are coupled to the antioxidative enzyme response. Therefore, it is important to consume a diet high in antioxidants, such as fruits and vegetables, to reduce the harmful effects of oxidative stress (Willet, 1994, Wang et al., 1996, Talcott et al., 2003, Lee et al., 2008).

Phenolic compounds, such as butylated hydroxyanisole (BHA), butylated hydroxy toluene (BHT), and *tert*-butylhydroquinone (TBHQ), have been widely used as synthetic antioxidants in the food industry for extending the shelf-life of foods that are susceptible to lipid oxidation. However, there are some arguments about the safety and adverse effects of synthetic antioxidants as food additives, and they do not always provide effective protection against in vitro oxidation. Therefore, there has been growing interest in natural antioxidants of plant origin because they have greater application in the food industry for increasing the stability and shelf-life of food products. Moreover, they also find use as nutraceuticals and phytoceuticals as they have significant impact on the status of human health (Suja et al., 2004, Obame et al., 2007).

Antioxidative activity can be expressed in terms of radical-scavenging ability. A rapid, simple, and inexpensive method to measure antioxidant capacity of food involves the use of the free radical, 1,1-diphenyl-2-picrylhydrazyl (DPPH). DPPH is widely used to test the ability of compounds to act as free radical scavengers or hydrogen donors, and to evaluate antioxidant activity of foods. It has also been used to quantify antioxidants in complex biological systems in recent years. The DPPH method can be used for solid or liquid samples and applies to the overall antioxidant capacity of the sample. A measure of total antioxidant capacity helps us to understand the functional properties of foods (Fukuda et al., 1981; Cerutii, 1985). The odd electron in the DPPH free radical gives a strong absorption maximum at 517 nm and is purple in color. The color turns from purple to yellow as the molar absorptivity of the DPPH radical at 517 nm reduces when the odd electron of DPPH radical becomes paired with a hydrogen from a free-radical-scavenging antioxidant to form the reduced DPPH-H. The resulting decolorization is stoichiometric with respect to number of electrons captured (Molyneux, 2004). Antioxidative activity has been expressed in various ways, including the percentage of the reagent used, the oxidation inhibition rate, and so on. An easier way to present antioxidative activity of foods would be to reference a common reference standard. One common reference standard, (S)-(-)-6-hydroxy-2,5,7,8-tetramethylchroman-2-carboxylic acid, also known as Trolox, serves this purpose.

In our study, the radical-scavenging effects (percentage of quenched radical) were determined for 34 kinds of citrus essential oils and 21 authentic compounds (Choi et al., 2000). The citrus fruit classification used here is based on the taxonomy of Swingle (1943), as shown in Table 6.1. The essential oil samples were prepared by means of the cold-pressing method. Trolox, a hydrophilic carboxylic acid derivative of α-tocopherol, was employed as a standard antioxidant to examine the radical-scavenging activities. Under a wide range of conditions and test systems, the antioxidant activity of Trolox proved to be superior to that of α-tocopherol. For example, Trolox is significantly more active than α-tocopherol in a bulk oil system, whereas in an oil-in-water emulsion α-tocopherol is significantly more active than Trolox.

The radical-scavenging activity, expressed as milligrams of Trolox equivalent per milliliter of each sample, was calculated by means of the following equation:

$$\text{mg of Trolox equiv} = (A-B)/(A-C)\times 25/1000\times 250.29/1000\times 1000/10\times D$$

where A is the peak height of the control, B is the peak height of the sample, C is the peak height of Trolox, 250.29 is the molecular weight of Trolox, and D is the dilution factor.

All the essential oils revealed scavenging effects on DPPH, ranging from 17.7 to 64.0%, as shown in Figure 6.1. There was weak radical-scavenging effect in the essential oils of oyu, daidai, and Valencia orange (17.7–19.1 %); the extent of the effect was weaker than that of Trolox. On the other hand, 31 kinds of citrus essential oils exhibited scavenging effects ranging from 21.6 to 64.0%, and their effects were comparable with or stronger than that of Trolox. On the basis of scavenging effects on DPPH, significant differences between these fruits were observed. Eureka lemon, Tahiti lime, and Ichang lemon showed the highest radical-scavenging effects (61.8–64.0%), followed by sudachi, yuko, yuzu, and

TABLE 6.1. *Citrus* genus samples for radical-scavenging activity

Number	Variety	Commom Name	Species[a]
1	*C. junos* Sieb. ex Tanaka	yuzu (Japan)	*C. ichangensis*
2	*C. junos* Sieb. ex Tanaka	yuza (Korea)	*C. ichangensis*
3	*C. junos* Sieb. ex Tanaka	mukakuyuzu or seedless yuzu	*C. ichangensis*
4	*C. inflata* Hort. ex Tanaka	michiyuzu	*C. ichangensis*
5	*C. sudachi* Hort. ex Shirai	sudachi	*C. ichangensis*
6	*C. yuko* Hort. ex Tanaka	yuko	*C. ichangensis*
7	*C. Wilsonii* Tanaka	Ichang lemon	*C. ichangensis*
8	*C. sphaerocarpa* Tanaka	kabosu	*C. ichangensis*
9	*C. tagumasudachi* Hort. ex Shirai	naoshichi	*C. ichangensis*
10	*C. aurantifolia* Swingle	Mexican lime	*C. aurantifolia*
11	*C. latifolia* Tanaka	Tahiti lime	*C. aurantifolia*
12	*C. bergamia* Risso var. *Fantastico*	bergamot (Italy)	*C. aurantifolia*
13	*C. bergamia* Risso var. *Balotin*	bergamot	*C. aurantifolia*
14	*C. limon* Burm. F. cv. *Eureka*	Eureka lemon	*C. limon*
15	*C. limon* Burm. F. cv. *Lisbon*	Lisbon lemon	*C. limon*
16	*C. grandis* Osbeck forma *Tosa*	Tosa-buntan	*C. grandis*
17	*C. grandis* Osbeck forma *Banhakuyu*	manhakuyu	*C. grandis*
18	*C. paradisi* Macfadyen	grapefruit	*C. paradisi*
19	*C. hassaku* Hort. ex Y. Tanaka	hassaku	*C. paradisi*
20	*C. natsudaidai* Hayata	natsudaidai	*C. paradisi*
21	*C. aurantium* Linn. var. Cyathifera Y. Tanaka	daidai	*C. aurantium*
22	*C.* sp.	kiyoookadaidai	*C. aurantium* (tentative)
23	C. *neo-aurantium* Tanaka	konejime	*C. aurantium*
24	*C. aurantium* Linn forma *Kabusu*	kabusu	*C. aurantium*
25	*C. sinensis* Osbeck forma *Valencia*	Valencia orange	*C. sinensis*
26	*C. sinensis* Osbeck var. Sanguinea Tanaka forma *Tarocco*	Tarocco orange	*C. sinensis*
27	*C. iyo* Hort. ex Tanaka	Iyokan	*C. sinensis*
28	*C. tamurana* Hort. ex Tanaka	Hyuganatsu	*C. sinensis*
29	*C. ujukitsu* Hort. ex Shirai	ujukitsu	*C. sinensis*
30	*C. ujukitsu* Marcov. Forma *Miyagawa-wase*	Satsuma mandarin	*C. reticulata*
31	*C. ujukitsu* Marcov. Forma *Imamura*	Satsuma mandarin	*C. reticulata*
32	*C. reticulata* Blanco cv. *F-2426*	ponkan	*C. reticulata*
33	*C. ozu* Hort. ex Y. Tanaka	oyu	unidentified
34	*Fortunella japonica* Swingle[b]	kumquat	*Fortunella japonica*

[a]Classified by Swingle.
[b]Another genus in the Rutaceae family comprising the *Citrus* genus.

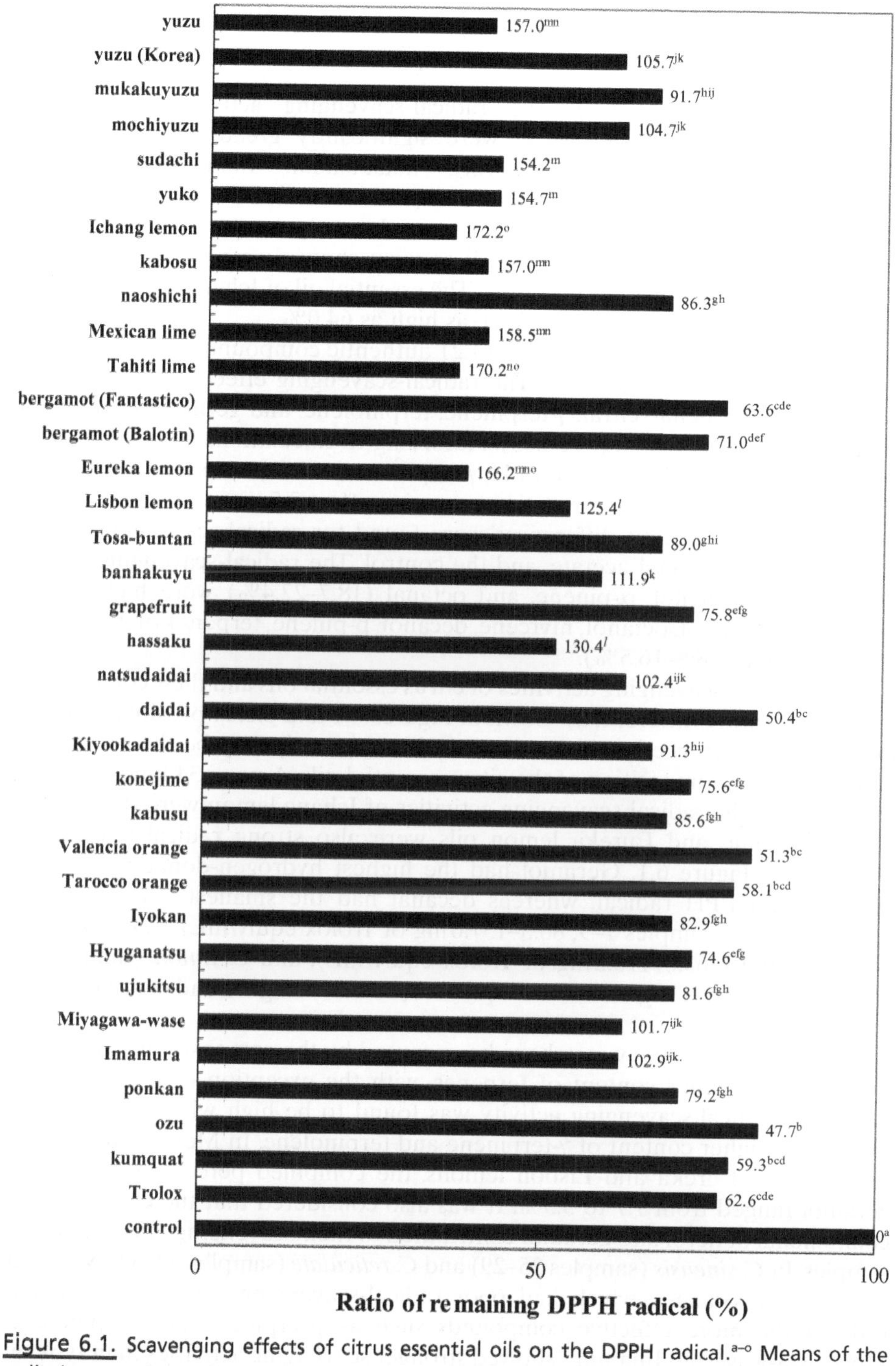

Figure 6.1. Scavenging effects of citrus essential oils on the DPPH radical.[a–o] Means of the radical-scavenging activity (mg of Trolox equiv/mL). Values with the same superscripts are not significantly different ($p < 0.05$).

Mexican lime (57.3–58.9%). The radical-scavenging activities of Lisbon lemon and hassaku (46.6–4.84%) were significantly greater than those of Miyagawa-wase (Satsuma mandarin), natsudaidai, Imamura (Satsuma mandarin), mochiyuzu, and Korean yuza (37.8–39.3%). The essential oils of Hyuganatsu, konejime grapefruit, ponkan, ujukitsu, Iyohan, kabusu, naoshichi, Tosa-buntan, Kiyookadaidai, and seedless yuzu showed scavenging effects on DPPH in the range from 27.7 to 34.1%. The essential oil of Ichang lemon showed the strongest radical-scavenging effect, as high as 64.0%.

The radical-scavenging activities of 21 authentic compounds of citrus essential oils are shown in Figure 6.2. The radical-scavenging effects of α-terpinene, nootkatone, citronellal, citral, γ-terpinene, terpinolene, and geraniol were much higher than that of Trolox ($p < 0.05$). According to calculations based simply on the decrease of peak height of DPPH, γ-terpinene (84.7%), terpinolene (87.4%), and geraniol (87.7%) have a radical-scavenging effect 3.5 times as strong as that of Trolox. No significant differences were found for radical-scavenging effects among decanal, geranyl acetate, and the control. The radical-scavenging effects of linalool, citronellol, α-pinene, and octanal (18.7–22.4%) were higher than those of α-terpineol, octanol, myrcene, decanol, β-pinene, terpen-4-ol, *p*-cymene, and *d*-limonene (8.8–16.5%).

The radical-scavenging activities of citrus essential oils and their components were significantly different, as shown in Figures 6.1 and 6.2. A possible explanation for the difference in efficiencies found in this study may be the substantial variation in the composition of the citrus essential oils. Among 34 kinds of citrus essential oils, the radical-scavenging activities of Ichang lemon were the highest, and Tahiti lime and Eureka lemon oils were also strong radical scavengers, as shown in Figure 6.1. Geraniol had the highest hydrogen-donating capacity against the DPPH radical, whereas decanal had the smallest. The family of *C. ichangenesis* (samples 1–9, 86.3–157.0 mg of Trolox equiv/mL), *C. aurantifolia* (samples 10–13, 63.6–170.2 mg of Trolox equiv/mL), and *C. limon* (samples 14 and 15, 125.4–166.2 mg of Trolox equiv/mL) showed higher radical-scavenging activities.

The higher efficiency may have been caused by the composition of essential oils having a higher content of terpenes, with the exception of limonene and myrcene. Radical-scavenging activity was found to be high when the terpenes included a higher content of γ-terpinene and terpinolene. In Mexican and Tahiti limes and in Eureka and Lisbon lemons, the combined percent of nerol and geraniol ranged from 1.7 to 3.5%. It was also considered that the characteristic components of nerol and geraniol contributed to their scavenging effects in these samples. In *C. sinensis* (samples 25–29) and *C. reticulate* (samples 30–32), Valencia and Tarocco oranges, which had poor radical-scavenging activities, contained little of the more effective compounds such as γ-terpinene and terpinolene. Miyagawa-wase and Imamura showed stronger scavenging activities than Iyokan, Hyuganatsu, and ujukitsu. Daidai, Valencia, and Tarocco oranges, ozu, and kumquat, in which γ-terpinene and terpinolene were almost 0%, form a group with the lowest DPPH radical-scavenging activity level. As those oils were mainly

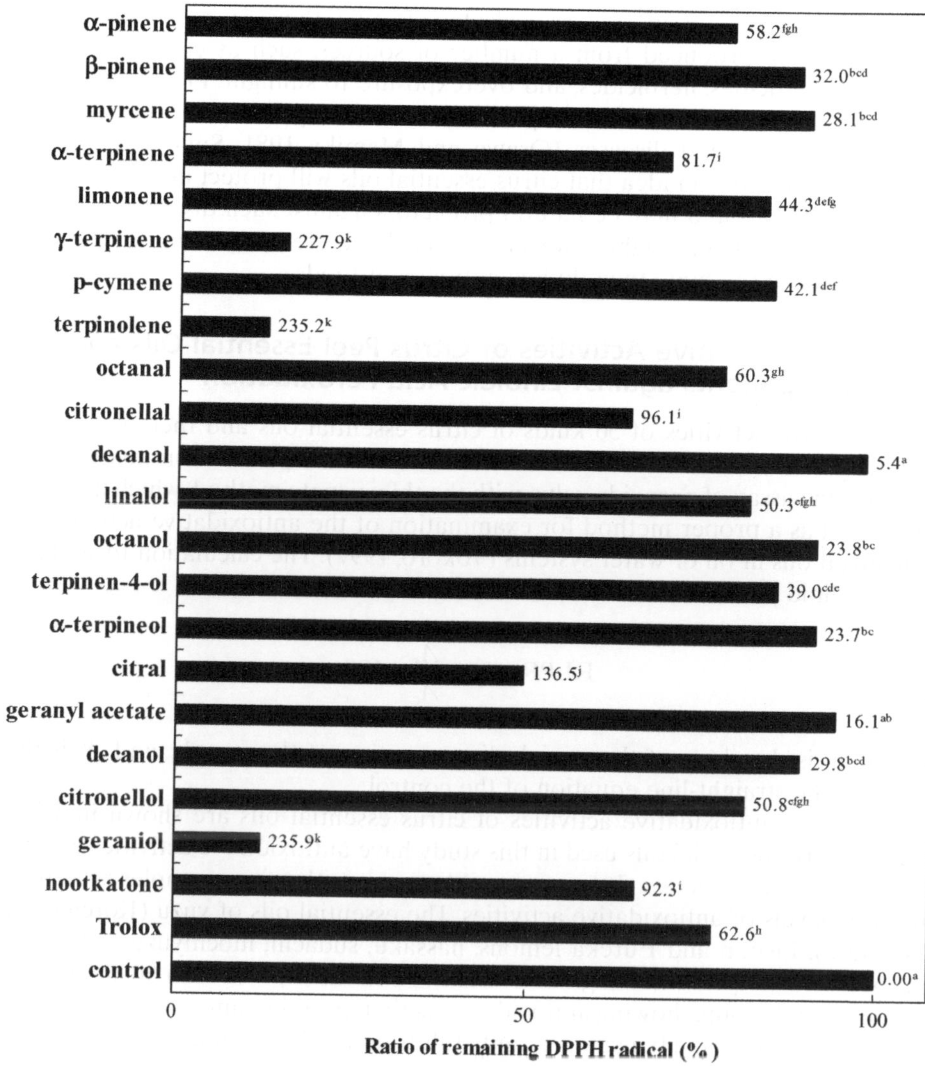

Figure 6.2. Scavenging effects of the authentic compounds relating to citrus essential oils on the DPPH radical.[a–k] Means of the radical-scavenging activity (mg of Trolox equiv/mL). Values with the same superscripts are not significantly different ($p < 0.05$).

composed of limonene in a proportion of >90%, it is considered that limonene would not play the principal role in determining the scavenging activity for the radical. Kiyokadaidai, banhakuyu, ujukitsu, and mochiyuzu were exceedingly abundant in myrcene compared with others, 63.7, 37.2, 28.3, and 20.6%, respectively. However, there was no direct correlation between the myrcene content and radical-scavenging activity. In each citrus essential oil, geraniol content was low; nevertheless, geraniol showed the highest radical-scavenging activity.

Antioxidants rein in free radicals by offering their own electrons. Free radicals can be produced from a number of sources, such as cigarette smoke, pollution, pesticides, herbicides, and overexposure to sunlight. Free radicals are responsible for inflammation, compromised immune systems, and degenerative and other age-related diseases (Osawa and Mamiki, 1981; Suja et al., 2004). These facts support an idea that citrus essential oils will protect against damage with free radicals and may be natural protectors against such diseases. It is reasonable to expect that high-antioxidant foods have greater potential to reduce free radicals in the body than do low-antioxidant foods.

6.1.2 Antioxidative Activities of Citrus Peel Essential Oils and Their Components against Linoleic Acid Peroxidation

Antioxidative activities of 30 kinds of citrus essential oils and their 14 components against linoleic acid oxidation were examined. The reaction mixture was used for the assay of peroxide value with the thiocyanate method, which has been suggested as a proper method for examination of the antioxidative activities of grapefruit oils in oil or water systems (Tokoro, 1997). The calculation formula of relative lipid peroxidation rate (RLPR) is as follows:

$$\mathrm{RLPR}\,(\%) = \frac{A_s}{A_c} \times 100$$

where A_s is the slope of the straight-line equation of the sample, and A_c is the slope of the straight-line equation of the control.

Relative antioxidative activities of citrus essential oils are shown in Table 6.2. All citrus essential oils used in this study have antioxidative activities against linoleic acid peroxidation. It seems possible to group the citrus samples according to three levels of antioxidative activities. The essential oils of yuzu (Korean and Japanese), Lisbon and Eureka lemons, hassaku, sudachi, mochiyuzu, yuko, and Tarocco orange presented high antioxidative activities, more than 90%. The oils of the second group, showing antioxidative activities in the range of 70–88% were bergamot (Italian), Hyuganatsu and Tahiti lime, Tosa-buntan, nastsudaidai, daidai, Valencia orange, Iyokan, Satsuma mandarin (*Miyagawa-wase*), ponkan, oyu, and kumquat. Other oils, such as Ichang lemon, bergamot (Japanese), grapefruit, kabusu, ujukitsu, and Satsuma mandarin, (*Imamura*) showed comparatively low antioxidative activities in the range of 49–60%.

It is possible to suggest that the species *C. limon*, *C. grandis*, *C. paradise*, and *C. reticulata* have high antioxidative activities. It has been previously reported that the inhibitory effects of citrus extracts on cyclooxygenase and lipoxygenase differed in citrus species; extract of citron and Eureka lemon showed selective inhibition effects on cyclooxygenase and those of yuzu and sudachi did so on lipoxygenase (Nogata et al., 1996). They also have shown that the inhibitory compounds on both enzyme metabolites were related to the citrus classification. Kawaii et al. (1999) also reported that the contents of 24 kinds of flavonoids in

TABLE 6.2. Relative lipid peroxidation rate of citrus essential oils

Citrus Essential Oil	RLPR[a] %
yuzu	2.6–3.3
seedless yuzu	50.3
sudachi	6.2–7.8
mochiyu	7.2
yuko	7.2
Ichang lemon	37.5
Mexican lime	35.1
Tahiti lime	25.1
bergamot (*Fantastico*)	11.7
bergamot (*Balotin*)	48.1
Eureka lemon	3.9–4.2
Lisbon lemon	3.6
Tosa-buntan	18.2
grapefruit	39.4
hassaku	5.9
natsudaidai	11.4
daidai	30–72
kabusu	39.7
Valencia orange	18.9
Tarocco orange	8.5–16.6
Iyokan	26.1
Hyuganatsu	11.7
ujukitsu	39.4
Satsuma mandarin (*Miyagawa-wase*)	25.1
Satsuma mandarin (*Imamura*)	37.1
ponkan	18.6
oyu	14.3
kumquat	17.6

[a]Relative lipid peroxidation rate.

the edible part of citrus fruits were related to the citrus classification. These results suggest that citrus essential oils may contain some constituents contributing to their different antioxidative activities among the species.

The 14 authentic compounds tested showed some antioxidative activities (Table 6.3). γ-Terpinene showed highly antioxidative activities, as much as 2.6% of relative lipid peroxidation rate (RLPR). The RLPRs of β-pinene, myrcene, α-terpinene and decanal were less than 10%. The RLPR of terpinolene was 18.6%. It was reported that terpinolene had an inhibitory effect on the oxidation of clove oil and nutmeg oil (Dorman et al., 2000). α-Pinene and citronellal were not as antioxidative, 26.1% and 42% of RLPR, respectively. The authentic flavor compounds showing high antioxidative activities have the isopentenyl group in their chemical structure. The conjugated double-bond and hydrophobicity of

TABLE 6.3. Relative lipid peroxidation rates of authentic compounds relating to flavor components in citrus essential oils

Authentic Compound	RLPR[a] %
α-pinene	26.1
β-pinene	8.8
myrcene	9.4
α-terpinene	9.4
limonene	12.1
γ-terpinene	2.6
terpinolene	18.6
octanal	12.4
citronellal	42
decanal	8.1
linalool	14
α-tocopherol	30.3
γ-tocopherol	30
δ-tocopherol	8.8

[a]Relative lipid peroxidation rate.

authentic flavor components, including octanal and decanal, seem to be important to antioxidation.

The essential oils of yuko, Lisbon and Eureka lemons, and sudachi were abundant in α-pinene and myrcene (1.5–3.1%, and 1.6–2.1%, respectively). Lemon oils were significantly abundant in β-pinene, accounting for about 12.5% of weight percent. Daidai, Tarocco orange, and oyu oils contained little α-terpinene, and their antioxidative activities were no higher than those of sudachi and lemons oils. The content of limonene, which is a major flavor component in citrus oils, ranged from 59 to 63% in Lisbon and Eureka lemons, yuko, and sudachi, and was 84.5, 85.7, and 81.1% in Tarocco orange, daidai, and oyu, respectively. Limonene is a monocyclic monoterpene with two isomers, L-limonene ((S)-(-)-limonene) and D-limonene ((R)-(+)-limonene). *l*-limonene exhibits a piney aroma and *d*-limonene smells like an orange. D-limonene is a stable, clear liquid at room temperature and is a major constituent in several citrus oils. It is commonly used as a flavor and fragrance additive in beverages, perfumes, and many processed foods. It is easily oxidized in moist air to carveol and carvone. Yuko oil was considerably rich in γ-terpinene and terpinolene (18.57 and 0.08%, respectively). The terpinolene contents in Lisbon and Eureka lemons and sudachi oils were significantly higher than those in daidai, Tarocco orange, and oyu oils. Mochiyu and hassaku, showing high antioxidative activities, contained much more monoterpene hydrocarbons in their essential oils. Weight percents of octanal in daidai and Tarocco orange were significantly as high as 0.76 and 1.44%, respectively. The percent of linalool was markedly high in sudachi (0.62%), but was significantly low in oyu (0.11%). Sudachi essential oil was unexpectedly abundant in citronellal, as much as 0.21%, of which RLPR was the highest (42%). High antioxidative activities of the citrus essential oils of lemon, yuko, and sudachi seem to result from the abundance of terpene hydrocarbons, γ-terpinene, β-pinene, and myrcene, because these authentic components showed high antioxidative activities.

Antioxidative activities of stored citrus oils were considerable. The antioxidative activities of Lisbon and Eureka lemons essential oils showed little difference between the stored and the fresh oils. The RLPRs of stored daidai, Tarocco orange, and oyu oils were 72, 16.6, and 28.7%, respectively, twice as high as those of fresh samples. The α-pinene contents of stored Lisbon lemon and yuko oils (2.43 and 3.66%, respectively) were significantly higher than in their fresh oils (2.19 and 3.13%, respectively). Both fresh and stored Lisbon lemon oils were abundant in γ-terpinene, as high as about 8.8 and 8.6%, respectively, of which RLPR was the lowest (2.6%). Myrcene and perpinolene were significantly more abundant in the stored yuko oil than in the fresh oil. β-Pinene contents in fresh Eureka and Lisbon lemon essential oils were more abundant than those in the stored ones (12.71 and 12.47%, respectively). The contents of limonene and α-pinene were not significantly different between stored and fresh essential oils, including daidai, Tarocco orange, and oyu. These results suggest that the composition of terpene compounds seems to be a major factor in the antioxidative activities of citrus essential oils.

6.1.3 Tocopherol Analysis of Citrus Peel Essential Oils

The tocopherol assays of citrus essential oils were carried out by the method described in Osuna-García et al. (1998). The tocopherol contents of these oils were determined and quantified by high-performance liquid chromatography monitored at 290 nm. The preliminary tocopherol assay was performed using standard α-tocopherol. Recovery in the assay was about 90% (Song et al., 2001).

The amounts of tocopherols in citrus essential oils are shown in Table 6.4. Each tocopherol content is given in μg per 100 mg of citrus essential oil. Mexican and Tahiti limes, Valencia orange, and yuzu essential oils were relatively abundant in tocopherols (about 0.4–0.6 μg of total tocopherol content). Mochiyu, Ichang lemon, natsudaidai, daidai, and kabusu essential oils contained little α-tocopherol. Lisbon lemon oil was abundant in γ-tocopherol, and daidai, hassaku, Valencia, and Tarocco orange oils in δ-tocopherol. The total tocopherol content of citrus essential oils usually depends on the level of α-tocopherol.

The correlation between total tocopherol contents and antioxidative activities of citrus essential oils was examined by statistical analysis. There was no significance in their relationship at the low level of correlation coefficient (0.0022). Correlation coefficients between each α-, γ-, and δ-tocopherol content and antioxidative activities of citrus essential oils were as low as 0.0058, 0.0530, and 0.0003, respectively. Thus it is suggested that the antioxidative activities of citrus essential oils are little related to their tocopherol contents.

TABLE 6.4. Tocopherol contents in citrus essential oils

Citrus Essential Oil	α-Tocopherol[a]	γ-Tocopherol[a]	δ-Tocopherol[a]	Total Amount
yuzu	0.384	0.001	0.385	0.385
seedless yuzu	0.149	0.001	0.150	0.150
sudachi	0.078	0.001	0.079	0.079
mochiyu	—	tr[b]	tr	tr
yuko	0.096	tr	0.096	0.096
Ichang lemon	—	0.001	0.026	0.026
Mexican lime	0.624	0.010	0.637	0.637
Tahiti lime	0.578	—	0.580	0.580
bergamot (*Fantastico*)	0.007	0.002	0.009	0.009
bergamot (*Balotin*)	0.036	0.001	0.037	0.037
Eureka lemon	0.098	0.008	0.106	0.106
Lisbon lemon	0.150	0.111	0.261	0.261
Tosa-buntan	0.230	0.003	0.233	0.233
grapefruit	0.195	0.002	0.197	0.197
hassaku	0.011	0.003	0.061	0.061
natsudaidai	—	0.010	0.016	0.016
daidai	—	0.005	0.062	0.062
kabusu	—	0.011	0.026	0.026
Valencia orange	0.391	—	0.424	0.424
Tarocco orange	0.032	0.002	0.071	0.071
Iyokan	0.006	0.003	0.009	0.009
Hyuganatsu	0.020	0.003	0.023	0.023
ujukitsu	0.007	0.002	0.009	0.009
Satsuma mandarin (*Miyagawa-wase*)	0.043	0.001	0.047	0.047
Satsuma mandarin (*Imamura*)	0.172	0.001	0.175	0.175
ponkan	0.171	0.005	0.176	0.176
oyu	0.016	—	0.016	0.016
kumquat	0.007	0.002	0.009	0.009

[a]Values are given in μg of tocopherol per 100 mg of citrus essential oil.
[b]Tr is less than 0.001 μg.

Standard samples of both α- and γ-tocopherol of 0.4 M (0.01 μmole in 25 ml of the test solution) were not as antioxodative, about 30% of RLPR; however, that of δ-tocopherol showed antioxidative activity as low as that of RLPR. Several extracts from sesame oil and sesamol showed lower antioxidative effects than γ-tocopherol as given in the previous report (Fukuda et al., 1985). On the other hand, tested solutions comprising an individual isomer of α-, γ-, and δ-tocopherol, which were preliminarily adjusted to the mean concentrations in citrus essential oils of 0.006 μM, 0.0002 μM, and 0.0002 μM, respectively, showed comparatively low antioxidative activities, although above 31% of RLPR. It has been reported that all constituents extracted from grapefruit oil as antioxidants showed higher antioxidative effects than α-tocopherol, even as high as BHT (Tokoro, 1997). These results suggest that the tocopherols enhance the antioxidative activities of citrus essential oils only slightly, the flavor components being primarily responsible for antioxidation. It is expected that citrus essential oils and their related flavor components may contribute to the prevention of oxidation in foods and inhibit lipid oxidation that results in chronic diseases in the body.

6.1.4 Other Antioxidative Studies of Citrus Fruits

Other compounds included in citrus fruits such as phenolic compounds, flavonoids, cumarins, and carotenoids, which have some inhibitory effects on cancer, may contribute to the antioxidative activities of citrus oils (Miyake et al., 1997, Yano, 1998; Kawaii et al., 1999, Rapisarda et al., 1999, Manthey, 2004).

Rapisarda et al. (1999) reported the antioxidant effectiveness as influenced by phenolic content of fresh oranges. Several fresh orange juices, obtained from five different *Citrus sinensis* (L.) Osbeck varieties (three pigmented varieties, Moro, Sanguinello, and Tarocco, and two blond varieties, Valencia late and Washington navel), were subjected to antioxidant profile determination for total polyphenols, flavanones, anthocyanins, hydroxycinnamic acids, and ascorbic acid. The antioxidant activity of these juices was then assessed by means of different in vitro tests. All orange juices tested showed an evident antioxidant effect. They reported the following: (1) the antioxidant efficiency of orange juices may be attributed, in a significant part at least, to their content of total phenols; (2) ascorbic acid seems to play a minor role; (3) the antioxidant activity of orange juices is related not only to structural features of phytochemicals contained in them, but also to their capability to interact with biomembranes; and (4) as to pigmented juices, their antioxidant efficiency appears to be widely influenced by the anthocyanin level. One could speculate that the supply of natural antioxidant phenols through daily consumption of orange juice might provide additional protection against in vivo oxidation of cellular molecules.

Nogata et al. (1996) reported the inhibitory activities of the albedo extracts of 42 species and cultivars of the genus *Citrus* and those of two *Fortunella* and one *Poncirus* species against rat platelet cyclooxygenase and lipoxygenase. Among the species investigated, the extract of Lumie (*Citrus lumia*) was shown to possess the highest inhibitory activity against cyclooxygenase (IC_{50} = 24 μg/mL), and that of Shuto (*Citrus aurantium*) was the highest against lipoxygenase (IC_{50} = 56 μg/mL). The albedo extracts of citrus from the same taxonomic group appeared to have similar inhibitory tendencies toward these enzymes. The flavedo extract of ripe Lumie inhibited cyclooxygenase to the same degree as the albedo, more than the pulp extract. The flavedo, pulp, and juice extracts of ripe Ponkan (*C. reticulata*) also inhibited lipoxygenase in addition to the albedo extract. Both the flavedo and albedo tissues were shown to be effective sources of inhibitory compounds against cyclooxygenase and lipoxygenase.

These results support the view that citrus fruits and their essential oils are highly available and may be active in the body as antioxidants and free radical scavengers. It is expected that citrus essential oils and their related flavor components may contribute to the prevention of oxidation in foods and inhibit lipid oxidation that results in chronic diseases in the body.

6.2 INHIBITORY FORMATION OF CARCINOGEN

Masayoshi Sawamura

There are many kinds of carcinogenic factors in everyday life. Physical factors are, for instance, radioactive rays such as α-, β-, and X-rays, cosmic rays, and ultraviolet and infrared rays. Chemical factors are aflatoxin, cycasin, and alkaloids from vegetable resources; nitrates, nitrates, and preservative chemicals from food additives; DDT, BHC, and PCB from chemical industries; asbestos, vanadium oxides, and chromates from minerals, and so forth. *N*-Nitroso compounds are also known as strong carcinogens. Table 6.5 shows carcinogenic and acute toxic activities of *N*-nitrosoamines (Nakamura and Tomita, 1992).

TABLE 6.5. Carcinogenesis and acute toxin of *N*-nitroso compouonds

Carcinogenicity log $(1/D_{50})$	*N*-Nitroso-	Carcinogenic Level		LD_{50}*2 mg/kg
		D_{50}*1	$\log(1/D_{50})$	
Very strong	diethylamine	0.00063	3.2	216–280
(>3.0)	methyl-2-chloroethylamine	0.00061	3.2	22
	metnylbenzylamine	0.00080	3.1	18
Strong	methylcyclohexylamine	0.0010	3.0	30
(2.1–3.0)	dimethylamine	0.0054	2.3	27–41
	di-*n*-propylamine	0.0088	2.1	480
Medium	piperidine	0.012	1.9	200
(1.1–2.0)	morphorine	0.011	1.9	282–320
	ethyl-2-hydroxyethylamine	0.016	1.8	7500
	di-*n*-butyllamine	0.025	1.6	1200
	methylaniline	0.025	1.6	
	n-butyl-4-hydroxybutylamine	0.031	1.5	1800
	pyrolidine	0.039	1.4	900
Weak	di-*n*-amylamine	0.26	0.6	1750
(≤1.0)	sarcosine	0.24	0.6	5000
	diethanolamine			5000
None	dicyclohexylamine	—	—	5000
	proline ethyl ester	—	—	5000

*1Minimum dose to cause cancer in 50% of tested rats (mol/kg body weight).
*2Minimum oral dose to cause LD_{50}.

Diethylamine, methyl-2-chloroethylamine, and methylbenzylamine are at the highest level, and dimethylamine also has a strong carcinogenicity. It may be said that higher levels of carcinogenic compounds show lower levels of toxic activity. Figure 6.3 shows the cancer induction mechanism from *N*-nitrosoamines. α-Carbon of nitrosodimethylamines is first oxidized by the P-450 enzyme from cytochrome to form α-hydroxide derivatives, which form aldehydes and diazohydroxides by heterogeneous or nonenzymatic reactions. Diazohydoxides are so unstable that they are decomposed into carbonium ions via alkyldiazonium. This reactive carbonium ion will finally alkylize DNA to cause necrosis, mutagenesis, or carcinogenesis (Nakamura and Tomita, 1992).

Citrus flavor is a favorite in most parts of the world, and the aroma essence is important in the food-flavoring, cosmetics, and perfume industries. According to longstanding customs, we generally consume meat, fish, and/or their processed forms together with vegetables. This pattern of dietary combination has long been considered to be good for health. However, these foods contain substantial

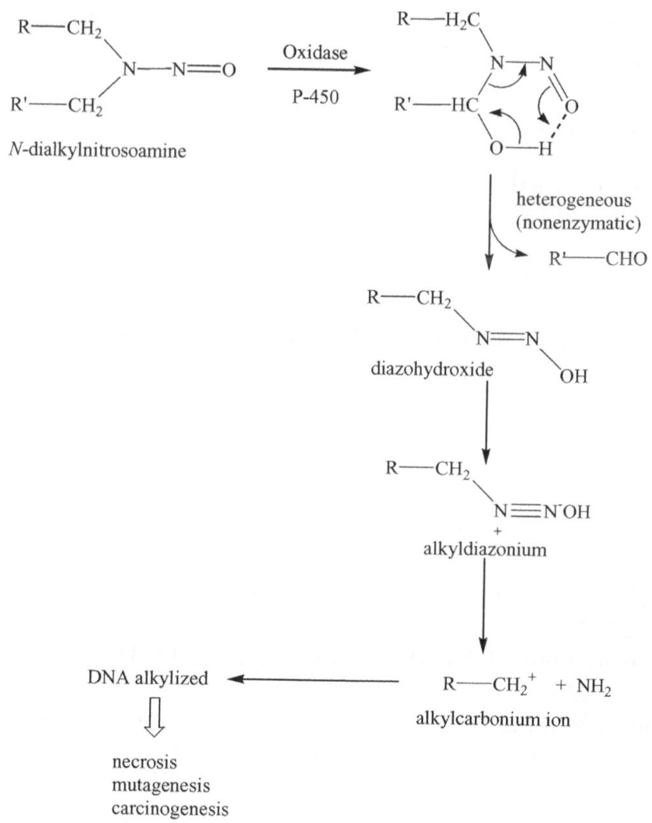

Figure 6.3. Metabolic activation of *N*-nitrosodialkylamine.

amounts of several kinds of amines and nitrates or nitrites. It is well-known that saliva is always a major source of nitrite for humans because the nitrates found in vegetables and other sources are readily converted by nitrate reductase in nature or in the human body (Vogtmann and Biedermann, 1985). Therefore, it is probable that nitrosoamines, including tertiary amines and quaternary ammonium compounds as well as secondary amines (Fiddler et al., 1972), would be formed in our organs during the process of digesting the diet or in blood after absorption. However, the food we consume in a usual meal also contains a number of foodstuffs that inhibit the formation of carcinogens, promote immunological functions, and supply nutrients. Besides, we possess natural defense mechanisms such as detoxification of potentially harmful compounds and immunological and biological responses. It is known that ascorbic acid and tocopherols, for instance, inhibit the formation of *N*-nitrosodimethylamine (NDMA) in vivo (Walters, 1981; Ohshima and Bartsch, 1981). In some cases, NDMA can be metabolized by peroxidase from horseradish (Stiborova et al., 1997). Citrus fruits are rich in essential oils, including terpene hydrocarbons, alcohols, aldehydes, and esters. It is not uncommon to consume the essential oils coincidentally when we eat fresh fruits or dishes seasoned with citrus fruits. Let us examine the effects of citrus essential oils and their components on the inhibition of formation of NDMA in vitro (Sawamura et al., 1999, 2005).

6.2.1 Experimental

The citrus samples used in the study are shown in Table 6.6. Essential oils were prepared by the cold-pressing method, as described in Chapter 2 (Section 2.5, Cold Pressing).

The assay for NDMA was performed by modifying the method used by Achiwa et al. (1997). Each 0.5 mL of 50 mM dimethylamine and sodium nitrite, the pH values of which were adjusted at 3.6 with 5% acetic acid in advance, and 10 μL of Tween 20 were mixed with 10 μL of essential oil or authentic compound in a brown vessel (3 mL) with a tightly screwed cap with an inner seal made of Teflon®. Water was used for the control instead of either essential oil or authentic compound. It was reported that Tween 20 was a good emulsifier in an O/W-type emulsion (Sirendi et al., 1998). Incubation was carried out for 24 h at 37°C with shaking at 50 strokes/min. After a 24-h period, the solutions were filtered through a 0.22-μL nitrate cellulose membrane prior to high-performance liquid chromatography (HPLC) injection. The measurement was triplicated. The wastes were treated with 2 N NaOH to break down NDMA.

The measurement of NDMA was carried out by HPLC. Absorbance was monitored at 220 nm. A reverse-phase column, Wakosil 5C18 (4.6 mm I.D. × 250 mm, Wako Pure Chemical Industries), was used. The column temperature was kept at 40°C, and 5% methanol was used isocratically as the mobile phase at 1.0 mL/min. All of the chemical reagents used for HPLC were of the highest purity from Wako Pure Chemical Industries. Water used in the experiment was Milli-Q. The incubation temperature for the NDMA assay was 37°C,

TABLE 6.6. Samples of *Citrus* genus

Number	Botanical Name	Common Name	Species[a]
1	*Citrus junos* Sieb. ex Tanaka	yuzu	*C. ichangensis*
2	*C. junos* Sieb. ex Tanaka	mukakuyuzu or seedless yuzu	*C. ichangensis*
3	*C. sudachi* Hort. ex Shirai	sudachi	*C. ichangensis*
4	*C. inflata* Hort. ex Tanaka	mochiyu	*C. ichangensis*
5	*C. yuko* Hort. ex Tanaka	yuko	*C. ichangensis*
6	*C. ozu* Hort. ex Y.Tanaka	oyu	*C. ichangensis*
7	*C. wilsonii* Tanaka	ichang lemon	*C. ichangensis*
8	*C. aurantifolia* Swingle	lime	*C. aurantifolia*
9	*C. latifolia* Tanaka	Tahiti lime	*C. aurantifolia*
10	*C. bergamia* Risso var. *Fantastico*	bergamot	*C. aurantifolia*
11	*C. bergamia* Risso var. *Balotin*	bergamot	*C. aurantifolia*
12	*C. limon* Burm. f. cv. *Eureka*	Eureka lemon	*C. limon*
13	*C. limon* Burm. f. cv. *Lisbon*	Lisbon lemon	*C. limon*
14	*C. grandis* Osbeck forma *Tosa*	Tosa-buntan	*C. grandisi*
15	*C. paradisi* Macfadyen	grapefruit	*C. paradisi*
16	*C. hassaku* Hort. ex Y. Tanaka	hassaku	*C. paradisi*
17	*C. natudaidai* Hayata	natsudaidai	*C. paradisi*
18	*C. aurantium* Linn. var. *Cyathifera* Y. Tanaka	daidai	*C. aurantium*
19	*C. aurantium* Linn. forma *Kabusu*	kabusu	*C. aurantium*
20	*C. sinensis* Osbeck forma *Valencia*	Valencia orange	*C. sinensis*
21	*C. sinensis* Osbeck var. *Sanguinea* Tanaka forma *Tarocco*	Tarocco orange	*C. sinensis*
22	*C. iyo* Hort. ex Tanaka	Iyokan	*C. sinensis*
23	*C. tamurana* Hort ex Tanaka	Hyuganatsu	*C. sinensis*
24	*C. ujukitsu* Hort. ex Shirai	ujukitsu	*C. sinensis*
25	*C. unshiu* Marcov. forma *Miyagawa-wase*	unshumikan or Satsuma mandarin	*C. reticulata*
26	*C. unshiu* Marcov. forma *Imamura*	unshumikan or Satsuma mandarin	*C. reticulata*
27	*C. reticulata* Blanco cv. *F-2426*	ponkan	*C. reticulata*
28	*Fortunella japonica* Swingle[b]	kinkan or kumquat	*Fortunella japonica*

[a]Classified by Swingle.
[b]Another genus in the Rutaceae family comprising the *Citrus* genus.

whereas the HPLC was carried out at 40°C, because we intended to reduce the analysis time to as short as possible. It was checked primarily that there was no different peak on each chromatogram regulated at 37° and 40°C.

6.2.2 Inhibitory Effect on the Formation of NDMA by Citrus Essential Oils

The formation of NDMA in the presence of citrus essential oils in model solutions was examined. The optimum pH of this reaction is ~3.5 to yield NDMA (Walters, 1981). The reactivity is extremely low at pH 1 and 2. The foodstuffs we eat pass successively through the stomach, duodenum, small intestine, and large intestine after mastication in the mouth. Some foods are even absorbed into the blood after digestion in each organ. Thus, the foodstuffs taken into the body are assumed to be in the pH range of 1–7. Considering the occurrence of carcinogens in the conditions in vivo, we preferred employing the optimum pH of 3.6 in this reaction.

The results are shown in Table 6.7. It was demonstrated that all kinds of citrus essential oils used in our experiment inhibited the formation of NDMA to some extent. The essential oils presenting an inhibition ratio between 20 and 50% were as follows: oyu; Tahiti lime; Eureka lemon; Tosa-buntan; grapefruit and hassaku; daidai; orange (*Tarocco*), and Hyuganatsu. The second category, with between 50 and 70% inhibition, included the following: seedless yuzu, sudachi, yuko, and ichang-lemon; lime, bergamot (*Balotin*), and Lisbon lemon; natsudaidai; kabosu; Valencia orange; Satsuma mandarin (*Imamura*); kumquat. The third category, with an inhibitory ratio of >70%, includes the following essential oils: yuzu and mochiyu; bergamot (*Fantastico*); Iyokan and ujukitsu; Satsuma mandarin (*Miyagawa-wase*); and ponkan. The essential oil of ujukitsu

TABLE 6.7. Inhibitory effect of citrus essential oils and their components on the formation of *N*-nitrosodimethylamine

Inhibition (%)	Citrus Essential Oils and Their Components
>70%	yuzu, mochiyu, yuko, ujukitusu, iyokan, ponkan, Satsuma mandarin (*Miyagawa-wase*), bergamot (*Fantastico*), kumquat myrcene, α-terpinene, terpinolene
50–70%	seedless yuzu, sudachi, yuko, ichang lemon, lime (*Mexican*), bergamot (*Balotin*), lemon (*Lisbon*), Tosa-buntan, grapefruit, kabuse, orange (*Valencia*), natsudaidai, hyuganatsu, unshu (*Imamura*)
	α-pinene, β-pinene, γ-terpinene, linalool, α-terpineol, citral
20–50%	oyu, hassaku, daidai, orange (*Tarocco*), lime (*Tahiti*), lemon (*Eureka*) grapefruit, hyuganatsu
	limonene, *p*-cymene, octanal, decanal, 1-octanol, terpinen-4-ol, geranyl acetate, geraniol, 1-decanol, citronellol, citronellal, nootkatone

showed an inhibition ratio as high as 85%. Although it seems to be difficult to find a relationship between species and inhibitory effect, it is clear that citrus essential oils affect the formation of NDMA.

6.2.3 Inhibitory Effects of the Formation of NDMA by Authentic Compounds

The results are shown in Table 6.7. Terpene hydrocarbons such as myrcene, α-terpinene, terpinolene, γ-terpinene, α-pinene, and β-pinene showed a ratio of inhibition of formation of NDMA >50%. However, the inhibitory ratio of limonene was 34% and that of *p*-cymene was only a few percent. The chemical structures of those compounds are given in Table 6.7. Myrcene, an open-chain monoterpene with three double bonds, presented the highest inhibition among all of the compounds examined, 87%. Most oxygenated compounds showed a slight inhibition, and ratios of terpinen-4-o1, 1-decanol, and nootkatone were almost 0%. The inhibitory ratios were ~65% in linalool and α-terpineol and ~50% in citral.

6.2.4 Inhibitory Effects of Essential Oils and Authentic Compounds

The major volatile compositions of cold-pressed oils are shown in Table 6.8. Ujukitsu (sample 24) and mochiyu (sample 4) were exceedingly abundant in myrcene compared with others, 28.3 and 20.6%, respectively. The inhibitory effect of myrcene on the formation of NDMA was the highest, as shown in Table 6.7. It is suggested that the inhibitory efficiency of most essential oils depends on composition. In the family of *C. ichangensis* (samples 1–7), except for oyu (sample 6), the higher efficiency may be caused by the composition of essential oils having a total of >10% myrcene, α-terpinene, and γ-terpinene. The higher efficiency of yuko (sample 5) may be caused by the composition of 21.3% γ-terpinene and 0.5% α-terpineol. In *C. aurantifolia* and *C. limon* (samples 8–13), the combined percent of β-pinene and γ-terpinene ranged from 12.4 to 31.1%. It is also considered that the characteristic composition of neral and geranial in limes and that of linalool and linalyl acetate in bergamots contributed to their inhibitory efficiency. As the essential oils of samples 16–28, except sample 24, were mainly composed of limonene in a proportion of ≥90%, limonene would play the principal role of inhibitory efficiency for these species. In addition to the limonene component, the inhibitory efficiency of the essential oils from samples 22–27 is likely to be further enhanced by a considerable amount of γ-terpinene and linalool. The essential oils of oyu (sample 6), hassaku (sample 16), daidai (sample 18), and Orange (*Tarocco*) (sample 21), which had poor inhibitory efficiencies, contained little of the more effective compounds such as α-terpinene, terpinolene, linalool, and α-terpineol. Kumquat (sample 28) showed a strong inhibition, although the component content was low except for limonene. Factors other than essential oil components that contribute to the inhibition of the formation of NDMA may exist. Achiwa et al. (1997) reported that the juices of lemon,

TABLE 6.8. Volatile components[a] of citrus essential oils

Compound	Sample[b]												
	1	2	3	4	5	6	7	8	9	10	11	12	13
α-pinene	1.8	1.8	1.6	0.3	3.3	0.7	3.3	3.6	3.2	1.6	1.3	2.3	2.6
β-pinene	0.7	0.7	0.5	0.1	1.8	*	1.8	13.4	13.0	8.9	6.8	10.5	14.0
myrcene	2.2	2.1	1.3	20.6	1.3	0.3	0.7	1.4	1.3	0.9	0.7	1.6	1.4
α-terpinene	0.2	0.3	1.4	*	0.3	0	2.4	0.3	0.3	0.2	0.1	*	*
limonene	78.1	78.1	69.1	77.2	66.6	93.9	68.8	50.5	52.2	38.8	24.3	69.7	64.6
γ-erpinene	9.3	9.1	7.5	0.8	21.3	*	16.0	17.7	17.0	8.3	5.6	8.2	10.3
p-cymene	0.4	0.4	0.4	*	0.2	*	*	0.1	0.1	0.3	*	*	*
terpinolene	0.4	0.5	0.3	*	0.9	*	0.7	0.7	0.7	0.3	0.2	0.3	0.4
octanal	*	*	*	0	0.1	0	0	*	*	0	*	*	0.1
citronellal	*	*	*	*	*	*	0	0.1	0.1	0	0	0.1	*
decanal	*	*	0.1	*	0.1	0	0	*	0.1	0.1	*	*	*
linalool	1.8	1.8	0.3	*	0.2	0.1	0.2	*	0.2	4.2	18.2	0.2	0.2
1-octanol	0	0	*	0	0.1	0	0	0	*	0	0	0	0
linalyl acetate	0	0	0	0	0	0	0	0	0	32.1	39.0	0	0
terpinen-4-o1	0	0	0	0	0.1	*	*	*	0	0.1	0.1	*	0
neral	*	0	0	*	0.1	*	*	1.0	1.2	0.2	0.2	1.1	0.6
α-terpineol	0.1	0.1	0.2	*	0.5	0.1	*	0.3	0.4	0.2	0.1	0.2	0.3
geranial	*	*	*	*	*	0	0	2.1	2.3	0.3	0	1.0	1.13
getanyl acetate	0	0	0	0	0	0	*	0.7	1.0	0.3	0.2	0.16	0.23
1-decanol	*	*	0	0	0	0	0	0	0	*	0	0	*
citronellol	0	0	0	0	0	*	0	*	0	0	*	*	*
nerol	0	0	0	0	0	*	*	0.1	0	*	0.1	*	*
geraniol	0	0	*	*	*	0	*	0.1	*	*	*	*	0.1
nootkatone	0	0	0	0	0	0	0	*	0	0.1	*	0	0

[a] Given in relative peak area percent.
[b] The sample number is coincident with that of Table 6.6.
[c] *, <0.1%.

Satsuma mandarin, and grapefruit demonstrated an NDMA inhibitory capacity. This suggested that ascorbic acid in those juices did not always play a major role in inhibition and that there existed other compounds that could cause inhibition. One of the factors may be the presence of some essential oil in those juices. Recently, terpenoids such as limonene, farnesol, geraniol, and perillyl alcohol have been reported to be effective in the inhibition of pancreatic or mammary cancer growth (Burke et al., 1997; Crowell, 1997; Gould, 1997; Nakaizumi et al., 1997). It was also reported that the administration of terpene hydrocarbons such as limonene and carvone to mice reduced the occurrence of cancer because of increased activity of glutathione *S*-transferase (Zheng et al., 1992a, 1992b). Terpenes and citrus essential oils containing high levels of them seem to have the potential to act through multiple mechanisms in the chemoprevention of

14	15	16	17	18	19	20	21	22	23	24	25	26	27	28
1.1	0.5	1.2	1.2	0.5	0.6	0.5	0.5	1.2	1.4	1.4	1.0	1.2	1.2	0.4
0.6	*c	0.4	0.3	0.7	0.9	*	*	0.3	0.8	0.4	0.2	0.3	0.3	*
1.2	1.3	1.8	1.7	1.6	1.7	1.8	1.8	1.8	1.8	28.3	1.8	1.8	1.8	1.8
0.1	0	0	0	0	0	0	0	0	*	0.1	0	0	0	0
75.3	83.1	89.8	90.2	94.7	92.0	95.8	96.6	88.2	84.5	59.2	90.6	89.7	89.9	96.7
4.9	0.1	5.6	4.9	0.1	0	*	*	5.4	7.5	7.6	3.5	4.6	4.6	0.1
0.1	0	*	0.1	0	0	0	0	0.1	*	0.1	0.2	0.2	0.1	*
0.4	*	0.2	0.2	*	*	*	*	0.2	0.3	0.3	0.2	0.2	0.2	*
0.2	0.5	0.1	0.3	0.1	0.2	0.3	0.1	0.1	*	*	0.1	*	0.2	*
0.2	0.1	*	0	0	0	*	*	*	0.2	*	*	*	0.1	0
0.4	0.5	0.1	0.2	0.1	0.1	0.1	0.1	0.1	*	0	0.1	0.1	0.1	*
0.2	0.2	0.1	0.1	0.2	1.1	0.4	0.3	1.3	1.3	0.7	0.4	0.3	0.6	0.1
0	0	0	*	0	0	*	*	*	*	0	0	0	*	0
0	0	0	0	0	0	0	0	0	0	0	0	0	0	0
0.1	0.2	*	*	0	0	*	0	*	*	*	*	*	0	0
0.1	0	*	*	*	0.1	0.1	*	*	*	0.1	*	0	*	0
0.1	0.1	0.1	0.1	*	0.1	0.1	0.1	0.1	0.1	0.1	0.1	0.1	0.1	*
0.2	0.1	0.1	0	*	0.1	0.1	0.1	0	0	0	0	0	*	0
0.1	0.1	*	0.1	0.1	0.1	0	*	0.1	*	*	*	0.1	*	0.1
0	0	0	0	0	0	0	0	0	0	0	0	0	0	0
*	*	*	0	*	0	*	*	*	*	0	*	*	*	0
*	0	0	0	*	0	*	*	0	0	0.1	0	0	*	0
*	*	0	0	*	0	*	0	0	0	*	0	0	0	0
0.4	0.1	*	*	0	0	0	0	0	0	0	*	0	0	0

cancers, although the mechanism of inhibition has not been clarified. Even if the inhibition of NDMA formation might not be cancer chemopreventative, it is substantially preferable in our diet to minimize the factors that act in the formation of carcinogens. Although the present study was carried out in a model solution, this is the first proof of inhibition of NDMA formation by citrus essential oils and their components. The present work also encompassed another functional property, that is, the inhibitory effects of citrus essential oils and terpenes on the formation of NDMA. This knowledge will contribute to improvement of our daily life and applications for food processing.

In conclusion, it was demonstrated that citrus essential oils inhibited the formation of NDMA in a given reaction medium and that the compositions of citrus essential oils were also related to the inhibitory efficiency.

6.2.5 Inhibitory Effect of Yuzu Essential Oil on the Formation of NDMA in Vegetables

As described so far, we have seen that citrus essential oils and their components had an inhibitory effect on the formation of NDMA in a model solution. In particular, the essential oil of yuzu (*Citrus junos* Tanaka), which is the most popular sour citrus fruit used for cuisine, dressing, and cosmetics in Japan, exhibits a high inhibitory effect on the formation of NDMA as shown in Table 6.7. The inhibitory effect of citrus essential oils in vegetable foods in the presence of saliva was further demonstrated.

N-Nitroso compounds are known as *strong carcinogens*. Among them, the ones that have been examined most are nitrosamines (Lijinsky, 1999). Nitrosamines are formed by *N*-nitrosation of secondary amines with nitrite in an acidic condition. The precursors commonly occur in a wide variety of foods. Secondary amines also occur in meats, cured meat products, and smoked fish. Nitrite is often added to foods such as hams and sausages as an antimicrobial or coloring substance (Kikugawa, 2003). Nitrate is a precursor of nitrite, and vegetable foods are a main source of nitrate (Vogtmann and Biedermann, 1985). The content of nitrate in crops depends on the species, genetic and environmental factors, and cultivation conditions. In certain crops, for instance, the levels are as high as 1000 mg/kg or more. The level of nitrites in plants and water, on the other hand, is commonly very low. It is well known that human saliva is a major source of nitrite (Vogtmann and Biedermann, 1985). About 75% of the nitrate taken into the body is excreted in urine and 25% is secreted in saliva. Twenty percent of the nitrate in saliva is readily reduced into nitrite by nitrate oxidoreductase (E. C. 1.6.6.1. NADH). WHO/FAO (1995) have suggested that the acceptable daily intakes (ADI) of nitrate and nitrite per kg of body weight are 3.7 and 0.6 mg, respectively. However, nitrate intake in Japan is about 1.5 times that of ADI. About 87% of the nitrate source is from vegetable foods (Sohn and Yoneyama, 1996), because the Japanese diet tends to be richer in vegetables than that of Europe, the United States, and other countries. It is reported that the mortality of Japanese by stomach cancer is higher than that of Europeans because of a large intake of nitrates from foods (Tanimura, 1980). Nevertheless, the probability of the development of cancer is statistically very low since substances that inhibit the formation of nitroso compounds, such as ascorbic acid, tocopherols, and polyphenols, are taken simultaneously from ordinary food (Kurechi et al., 1980; Mirvish, 1986; Wu et al., 1993). It is reported that the extracts from persimmon (*Diospyros kaki* Thunb.), knotweed (*Polygonum longisetum*), and Japanese-aucuba (*Aucuba japonica*) remarkably inhibited mutagenicity by the C-nitro and C-nitroso compounds formed by the reaction of sorbic acid and sodium nitrite (Achiwa, et al., 1996). The consumption of whole strawberry, kale juice, and garlic juice has been reported to be effective in the inhibition of *N*-nitrosodimethylamine (NDMA) (Chung et al., 2002). Terpene hydrocarbons such as limonene and carvone reduced the occurrence of cancer in mice due to activation of glutathione *S*-transferase (Zheng, et al., 1992a, b). It is also reported that limonene, one of the major volatile components of citrus essential oils, possessed anticarcinogenesis against mammary, lung, stomach, and skin cancers (Gould, 1997; Nakaizumi et al., 1997). In this section, the inhibitory effects of vegetable foods and citrus essential oils in the presence of saliva and the mechanism inhibitory effects of terpene hydrocarbons in citrus essential oils on the formation of NDMA will be described.

6.2.6 Assay for NDMA and Its Derivatives

Preparation of Vegetable Samples for NDMA Assay. Thirty-one kinds of vegetable samples used in this study, including leaves, roots, seeds, fruits, herbs, and mushrooms, were purchased at the market as shown in Table 6.9. Each sample (100 g) was treated with a juicer for 1 min. The juice was centrifuged at 9000 *g* for 10 min at 5°C. The supernatant (25 mL) was adjusted to pH 3.6 with an aqueous solution of 10% acetic acid and then diluted to 100 mL with Milli-Q water. The dilute was filtered through a 0.2-μm membrane filter. These vegetable extracts were used for the NDMA assay. The saliva from three donors in our laboratory, who were in good health and nonsmokers, was sampled, mixed together, and immediately kept in ice until it was used in the experiment.

Determination of Nitrite and Nitrate. The contents of nitrite and nitrate in the 31 vegetable samples were determined by HPLC according to the method of Kunugi et al. (1983). 2,6-Xylenol was used as an internal standard.

LC-MS. A Shimadzu system of LC-10 AD HPLC coupled with an LC-MS 2010 mass spectrometer was used for LC-MS. A Cosmosil 5C18 column (3.0 mm I.D. × 150 mm, Nacalai Tesque, Tokyo) was used. The column temperature was kept at 37°C. An aqueous solution of 5% methanol was used as mobile phase at 0.8 mL/min. The analytical conditions for LC-MS 2010 were as follows: nitrogen gas flow rate, 1.5 L/min; CDL temperature, 250°C; block temperature, 200°C; detector voltage, 1.5 kV; mode, ESI; probe voltage, 4.5 kV; scan, 40–1500 m/z.

6.2.7 Effects of Vegetable Extracts on NDMA Formation with or without Yuzu Oil

The effects of vegetable extracts in a given model on the formation of NDMA with or without yuzu oil were investigated. The results are shown in Table 6.10. The inhibition ratio was calculated using the following equation:

$$\text{Inhibition ratio (\%)} = 100\% - (\text{percent of NDMA formation})$$

Most vegetable extracts used in the present study little affected the inhibition of NDMA formation. Celery, Chinese cabbage, and salad parsley slightly inhibited the formation of NDMA to the extents of 1%, 4%, and 4%, respectively.

TABLE 6.9. Vegetable samples

Tissue	Common Name	Botanical Name
Leaves	Cabbage	*Brassica oleracea* L. var. *capitata* L.
	Celery	*Apium graveolens* L. var. *dulce* DC.
	Chinese cabbage	*Brassica campestris* L.
	Komatsuna	*Brassica campestris* L.
	Lettuce	*Lactuca sativa* L.
	Mitsuba (Japanese horwort)	*Cryptotaenia japonica* Makino
	Potherb mustard	*Brassica rapa* var. *lancinifolia*
	Spinach	*Spinacia oleracea* L.
Roots	Carrot	*Daucus carota* L.
	Carrot *(kintoki)*	*Daucus carota* L.
	Garlic	*Allium sativum* L.
	Ginger	*Zingiber officinale* Rosc.
	Lotus (root)	*Nelumbo nucifera* Gaertn
	Onion (white)	*Allium cepa* L.
Seeds	Bean sprouts	*Vigna radiata* Wilcz.
	Peas	*Pisum sativum* L.
Fruits	Bitter gourd (Balsam pear)	*Momordica charantia* L.
	Cucumber	*Cucumis sativus* L.
	Eggplant	*Solanum melongena* L.
	Sweet pepper	*Capsicum annum* L.
	Tomato	*Licopersicon esculentum* Mill
Herbs	Coriander	*Coriandrum sativum* L.
	Dill	*Anethum graveolen* L.
	Italian parsley	*Petroselinum sativum* Hoffm.
	Lemon balm	*Melissa offisinalis* L.
	Mint	*Mentha sp.*
	Rocket	*Eruca vesicaria sativa* Mill
	Salad parsley	*Petroselinum sativum* Hoffm.
	Thyme	*Thymus vulgaris* L.
Mushrooms	Hen of the wood	*Grifola frondosa* (Dicks: Fr.) S. F. Gray
	Shiitake mushroom	*Lentinus edodes* (Berk.) Sing.

There was no significant inhibitory effect of NDMA in cabbage and carrot (*kintoki*) ($P < 0.05$). The other 26 kinds of vegetable extracts even accelerated the formation of NDMA. The vegetables that presented the formation ratio of NDMA from 101 to 110% were mitsuba, potherb mustard, carrot, bean sprouts, bitter gourd, cucumber, sweet pepper, Italian parsley, and mint. The vegetables with effects ranging from 110 to 120% of NDMA formation ratio were as follows: komatsuna, lettuce, spinach, ginger, onion (white), peas, eggplant, tomato, lemon balm, thyme, and shiitake mushroom. The vegetables with effects increasing the

TABLE 6.10. Contents of nitrate, nitrite, and ascorbic acid in vegetable samples, and the formation of NDMA in vegetable extracts with or without yuzu oil and saliva

Samples	Contents[a]			NDMA formation (%)[b]			
	Nitrate	Nitrite	Ascorbic Acid	Absence of Saliva[c]		Presence of Saliva[d]	
	mg/100 g	μg/100 g	mg/100 g	Juice Alone	Yuzu Oil Added	Juice Alone	Yuzu Oil added
Cabbage	158 ± 1.7	230 ± 1.0	34 ± 1.7	100 ± 1.5	34 ± 0.4	103 ± 1.4	28 ± 0.4
Celery	210 ± 2.0	100 ± 1.7	1 ± 0.2	99 ± 2.2	26 ± 0.5	96 ± 0.7	27 ± 1.1
Chinese cabbage	159 ± 2.6	630 ± 2.4	11 ± 1.0	96 ± 2.6	35 ± 1.3	107 ± 2.3	32 ± 0.9
Komatsuna	484 ± 1.7	750 ± 2.6	29 ± 1.7	117 ± 2.2	26 ± 1.9	101 ± 2.7	36 ± 2.2
Lettuce	81 ± 2.0	360 ± 1.7	2 ± 0.2	115 ± 1.3	37 ± 0.4	92 ± 2.1	24 ± 0.3
Mitsuba	560 ± 1.8	230 ± 1.8	2 ± 0.3	105 ± 1.7	25 ± 0.2	91 ± 0.8	29 ± 0.4
Potherb mustard	535 ± 1.6	650 ± 2.0	18 ± 1.4	106 ± 1.0	28 ± 0.7	100 ± 2.6	31 ± 1.1
Spinach	123 ± 1.1	710 ± 2.5	65 ± 1.2	114 ± 2.7	37 ± 1.1	99 ± 1.5	28 ± 1.1
Carrot	9 ± 0.8	70 ± 1.1	6 ± 0.5	110 ± 2.6	22 ± 1.6	115 ± 1.0	25 ± 0.1
Carrot (*kintoki*)	14 ± 0.8	180 ± 1.9	10 ± 0.9	101 ± 1.7	34 ± 0.8	94 ± 0.5	29 ± 0.9
Garlic	3 ± 0.3	10 ± 0.9	5 ± 0.4	124 ± 0.7	35 ± 0.5	114 ± 2.4	27 ± 1.5
Ginger	10 ± 0.4	20 ± 0.9	0.4 ± 0.03	113 ± 2.3	41 ± 1.6	114 ± 1.2	35 ± 1.9
Lotus (root)	7 ± 0.3	10 ± 0.2	30 ± 1.7	138 ± 1.5	39 ± 1.2	124 ± 1.7	44 ± 1.1
Onion (white)	6 ± 0.2	10 ± 0.4	6 ± 0.2	115 ± 2.2	46 ± 0.7	99 ± 1.4	31 ± 0.2
Bean sprouts	5 ± 0.3	30 ± 1.0	3 ± 0.2	110 ± 1.8	41 ± 0.7	91 ± 1.0	26 ± 0.8
Peas	15 ± 0.7	210 ± 2.4	25 ± 0.7	112 ± 0.8	26 ± 0.2	92 ± 2.6	24 ± 0.7
Bitter gourd	84 ± 1.0	250 ± 1.6	48 ± 0.7	109 ± 2.0	36 ± 0.4	119 ± 1.4	33 ± 0.9
Cucumber	66 ± 0.8	150 ± 1.2	5 ± 0.2	102 ± 1.1	28 ± 0.8	84 ± 2.2	25 ± 0.1
Eggplant	8 ± 0.2	130 ± 2.2	4 ± 0.3	115 ± 1.2	34 ± 0.2	104 ± 1.0	32 ± 1.0
Sweet pepper	42 ± 0.9	90 ± 1.7	49 ± 1.1	102 ± 1.4	27 ± 0.9	110 ± 1.8	36 ± 1.9

TABLE 6.10. *Continued*

Samples	Contents[a]			NDMA formation (%)[b]			
	Nitrate	Nitrite	Ascorbic Acid	Absence of Saliva[c]		Presence of Saliva[d]	
	mg/100 g	μg/100 g	mg/100 g	Juice Alone	Yuzu Oil Added	Juice Alone	Yuzu Oil added
Tomato	50 ± 1.5	40 ± 1.1	5 ± 0.1	115 ± 0.8	45 ± 0.6	113 ± 1.3	39 ± 1.4
Coriander	457 ± 1.1	110 ± 1.7	0.4 ± 0.01	136 ± 0.9	56 ± 1.1	121 ± 1.0	46 ± 0.8
Dill	11 ± 0.8	20 ± 1.1	0.3 ± 0.01	129 ± 1.2	48 ± 1.9	109 ± 0.6	50 ± 0.5
Italian parsley	404 ± 1.1	10 ± 0.9	0.4 ± 0.01	106 ± 2.4	49 ± 1.2	113 ± 1.9	44 ± 1.4
Lemon balm	336 ± 1.1	490 ± 2.5	3 ± 0.2	115 ± 2.0	58 ± 1.0	103 ± 1.4	41 ± 1.0
Mint	581 ± 2.5	50 ± 1.0	0.4 ± 0.01	104 ± 1.3	43 ± 0.5	108 ± 1.0	45 ± 0.7
Rocket	471 ± 2.2	50 ± 1.7	23 ± 0.9	136 ± 1.7	51 ± 1.0	94 ± 1.7	32 ± 0.4
Salad parsley	460 ± 1.7	150 ± 1.6	1 ± 0.04	96 ± 1.6	35 ± 0.3	97 ± 0.5	37 ± 0.8
Thyme	20 ± 1.5	160 ± 1.6	0.5 ± 0.04	120 ± 1.1	59 ± 0.7	145 ± 0.5	62 ± 0.4
Hen of the wood	8 ± 0.3	10 ± 0.6	3 ± 0.2	133 ± 1.7	43 ± 0.6	145 ± 1.0	42 ± 0.3
Shiitake mushroom	10 ± 0.5	10 ± 0.3	7 ± 0.2	117 ± 1.3	50 ± 0.6	109 ± 0.7	57 ± 0.3

[a,b]Values are mean ± SD (standard deviation) of triplicates/treament.
[c]Compared with Milli-Q water control 1, which is 100% NDMA formation.
Control 1: A mixture of 0.5 mL of dimethylamine (25 mM), 0.5 mL of sodium nitrite (25 mM), 0.1 mL of Tween 20 (6.55%), and 0.21 mL of Milli-Q water. The total volume came to 1.31 mL.
[d]Compared with Milli-Q water control 2, which is 100% NDMA formation.
Control 2: A mixture of 0.4 mL of dimethylamine (31.25 mM), 0.4 mL of sodium nitrite (31.25 mM), 0.1 mL of Tween 20 (6.55%), 0.2 mL of saliva, and 0.21 mL of Milli-Q water. The total volume was 1.31 mL.

ratio of NDMA from 120 to 140% were garlic, lotus (root), coriander, dill, rocket, and hen of the wood. Achiwa et al. (1997) reported that vegetable juices inhibited the formation of NDMA in the range between 0 and 50%. In our study, among the 21 kinds of vegetable extracts, celery and Chinese cabbage presented a ratio of NDMA formation less than 100%, and the other vegetable extracts exceeded 100%. Most herbs have been used as medicinal plants for thousands of years, primarily as a remedy or antiseptic for digestive disorders. There have been few studies about the effect of herbs on the formation of NDMA. The authors then examined 8 species of herbs, including coriander, dill, Italian parsley, lemon balm, mint, rocket, salad parsley, and thyme. As shown in Table 6.10, only salad parsley slightly inhibited the formation of NDMA. The other herb samples, however, increased the formation of NDMA (104–136%). Two kinds of mushroom samples, hen of the wood and shiitake mushroom, also formed high amounts of NDMA (117 and 133%), as shown in Table 6.10. Neither of the two mushrooms had an inhibitory effect on the formation of NDMA.

The addition of yuzu oil to the reaction mixture containing the vegetable extracts showed high inhibitory effects on the formation of NDMA. The extent of inhibition in the presence of yuzu oil was between 78 and 41%. The vegetables having an inhibitory effect of more than 70% were celery, komatsuna, mitsuba, potherb mustard, carrot, peas, cucumber, and sweet pepper. The vegetables that presented the inhibition ratio of 70 to 60% were cabbage, Chinese cabbage, lettuce, spinach, carrot (*kintoki*), garlic, lotus (root), bitter gourd, eggplant, and salad parsley. Ginger, bean sprouts, onion (white), tomato, dill, Italian parsley, mint, hen of the wood, and shiitake mushroom had inhibitory effects ranging from 50 to 60%. Coriander, lemon balm, rocket, and thyme showed inhibition ratios of more than 40%. From these results, each of the vegetable samples presented the inhibitory effect remarkably when yuzu oil was added. As shown in Table 6.10, among the 31 kinds of vegetable samples, for instance, lotus (root), having a high formation ratio of NDMA, as much as 138%, presented a considerable inhibition by addition of yuzu oil. The formation ratio of NDMA by lotus with yuzu oil was 39%, which was only about one-third of the NDMA formation ratio without yuzu oil. The previous study indicated that yuzu oil presented a higher inhibition ratio of more than 70% (Sawamura, et al., 1999). It was found that the mixture of yuzu oil and vegetable samples highly inhibited NDMA formation, although the inhibitory effect on NDMA formation was not found in vegetable samples alone.

6.2.8 Effects of Vegetable Extracts with Yuzu Oil and Saliva on the Formation of NDMA

The effects of vegetable extracts with saliva on the NDMA formation are shown in Table 6.10. Among the 31 kinds of vegetable extracts, cucumber showed a strong inhibitory effect of NDMA formation (as much as 16%). Celery, lettuce, mitsuba, spinach, carrots (*kintoki*), onion (white), bean sprouts, peas, rocket, and salad parsley presented low inhibitory effects of NDMA (less than 10%). The other vegetable extracts enhanced the formation of NDMA to some extent. The vegetables that presented a formation ratio of NDMA from 101 to 120% were as follows: cabbage, Chinese cabbage, komatsuna, carrot, garlic, ginger, bitter gourd, eggplant, sweet pepper, tomato, dill, Italian parsley, lemon balm, mint, and shiitake mushroom. Lotus (root), coriander, thyme, and hen of the wood increased the formation of NDMA in the range of 120 to 145%. However, each vegetable extract effectively inhibited the formation of NDMA in the presence of yuzu oil. The inhibition ratio of NDMA formation in vegetable extracts and yuzu oil was from 38 to 76%. The vegetables presenting an inhibition ratio of NDMA formation of more than 70% were cabbage, celery, lettuce, mitsuba, spinach, carrot, carrot (*kintoki*), garlic, bean sprouts, peas, and cucumber, and the vegetables with an inhibition ratio between 60 and 70% were Chinese cabbage, komatsuna, potherb mustard, ginger, onion (white), bitter gourd, eggplant, sweet pepper, tomato, rocket, and salad parsley. Thyme showed a low inhibition ratio of 38% even in the presence of yuzu oil. However, the formation ratio of NDMA was as high as 145% in the absence of yuzu oil (Table 6.10). These results suggest that all the vegetable extracts used in this study had an inhibitory effect against the formation of NDMA when yuzu oil was added. Yuzu oil, in other words, does not lose its inhibitory function even in the presence of saliva.

In Table 6.10, the information about the inhibitory effect of yuzu oil in vegetable extracts on NDMA formation in the absence or presence of saliva can be independently obtained. The data for NDMA formation ratio in the absence of saliva could not be directly compared with those in the presence of saliva, because the basic peak areas were different between control 1 and control 2. In order to elucidate the NDMA formation in vegetable extracts in the presence of saliva, the effect of saliva on NDMA formation in vegetable extracts was investigated. It was demonstrated that the formation ratio of NDMA in each vegetable extract was in the range of 106 to 148% compared to control as long as saliva was present. The percentage was figured out as follows: The peak area of juice with saliva was divided by that of juice without saliva (the data are not shown here). In the case of eggplant, for example, the estimate was 106%, while in the case of hen of the wood, it was 148%. These estimations suggest that saliva can promote the formation of NDMA in vegetable extracts.

In this study, it was intact saliva that was added into the reaction mixture for NDMA formation. To examine the effect of bacteria in saliva on the NDMA formation, the saliva samples were filtered through a 0.2-μm membrane filter (Millipore, Tokyo) for removal of bacteria before being added into the reaction mixture. The results indicated that the formation of NDMA increased in the presence of intact saliva samples to the extent of 1.4 times that of the filtered saliva samples. Therefore, it is suggested that the increase in NDMA formation in the vegetable samples with saliva is caused by the reduction of nitrate by bacteria in saliva.

6.2.9 Effect of Ascorbic Acid, Nitrite, Nitrate, and Saliva on the Formation of NDMA

Ascorbic Acid. The contents of ascorbic acid in the 31 vegetable samples ranged from 0.3 to 65.0 mg/100 g, as shown in Table 6.10. Particularly, the contents of ascorbic acid in the herb samples such as Italian parsley, coriander, mint, thyme, and dill were less than 1 mg/100 g. The effect of ascorbic acid on NDMA formation is shown in Figure 6.4. The inhibition of NDMA formation depended on the concentration of ascorbic acid. These results are consistent with the reports that ascorbic acid can inhibit NDMA formation (Kurechi et al., 1980; Mirvish, 1986; Wu et al., 1993). However, the amount of ascorbic acid equivalent to that in vegetables little affected the inhibition of NDMA formation. Spinach contained the highest amount of ascorbic acid (65 mg/100 g) among the vegetable samples, but this level affected only 10% inhibition of NDMA formation.

Nitrite. The nitrite contents of the 31 vegetables were between 10 and 750 μg/100 g, as shown in Table 6.10. It is known that the rate of formation of nitrosamines is proportional to the square of nitrite concentration (Lijinsky, 1999). Although the amount of nitrite equivalent to that analyzed in the vegetables was added to the reaction mixture, there was little increase in NDMA. The results indicated that a small amount of nitrite (10–750 μg/100 g) in vegetables did not affect the formation of NDMA. It is considered that nitrite in vegetables is not a main factor that conducts the formation of NDMA. It is reported that a minor part of nitrite source results from nitrite-containing foods such as preserved meat and certain vegetables, but such a level is generally very low (Gangolli et al., 1994). The main source of nitrite results from the reduction of nitrate into nitrite by oral bacteria (Stephany and Schuller, 1980; Walters and Smith, 1981).

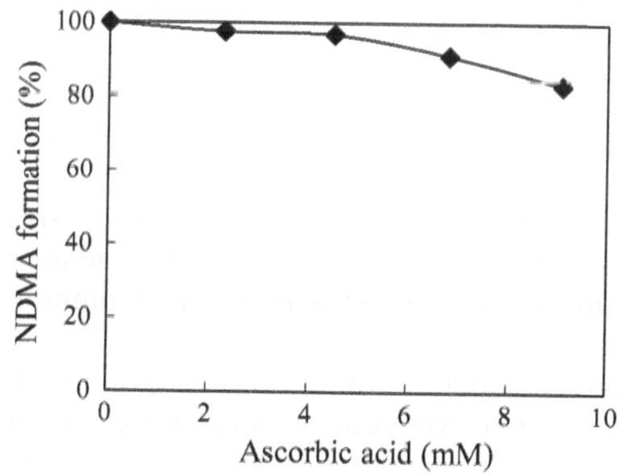

Figure 6.4. Effect of ascorbic acid on NDMA formation.

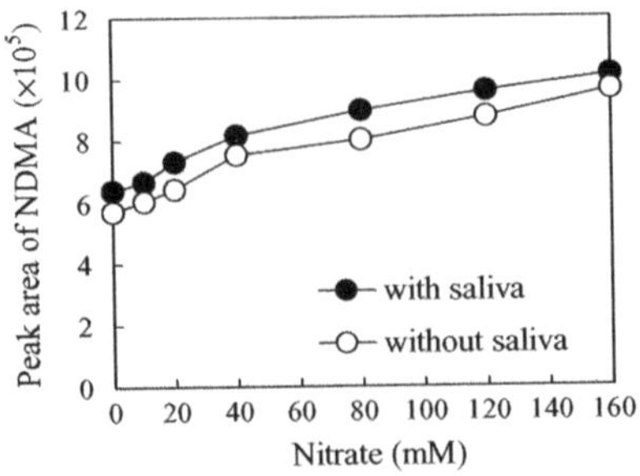

Figure 6.5. Effect of saliva on NDMA formation in nitrate.

Nitrate. The contents of nitrate in the 31 vegetables were between 3 and 581 mg/100 g, as shown in Table 6.10. The leafy vegetables and most herbs, such as cabbage, celery, Chinese cabbage, komatsuna, mitsuba, potherb mustard, spinach, coriander, Italian parsley, lemon balm, mint, rocket, and salad parsley, had a high level of nitrate (more than 100 mg/100 g). The effect of nitrate on NDMA formation is shown in Figure 6.5 by an open-circle mark. The formation of NDMA increased with a small increase in the concentration of nitrate.

Saliva. The effect of saliva on NDMA formation in nitrate was examined, as shown in Table 6.10. NDMA was increasingly formed in the presence of saliva more than in its absence.

Sawamura et al. (2005) showed that saliva enhanced the formation of NDMA in vegetable extracts as described above. Therefore, the increased formation of NDMA with saliva may be caused by the reduction of nitrate from vegetables by oral bacteria. This is an additional indication that saliva is a major source of nitrite for humans.

6.2.10 Inhibitory Mechanism of the Formation of NDMA by Terpene Hydrocarbons

The reaction of dimethylamine with nitrite is conducted by electrophilic substitution to form NDMA. The N atom on HNO_2 is so electrophilic that it attacks the N atom on dimethylamine, the electron density of which is apt to increase with two alkyl groups. It is considered that hydrocarbons consisting of two or three double bonds such as α-terpinene, γ-terpinene, terpinolene, and myrcene would compete with dimethylamine to react with nitrite. Common terpene hydrocarbons such as terpinolene, α-terpinene, myrcene, and limonene were examined on NDMA formation. The effect of these four compounds on NDMA formation is illustrated in Figure 6.6. Myrcene, α-terpinene, and terpinolene had an inhibitory effect of more than 80%. Limonene showed a low inhibitory effect, as much as 38%. These results were similar to those of previous studies (Sawamura et al., 1999).

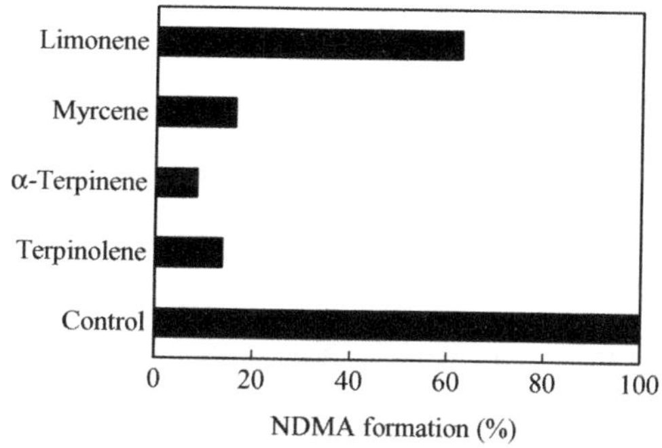

Figure 6.6. Effect of terpene hydrocarbons on NDMA formation.

In order to obtain information on the inhibition mechanism of NDMA formation, α-terpinene, one of the terpene compounds, was further investigated. The result is shown in Figure 6.7. The addition of α-terpinene to the reaction media developed one new compound (peak 6 in Figure 6.7 (C)), whose retention time was 37.6 min. It is considered possible that this compound could be an α-terpinene derivative that substitutes for NDMA. The behavior of formation of the α-terpinene derivative was further examined after 0.1 mL of α-terpinene was added to the model solution for NDMA formation. The result is shown in Figure 6.7 (D). The formation of the α-terpinene derivative (peak 6 in Figure 6.7 (D)) considerably increased as compared to that described in Figure 6.7 (C). These results indicated that the α-terpinene derivative not only was formed by the reaction between α-terpinene and nitrite, but also increased with an increase in the concentration of α-terpinene in the model solution for NDMA formation. It is considered that the decrease of NDMA formation in the presence of terpene hydrocarbons is due to the formation of terpene derivative by the reaction of terpene hydrocarbons with nitrite. Peak 6 was repeatedly isolated by HPLC. The isolated substance was concentrated under vacuum with a stream of nitrogen. This unknown sample was analyzed by LC-MS. The MS spectrum of α-terpinene derivative is shown in Figure 6.8. The peak of *m/z* 217 is most likely to be the relating compound of the α-terpinene derivative. When we assume the *m/z* 217 compound is bound with sodium, the molecular weight of the α-terpinene derivative would be 194. It is considered that the compound consisting of two or three double bonds such as α-terpinene, terpinolene, and myrcene would compete with dimethylamine to react with the nitrite (Sawamura, et al., 1999). α-Terpinene (0.01 mL) added to 1.31 mL of the model solution amounts to 63 μmol, and 0.5 mL of nitrite added to 1.31 mL of the model solution amounts to 12.5 μmol. Therefore, it is supposed that the reaction of nitrite with α-terpinene would make a compound with the nitroso group in the model solution for NDMA formation. Accordingly, the chemical structure of α-terpinene derivative is postulated in Figure 6.9. It is a monocyclic and unsaturated compound with two nitroso groups.

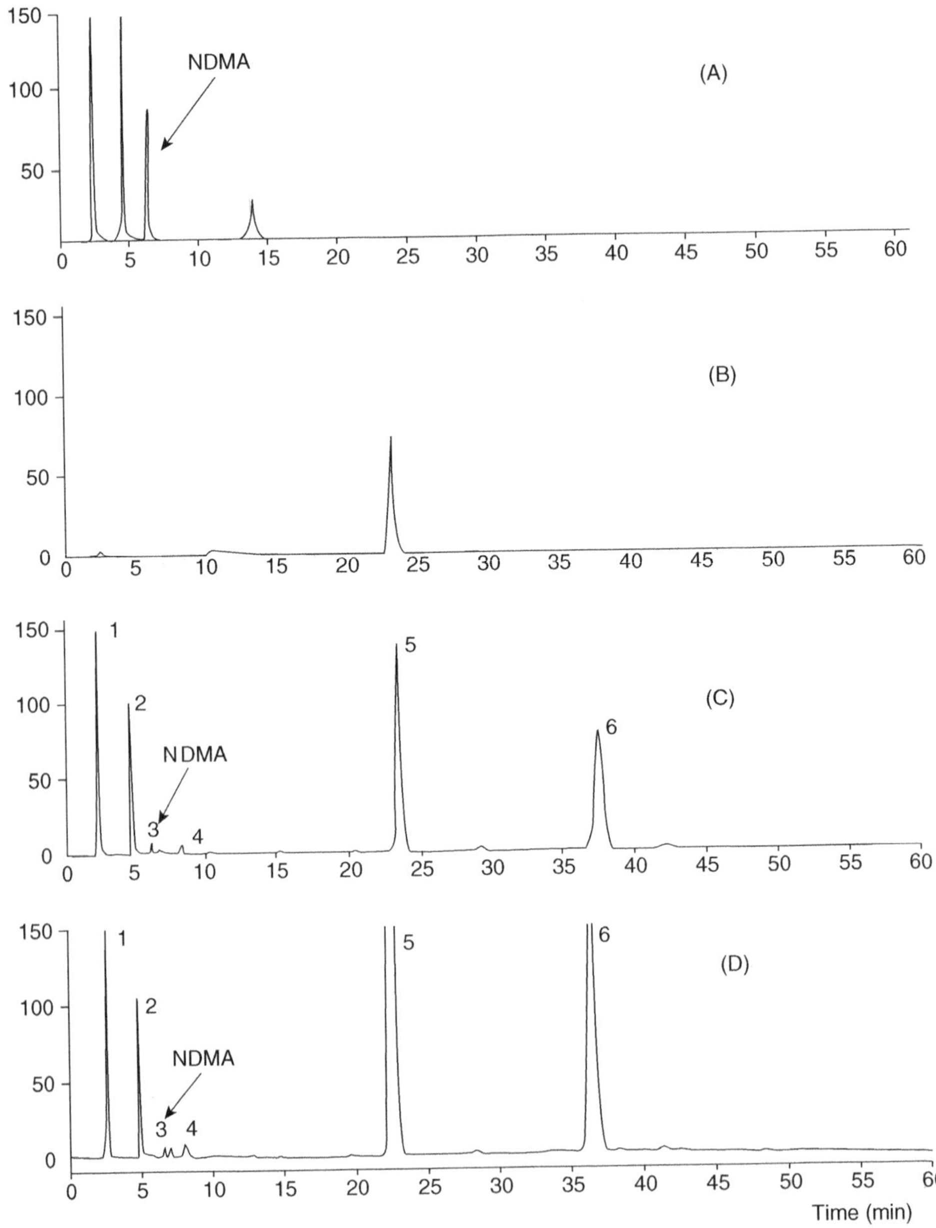

Figure 6.7. Chromatograms for NDMA formation with or without α-terpinene. (A) Control for NDMA formation. (B) α-Terpinene alone. (C) α-Terpinene (0.01 mL) for NDMA formation. (D) α-Terpinene (0.1 mL) for NDMA formation. Peak No. 1: nitrite. Peak No. 2: acetic acid.

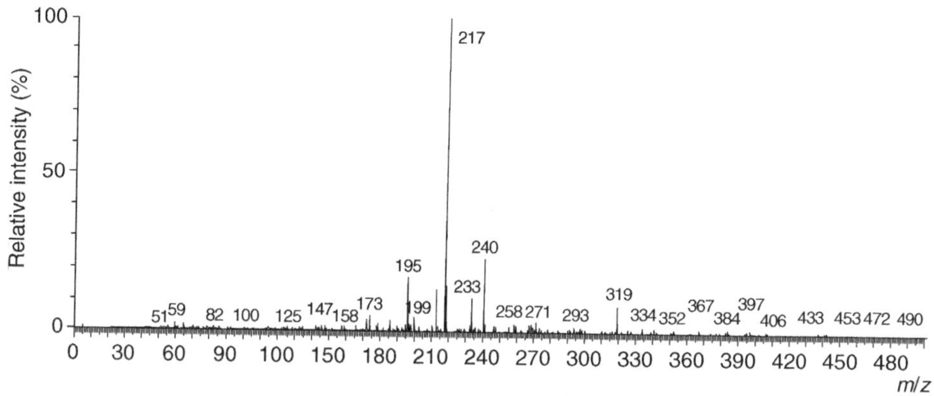

Figure 6.8. MS spectrum of α-terpinene derivative.

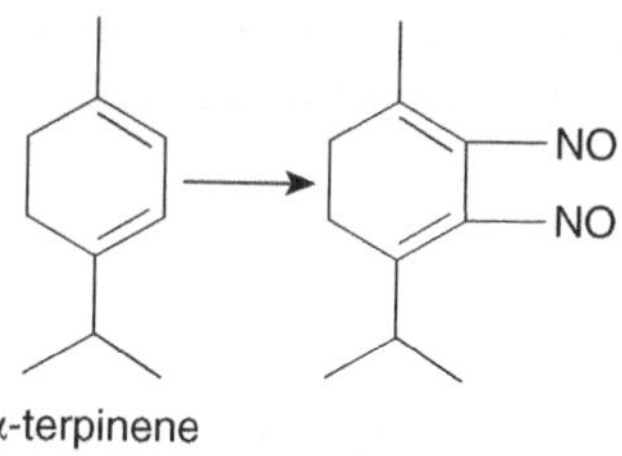

Figure 6.9. Postulated chemical structure of α-terpinene derivative.

In conclusion, the inhibitory effect of yuzu (*Citrus junos* Tanaka) essential oil on the formation of *N*-nitrosodimethylamine (NDMA) in the presence of vegetables (31 species) or saliva was elucidated. Most vegetable extracts enhanced the formation of NDMA. However, the formation ratio of NDMA in vegetable extracts was decreased by yuzu oil in the range of 59 to 22%. In the presence of yuzu oil and saliva, its ratio ranged between 62 and 24%. These results indicated that yuzu oil inhibited the formation of NDMA even in vegetables and saliva. The contents of ascorbic acid, nitrate, and nitrite in the 31 vegetable species were 0.3–65 mg/100 g, 3–581 mg/100 g, and 10–750 μg/100 g, respectively. Ascorbic acid and nitrite had little effect on the inhibition or formation of NDMA at their intact levels. Nitrate accelerated the formation of NDMA, and the addition of saliva further enhanced it. The mechanism of inhibition of NDMA formation by α-terpinene was studied. It was assumed from the results of LC-MS that a new compound formed by the reaction of α-terpinene with nitrite would be a derivative of α-terpinene with dinitroso groups. The molecular weight of this compound was 194. It is suggested that terpene hydrocarbons in citrus essential oils would contribute to the decrease of NDMA formation.

6.3 ANTIMICROBIOLOGY

Hee-Sun Song

Anitimicrobial activity is an important functional property of herb plants because they appear to play a defensive role against invading pathogens, including bacteria, fungi, and viruses. Among various herb essential oils, antimicrobial activities of citrus essential oils have been steadily studied for industrial use as natural preservatives. Since the antibacterial effect of citrus oil was reported by Brock and Ketchum (1951), many researchers have tried to assay antimicrobial activities of various citrus oils. The oils of orange, lemon, grapefruit, mandarin, and bergamot have been most often focused on as citrus samples for the examination of antimicrobial activities, though there are a lot of citrus species cultivated in the world.

The summary of antimicrobial activities of citrus oils is presented in Table 6.11; these were classified according to the species of citrus fruit, including orange, bergamot, lemon, mandarin, and grapefruit. The antimicrobial activities of volatile compounds such as limonene, linalool, and thymol were summarized in Table 6.12. As shown in Tables 6.11 and 6.12, the summary consists of oil type or compound, species of microorganism, and assay method.

6.3.1 Micro-organisms

Antimicrobial activities of citrus essential oils have been investigated on various microorganisms including yeast, fungi, and bacteria. *Penicillium digitatum* and *Penicillium italicum* are known as harmful postharvest pathogens of citrus fruit. Though these fungi infect the fruit through micro-injuries produced in the flavedo during harvesting and processing, citrus oils such as lemon, grapefruit, mandarin, and orange or terpene components have been suggested to play a role of antifungal activity in the pathogenic process of citrus fruit (Norman et al., 1967; McCalley and Torres-Grifol, 1992; Caccioni et al., 1998). The other postharvest pathogens such as *Botryodiplodia theobromae*, *Alternaria alternate*, and *Phaeoramularia angolensis* were used for the assay of antifungal activity of citrus oils (Kuate et al., 2006; Sharma and Tripathi, 2006). Other fungal species related to the spoilage of bakery products were used for the examination of functional properties of citrus oils: *Eurotium amstelodami*, *Eurotium herbariorum*, *Eurotium rubrum*, *Eurotium repens*, *Penicillium corylophilum*, *Aspergillus niger*, and *Aspergillus flavus* (Guynot et al., 2003). *Aspergillus niger* is a common fungus causing deterioration of food and food materials together with *Penicillium chrysogenum* and *Penicillium verrucosum* (Sharma and Tripathi, 2006; Viuda-Martos et al., 2008). Human pathogenic fungi causing dermatophyte infection or tinea pedis (Athlete's foot) infection were also focused on: *Trichophyton spp*, *Microsporum canis*, *Pityrosporum ovale*, and *Epidermophyton floccosum* (Jo et al., 2004; Shin and Lim, 2004; Johann et al., 2007; Sanguinetti et al., 2007).

Among yeasts, *Candida spp* such as *Candida albicans* have been especially used on the microbial assay; these are a sort of human skin–resident pathogen

TABLE 6.11. Antimicrobial activities of citrus oils

Species: *Citrus sinensis* (Orange)				
Common Name/Oil Type	Antibiological Activity		Assay	Ref
Washington navel, Ovale, Sanguinello, Tarocco, Moro, Valencia/peel HD oil	Fungi (post-harvest pathogen)	*Penicillium digitatum, Penicillium italicum*	Mycelial weight	3
Essential oil (F.D. Copelans & Sons, Ltd., London, UK)	Fungi (deterioration of bakery products)	*Eurotium amstelodami, Aspergillus niger, Penicillium corylophilum*	Disc diffusion method	9
Peel: Hexane extract, wax extract	Fungi: dermatophytes from human (high effect)	*Trichophyton mentagrophytes, Microsorum canis*	Disc diffusion method, MIC	12
Orange, Musambi/peel HD oil	Fungi	*Aspergillus niger, Botryodiplodia theobromae, Alternaria alternata, Cladosporium fluvum, Botrytis cinerea, Penicillium expansum, Ulocladium chartarum, Alternaria mali, Penicillium chrysogenum, Cladosporium cladosporiodes, Myothecium roridum, Ulocladium sp.*	MIC, agar diffusion method, mycelial weight	22
Peel CPO (Ravetllat Aromatics)	Food-pathogenic fungi	*Aspergillus niger* (effect), *Aspergillus flavus, Penicillium chrysogenum, Penicillium verrucosum*	Agar dilution method	27
Essential oil (F.D. Copeland & Sons)	Foodborne pathogene (no or mild effect)	*Esherichia coli, Staphylococcus aureus, Listeria monocytogenes, Salmonella enteritidis, Campylobacter jejuni*	Agar well technique	25
Essential oil	Gram-positive bacteria	*Bacillus subtilis*		26
CPO: Terpeneless, fivefold, singlefold, aqueous aroma	Bacteria	*Samolnella spp* (Terpeneless CPO is most effective)	Population reduction assay	19
Peel stripper oil	Ethanolgenic bacterium	*Zymomonas mobilis*	MIC	28

TABLE 6.11. *Continued*

Species: *Citrus aurantifolia*				
Bergamot (*Citrus bergamia* Risso/*Citrus aurantitum* var. *bergamia*)				
Common Name/Oil Type	Antibiological Activity		Assay	Ref
Fruit HD oil	Fungi: tinea infection	*Trichophyton erinacei, T. mentagrophytes, T. rubrum, T. tonsurans, T. schoenleinii, T. soudanense*	Disc diffusion method, MIC	23
Bergamot (Consorzio del Bergamotto, Italy) Natural essence (pressed oil), HD oil, furanocoumarin-free oil	Fungi: dermatophytes	*Trichophyton mentagropytes, T. rubrum, T. interdigitale T. tonsurans, Mycrosporum canis, M. gypseum, Epidermophyton floccosum*	Dilution broth method, MIC	21
	Yeast	*Candida albicans, Candida glabrata, Candida krusei Cnadida tropicalis. Candida parapsilosis*	MIC	20
Essential oil (Sunspirit Oils Pty, Ltd., Australia)	Yeast	*Candida albicans* (effective)	MIC, agar dilution method	10
	Bacteria	*Acinetobacter baumanii, Aeromonas sobria, Escherichia coli* (effective)		
Essential oil	Bacteria	*Listeria monocytogenes, Staphylococcus aureus, Bacillus cereus, Escherichia coli* O157, *Campylobacter jejuni*	Disc diffusion method	6
	Bacteria	*Arcobacter butzleri* (effective i*n vitro* and on food)		7
Peel fraction: flavonoid	Gram-negative bacteria	*Escheichia coli, Pseudomonas putida, Salmonella enterica*	MIC	14
Lime				
Essential oil (F.D. Copeland & Sons)	Foodborne pathogene	*Esherichia coli Salmonella enteritidis*	Agar well technique	25

TABLE 6.11. *Continued*

		Lime		
Sunspirit Oils Pty, Ltd., Australia	Bacteria	*Acinetobacter baumanii* (effective), *Aeromonas sobria* (effective)	MIC, agar dilution method	10
Extract (used locally in cough mixtures)	Upper respiratory tract bacterial pathogens	*Escherichia coli* (effective), *Staphylococcus aureus, Streptococcus feacalis, Klebsiella pneumoniae* *Pseudomonas aeruginosa, Salmonella spp, Shigella dysenteriae, Candida albicans* (yeast)	Patched-hole and agar diffusion method	1
Fruit HD oil	Anaerobic bacteria	*Staphylococcus aureus, Salmonella paratyphi, Shigella flexnerii, Streptococcus feacalis, Citrobacter spp, Serratia spp, Klebsiella pneumoniae, Pseudomonas aeruginosa, Escherichia coli* (effective)	MIC, Agar diffusion method	2
	Aerobes	*Bacteroides spp, Porphyromonas spp, Clostridium spp*		
	Yeast, fungi	*Candida albicans, Aspergilus niger*		
		Species: *Citrus limon* (Lemon)		
Common Name/Oil Type	Antibiological Activity		Assay	Ref
Femminello/ peel: HD oil	Fungi (good effect)	Penicillium digitatum, Penicillium italicum	Mycelial weight	3
Peel oil	Fungi	Epidermophyton floccosum, Microsporum gypseum, Trichophyton mentagropytes	MIC	15
Essential oil (F.D. Copelans & Sons, Ltd., London, UK)	Fungi: causing deterioration of bakery products	Eurotium herbariorum, Eurotium repens, Aspergillus flavus, Aspergillus niger, Penicillium corylophilum	Disc diffusion method	9
Peel: Hexane extract, wax extract	Fungi: dermatophytes	Trichophyton mentagrophytes, Microsorum canis (high effect in hexane extract)	Disc diffusion method, MIC	12
Peel CPO (Ravetllat Aromatics)	Fungi: foodpathogen	Aspergillus niger, Aspergillus flavus, Penicillium chrysogenum., Penicillium verrucosum	Agar dilution method	27

TABLE 6.11. *Continued*

Species: *Citrus limon* (Lemon)				
Common Name/Oil Type	Antibiological Activity		Assay	Ref
Essential oil (F.D. Copeland & Sons)	Bacteria: foodborne pathogene	Staphylococcus aureus	Agar well technique	25
Sunspirit Oils Pty. Ltd., Australia	Bacteria	Aeromonas sobria (effective), Candida albicans (yeast), Enterococcus faecalis, Staphylococcus aureus	MIC, Agar dilution method	5, 10
Essential oil, concentrated juice, fresh & dehydrated peel	Bacteria: cholera	Viibrio cholerae O1	Agar dilution method and exposure time	4
Essential oil (combination benzethonium chloride)	Bacteria: synergistic activity for healthcare hand rub	Staphylococcus aureus	Microbial count	24

Species: *Citrus unshiu*, *Citrus deliciosa* (mandarin)				
Common Name/Oil Type	Antibiological Activity		Assay	Ref
Avana/peel HD oil	Fungi (good)	Penicillium digitatum, Penicillium italicum	Mycelial weight	3
Sunspirit Oils Pty. Ltd., Australia	Yeast	Candida albicans	MIC, Agar dilution method	10
Essential oil (F.D. Copelans & Sons, Ltd., London, UK)	Fungi: causing deterioration of bakery products	Aspergillus flavus, Aspergillus niger, Penicillium corylophilum	Disc diffusion method	9
Peel HD oil	Fungi: Human skin- resident (high effect)	Candida albicans, Aspergillus niger	Dried weight method	11
	Fungi: Athlete's foot (high effect)	Trichophyton rubrum, Trichophyton mentagrophytes, Pityrosporum ovale		

TABLE 6.11. *Continued*

Species: *Citrus unshiu*, *Citrus deliciosa* (mandarin)				
Common Name/Oil Type	Antibiological Activity		Assay	Ref
Peel: Hexane extract, wax extract	Fungi: dermatophytes (high activity)	Trichophyton mentagrophytes, Microsorum canis	Disc diffusion method, MIC	12
Peel CPO (Ravetllat Aromatics)	Fungi: food pathogen	Aspergillus flavus (effective), Aspergillus niger, Penicillium chrysogenum, Penicillium verrucosum	Agar dilution method	27
Peel HD oil	Bacteria: human skin-resident	Bacillus subtilis, Staphylococcus aureus, Escherichia coli	Colony count, dried weight method	12
Peel oil	Inhibition of anaerobic digestion (methane fermentation)			16

Species: *Citrus paradisi* (grapefruit)				
Common Name/Oil Type	Antibiological Activity		Assay	Ref
Marsh seedless, red blush/peel HD oil	Fungi (good effect)	Penicillium digitatum, Penicillium italicum	Mycelial weight	3
Essential oil (F.D. Copelans & Sons, Ltd., London, UK)	Fungi: causing deterioration of bakery products	Eurotium amstelodam, Eurotium herbariorum, Eurotium repens, Aspergillus niger, Penicillium corylophilum	Disc diffusion method	9
Peel oil	Fungi: citrus leaf and fruit spot disease	Phaeoramularia angolensis	Sportulation	13
Peel CPO (Ravetllat Aromatics)	Fungi: food pathogen	Penicillium chrysogenum (effective), Penicillium verrucosum (effective), Aspergillus niger, Aspergillus flavus	Agar dilution method	27
Essential oil (F.D. Copeland & Sons)	Bacteria: foodborne pathogene (no or mild effect)	Esherichia coli, Staphylococcus aureus, Listeria monocytogenes, Salmonella enteritidis, Campylobacter jejuni	Agar well technique	25

TABLE 6.11. *Continued*

Species: *Citrus paradisi* (grapefruit)				
Common Name/Oil Type	Antibiological Activity		Assay	Ref
Sunspirit Oils Pty. Ltd., Australia	Bacteria	Aeromonas sobria, (effective), Staphylococcus aureus, Candida albicans (yeast, effective),	MIC, Agar dilution method	10
Species: *Citrus aurantium* (Bitter Orange)				
Common Name/Oil Type	Antibiological Activity		Assay	Ref
Peel HD oil	Fungi (good effect)	Penicillium digitatum, Penicillium italicum	Mycelial weight	4
Sunspirit Oils Pty. Ltd., Australia	Bacteria	Aeromonas sobria (effective), Staphylococcus aureus, Candida albicans (yeast , effective)	MIC, agar dilution method	10
Essential oil	Bacteria (high effect)	Campylobacter jejuni	MIC	8
Species: *Citrus grandis* Osbeck (Buntan)				
Peel extract, albedo tissue methanol extract	Bacteria	Staphylococcus aureus, Bacillus subtilis, Bacillus cereus, Salmonella enteritidis, Escherichia coli	Disc diffusion method, MIC	17, 18
Species: *Citrus maxima* (Pummelo)				
Peel oil	Fungi: citrus leaf and fruit spot disease	Phaeoramularia angolensis	Radial growth	13
Species: *Citrus sinensis* × Poncirus trifoliata (Citrange)				
Carrizo, Troyer/ peel HD oil	Fungi (high effect)	Penicillium digitatum, Penicillium italicum	Mycelial weight	3

References:
1: Adeleye and Opiah, 2003; 2: Aibinu et al., 2007; 3: Caccioni et al., 1998; 4: De Castillo et al., 2000; 5: Dutta et al., 2007; 6: Fisher and Phillips, 2006; 7: Fisher, et al. 2007; 8: Friedman et al., 2002; 9: Guynot et al., 2003; 10: Hammer et al., 1999; 11: Jo et al., 2004; 12: Johann et al., 2007; 13: Kuate et al., 2006; 14: Mandalari et al., 2007; 15: Misra et al., 1998; 16: Mizuki et al., 1990; 17: Mokbel et al., 2006; 18: Mokbel and Suganuma, 2006; 19: Parish et al., 2003; 20: Romano, 2005; 21: Sanguinetti et al., 2007; 22: Sharma and Tripathi, 2006, 2008; 23: Shin and Lim, 2004; 24: Shintre et al., 2006; 25: Smith-Palmer et al., 1998; 26: Subba et al., 1967; 27: Viuda-Martos et al., 2008; 28: Wilkins, 2007.

TABLE 6.12. Antimicrobical activities of volatile compounds

Compound		Antibiological Activity		Assay	Ref
1	Limonene	Bacteria	*Citrobacter freundii, Clostidium sporogenes, Enterobacter aerogenes, Erwinia carotovora, Escherichia coli, Flavobacterium suaveolens, Klebsiella pneumoniae, Moraxella sp., Proteus vulgaris, Salmonella pullorum, Serratia marcescens, Yersinia enterocolitica*	Agar diffusion assay	1
2	α-Pinene		*Citrobacter freundii, Clostidium sporogenes, Enterococcus faecalis, Erwinia carotovora, Escherichia coli, Flavobacterium suaveolens, Klebsiella pneumoniae, Micrococcus luteus, Moraxella sp., Proteus vulgaris, Salmonella pullorum, Staphylococcus aureus, Yersinia enterocolitica*		
3	β-Pinene		*Acinetobacter calcoacelica, Aeromonas hydrophila, Alcaligenes faecalis, Beneckea nalriegens, Brocothrix thermosphacta, Citrobacter freundii, Clostidium sporogenes, Enterococcus faecalis, Escherichia coli, Flavobacterium suaveolens, Klebsiella pneumoniae, Micrococcus luteus, Moraxella sp., Proteus vulgaris, Pseudomonas aeruginosa, Salmonella pullorum, Serratia marcescens, Staphylococcus aureus, Yersinia enterocolitica*		
4	Sabinene		*Acinetobacter calcoacelica, Alcaligenes faecalis, Bacillus subtilis, Beneckea nalriegens, Brevibacterium linens, Brocothrix thermosphacta, Citrobacter freundii, Enterobacter aerogenes, Klebsiella pneumoniae*		
5	α-Terpinene		*Beneckea nalriegens, Brevibacterium linens, Citrobacter freundii, Clostidium sporogenes, Erwinia carotovora, Escherichia coli, Klebsiella pneumoniae, Lactobacillus plantarum, Moraxella sp., Proteus vulgaris, Pseudomonas aeruginosa, Salmonella pullorum*		

TABLE 6.12. *Continued*

Compound			Antibiological Activity	Assay	Ref
6	δ-3-Carene		*Acinetobacter calcoacelica, Aeromonas hydrophila, Alcaligenes faecalis, Bacillus subtilis, Beneckea nalriegens, Brevibacterium linens, Clostidium sporogenes, Enterococcus faecalis, Enterobacter aerogenes, Erwinia carotovora, Escherichia coli, Flavobacterium suaveolens, Klebsiella pneumoniae, Micrococcus luteus, Moraxella sp., Proteus vulgaris, Pseudomonas aeruginosa, Salmonella pullorum, Serratia marcescens, Staphylococcus aureus, Yersinia enterocolitica*		
7	Linalool	Bacteria	*Acinetobacter calcoacelica, Aeromonas hydrophila, Alcaligenes faecalis, Bacillus subtilis, Beneckea nalriegens, Brevibacterium linens, Brocothrix thermosphacta, Citrobacter freundii, Clostidium sporogenes, Enterococcus faecalis, Enterobacter aerogenes, Erwinia carotovora, Escherichia coli, Flavobacterium suaveolens, Klebsiella pneumoniae, Lactobacillus plantarum, Micrococcus luteus, Moraxella sp., Proteus vulgaris, Salmonella pullorum, Serratia marcescens, Staphylococcus aureus, Yersinia enterocolitica*	Punched-hole/disc diffusion assay	1
			Arcobacter butzleri (highly effective in vitro & on food)		3
			Listeria monocytogenes, Staphylococcus aureus, Bacillus cereus, Escherichia coli O157, Campylobacter jejuni		2
8	Geraniol	Bacteria	*Acinetobacter calcoacelica, Aeromonas hydrophila, Alcaligenes faecalis, Bacillus subtilis, Beneckea nalriegens, Brevibacterium linens, Brocothrix thermosphacta, Citrobacter freundii, Clostidium sporogenes, Enterococcus faecalis, Enterobacter aerogenes, Erwinia carotovora, Escherichia coli, Flavobacterium suaveolens, Lactobacillus plantarum, Micrococcus luteus, Moraxella sp., Proteus vulgaris, Pseudomonas aeruginosa, Salmonella pullorum, Serratia marcescens, Staphylococcus aureus, Yersinia enterocolitica*	Agar diffusion assay	1

TABLE 6.12. *Continued*

Compound			Antibiological Activity	Assay	Ref
			E. coli O157:H7, *Listeria monocytogenes, Salmonella enterica*	MIC	4
		Fungi	Tinea infection pathogen: *Trichophyton erinacei, T. mentagrophytes, T. rubrum, T. tonsurans, T. schoenleinii, T. soudanense*	MIC	7
9	Nerol	Bacteria	*Acinetobacter calcoacelica, Aeromonas hydrophila, Alcaligenes faecalis, Bacillus subtilis, Beneckea nalriegens, Brevibacterium linens, Brocothrix thermosphacta, Citrobacter freundii, Enterobacter aerogenes, Erwinia carotovora, Escherichia coli, Flavobacterium suaveolens, Lactobacillus plantarum, Micrococcus luteus, Pseudomonas aeruginosa, Serratia marcescens, Staphylococcus aureus, Yersinia enterocolitica*	Agar diffusion assay	1
10	Citronellol	Fungi	Tinea infection pathogen: *Trichophyton erinacei, T. mentagrophytes, T. rubrum, T. tonsurans, T. schoenleinii, T. soudanense*	MIC	7
11	Carvacrol	Bacteria (high effect)	*Acinetobacter calcoacelica, Aeromonas hydrophila, Alcaligenes faecalis, Bacillus subtilis, Beneckea nalriegens, Brevibacterium linens, Brocothrix thermosphacta, Citrobacter freundii, Clostidium sporogenes, Enterococcus faecalis, Enterobacter aerogenes, Erwinia carotovora, Escherichia coli, Flavobacterium suaveolens, Klebsiella pneumoniae, Lactobacillus plantarum, Micrococcus luteus, Moraxella sp., Proteus vulgaris, Pseudomonas aeruginosa, Salmonella pullorum, Serratia marcescens, Staphylococcus aureus, Yersinia enterocolitica*	Agar diffusion assay	1, 6
		Bacteria	*Campylobacter jejuni, E. coli* O157:H7, *Listeria monocytogenes, Salmonella enterica*	MIC	4
		Bacteria (high effect)	*Staphylococcus aureus, Pseudomonas aeruginosa* Render bacterial cell membranes permeable	MIC	5

TABLE 6.12. *Continued*

Compound			Antibiological Activity	Assay	Ref
12	Thymol	Bacteria (high effect)	*Acinetobacter calcoacelica, Aeromonas hydrophila, Alcaligenes faecalis, Bacillus subtilis, Beneckea nalriegens, Brevibacterium linens, Brocothrix thermosphacta, Citrobacter freundii, Enterococcus faecalis, Enterobacter aerogenes, Erwinia carotovora, Escherichia coli, Flavobacterium suaveolens, Klebsiella pneumoniae, Lactobacillus plantarum, Micrococcus luteus, Moraxella sp., Proteus vulgaris, Pseudomonas aeruginosa, Salmonella pullorum, Serratia marcescens, Staphylococcus aureus, Yersinia enterocolitica*	Agar diffusion assay	1
			Campylobacter jejuni, E. coli O157:H7, *Listeria monocytogenes, Salmonella enterica*	MIC	4
			Staphylococcus aureus, Pseudomonas aeruginosa	MIC	5
			Render bacterial cell membranes permeable		
		Fungi	Tinea infection pathogen: *Trichophyton erinacei, T. mentagrophytes, T. rubrum, T. tonsurans, T. schoenleinii, T. soudanense*	MIC	7
13	Eugenol	Bacteria	*Acinetobacter calcoacelica, Aeromonas hydrophila, Alcaligenes faecalis, Bacillus subtilis, Beneckea nalriegens, Brevibacterium linens, Brocothrix thermosphacta, Citrobacter freundii, Clostidium sporogenes, Enterococcus faecalis, Enterobacter aerogenes, Erwinia carotovora, Escherichia coli, Flavobacterium suaveolens, Klebsiella pneumoniae, Lactobacillus plantarum, Micrococcus luteus, Moraxella sp., Proteus vulgaris, Pseudomonas aeruginosa, Salmonella pullorum, Serratia marcescens, Staphylococcus aureus, Yersinia enterocolitica*	Agar diffusion assay	1
			Campylobacter jejuni, E. coli O157:H7, *Listeria monocytogenes, Salmonella enterica*	MIC	4

TABLE 6.12. *Continued*

Compound			Antibiological Activity	Assay	Ref
14	Terpinen-4-ol	Bacteria	*Acinetobacter calcoacelica, Aeromonas hydrophila, Alcaligenes faecalis, Bacillus subtilis, Beneckea nalriegens, Brevibacterium linens, Brocothrix thermosphacta, Citrobacter freundii, Clostidium sporogenes, Enterococcus faecalis, Enterobacter aerogenes, Erwinia carotovora, Escherichia coli, Flavobacterium suaveolens, Klebsiella pneumoniae, Lactobacillus plantarum, Micrococcus luteus, Moraxella sp., Proteus vulgaris, Pseudomonas aeruginosa, Salmonella pullorum, Serratia marcescens, Staphylococcus aureus, Yersinia enterocolitica*	Agar diffusion assay	1
15	α-Terpineol	Bacteria	*Acinetobacter calcoacelica, Aeromonas hydrophila, Alcaligenes faecalis, Bacillus subtilis, Beneckea nalriegens, Brevibacterium linens, Brocothrix thermosphacta, Citrobacter freundii, Enterococcus faecalis, Enterobacter aerogenes, Erwinia carotovora, Escherichia coli, Flavobacterium suaveolens, Klebsiella pneumoniae, Lactobacillus plantarum, Micrococcus luteus, Moraxella sp., Proteus vulgaris, Pseudomonas aeruginosa, Salmonella pullorum, Serratia marcescens, Staphylococcus aureus, Yersinia enterocolitica*	Agar diffusion assay	1
16	Farnesol	Bacteria	*Staphylococcus aureus* (Synergistic activity in combination with benzethonium chloride for health-care hand rub)	Microbial count	8
17	*Cis/trans* citral	Bacteria	*Acinetobacter calcoacelica, Aeromonas hydrophila, Alcaligenes faecalis, Bacillus subtilis, Beneckea nalriegens, Brevibacterium linens, Brocothrix thermosphacta, Citrobacter freundii, Clostidium sporogenes, Enterococcus faecalis, Enterobacter aerogenes, Erwinia carotovora, Escherichia coli, Flavobacterium suaveolens, Klebsiella pneumoniae, Lactobacillus plantarum, Micrococcus luteus, Moraxella sp., Proteus vulgaris, Pseudomonas aeruginosa, Salmonella pullorum, Serratia marcescens, Staphylococcus aureus, Yersinia enterocolitica*	Punched-hole/disc diffusion assay, MIC	1, 3

TABLE 6.12. *Continued*

Compound			Antibiological Activity	Assay	Ref
			Arcobacter butzleri (In vitro & on food)		
			Listeria monocytogenes, Staphylococcus aureus, Bacillus cereus, Escherichia coli O157, Campylobacter jejuni		2, 4
		Fungi	Citrus postharvest pathogens (*Penicillium digitatum, Gerotrichum candidum)*	MIC	9
	Geranial	Fungi	Citrus postharvest pathogens (*Penicillium digitatum, Gerotrichum candidum)*		
	Neral		Citrus postharvest pathogens (*Gerotrichum candidum*)		
18	Perilaldehyde	Bacteria	*Campylobacter jejuni, E. coli* O157:H7, *Listeria monocytogenes, Salmonella enterica*	MIC	4
19	Geranyl acetate	Bacteria	*Acinetobacter calcoacelica, Aeromonas hydrophila, ,Alcaligenes faecalis, Bacillus subtilis, Beneckea nalriegens, Brevibacterium linens, Brocothrix thermosphacta, Citrobacter freundii, Clostidium sporogenes, Enterococcus faecalis, Enterobacter aerogenes, Erwinia carotovora, Escherichia coli, Flavobacterium suaveolens, Klebsiella pneumoniae, Lactobacillus plantarum, Micrococcus luteus, Moraxella sp., Proteus vulgaris, Pseudomonas aeruginosa, Salmonella pullorum, Serratia marcescens, Staphylococcus aureus, Yersinia enterocolitica*	Agar diffusion assay	1
			Campylobacter jejuni	MIC	4
20	Menthone	Bacteria	*Acinetobacter calcoacelica, Aeromonas hydrophila, Alcaligenes faecalis, Bacillus subtilis, Beneckea nalriegens, Brocothrix thermosphacta, Citrobacter freundii, Clostidium sporogenes, Enterobacter aerogenes, Erwinia carotovora, Escherichia coli, Flavobacterium suaveolens, Klebsiella pneumoniae, Lactobacillus plantarum, Micrococcus luteus, Moraxella sp., Proteus vulgaris, Salmonella pullorum, Serratia marcescens, Staphylococcus aureus, Yersinia enterocolitica*	Agar diffusion assay	1

TABLE 6.12. *Continued*

Compound			Antibiological Activity	Assay	Ref
21	(-)-Thujone	Bacteria	*Acinetobacter calcoacelica, Aeromonas hydrophila, Alcaligenes faecalis, Bacillus subtilis, Beneckea nalriegens, Brevibacterium linens, Brocothrix thermosphacta, Citrobacter freundii, Clostidium sporogenes, Enterococcus faecalis, Enterobacter aerogenes, Erwinia carotovora, Escherichia coli, Flavobacterium suaveolens, Klebsiella pneumoniae, Lactobacillus plantarum, Micrococcus luteus, Moraxella sp., Proteus vulgaris, Pseudomonas aeruginosa, Salmonella pullorum, Serratia marcescens, Staphylococcus aureus, Yersinia enterocolitica*	Agar diffusion assay	1
22	1,8-Cineol	Fungi	Tinea infection pathogen: *Trichophyton erinacei, T. mentagrophytes, T. rubrum, T. tonsurans, T. schoenleinii, T. soudanense*	MIC	7

Reference:
1: Dorman and Deans, 2000; 2: Fisher and Phillips, 2006; 3: Fisher et al., 2007; 4: Friedman et al., 2002; 5: Lambert et al., 2001; 6: Ogawa and Isshiki, 1996; 7: Shin and Lim, 2004; 8: Shintre et al., 2006; 9: Wuryatmo et al., 2003.

causing Candida disease (Hammer et al., 1999; Adeleye and Opiah, 2003; Jo et al., 2004; Romano et al., 2005).

Among many species of bacteria strains, foodborne bacteria causing food poisoning have been commonly used for investigation of the anitbacterial potential of citrus oils. Those foodborne bacteria are *Escherichia coli*, *Staphylococcus spp*, *Listeria monocytogenes*, *Salmonella spp*, *Camphylobacter jejuni Bacillus subtilis*, *Streptococcus feaclis*, *Klebsiella pneumoniae, Pseudomonas spp*, *Shigella dysenteriae*, *Vibrio spp*, and so on. *Camphylobacter jejuni* is known to be the most resistant of the bacteria investigated for plant essential oils including citrus oils (Smith-Palmer et al., 1998).

6.3.2 Methods for Assessment of Antimicrobial Effects

The disc diffusion method or agar diffusion method have been often used for antibiotic screening in vitro, and minimum inhibitory concentrations (MIC) such as the agar dilution method and broth dilution method for observation of visible growth, optical density, and measurement of absorbance or visible counts of microbials (Burt, 2004; Fisher and Phillips, 2006). The major problem in the application of essential oil for antibiotic assay is the hydrophobic nature of essential oil, which makes them insoluble in water-based media. For the solution of these problems, the use of emulsifiers such as Tween 20 or 80 has been tried together with use of organic chemicals such as acetone, polyethylene glycol, or ethanol (Smith-Palmer et al., 1998; Burt, 2004; Fisher and Phillips, 2008).

6.3.3 Antimicrobial Activity of Citrus Oil

Citrus oils have been trusted to have functional properties against microorganisms like other herb oils, addition to having a long history of local aromatherapy. The antimicrobial effect of citrus peel oil was first examined by using pathogen strains in the laboratory in 1951. This report was related to the inhibition of the growth of *M. tuberculosis*, infecting humans (Brock and Ketchum, 1951). However, the species of citrus was not presented in this report. In 1967, antimicrobial effects of lemon and orange oils were reported. The microbial organism used was gram positive and negative bacteria, and orange oil was more effective in the inhibition of growth of those bacteria than was lemon oil (Subba et al., 1967). Mizuki et al. (1990) emphasized the antimicrobial activity of citrus peel oil itself, not the other substances from peel or fruit. In their research, mandarin (*Citrus unshiu*) peel oil significantly inhibited methane fermentation in anaerobic digestion. However, mandarin peel did not inhibit methane fermentation after removal of peel oil by steam distillation or aeration. The fungitoxic activities of the hydrodistilled oils of sweet oranges (*Citrus sinensis*), bitter orange (*Citrus aurantium*), mandarin (*Citrus deliciosa*), grapefruits (*Citrus paradisi*), citranges (*Citrus sinensis* × *Poncirus trifoliate*), and lemon (*Citrus limon*) were examined against postharvest pathogens, *Penicillium digitatum* and *Penicillium italicum* (Caccioni et al., 1998). These citrus oils showed inhibition effects on the growth of postharvest pathogens; citrange oils were especially active.

Although citrus oils show antimicrobial activity against various microorganisms, the power of the activity seems not to be stronger than that of the other plant oils (Smith-Palmer et al., 1998; Cowan, 1999; Hammer et al., 1999; Guynot et al., 2003). Smith-Palmer et al. (1998) and Hammer et al. (1999) investigated the antimicrobial properties of 21–52 plant essential oils, including grapefruit, lemon, lime, mandarin, bergamot, and orange, against general foodborne pathogens and gram-positive and gram-negative bacteria. In the results, citrus oils showed mild inhibition effects. In the examination of bactericidal activity levels of 96 essential oils, bitter orange oils had inhibition effects only against *C. jejuni* (Friedman et al., 2002).

The condition and type of citrus oils were regarded as important factors in the examination of antimicrobial activity (Parish et al., 2003; Romano et al., 2005; Sanguinetti et al., 2007). Antifungal effects of some citrus oils are changeable according to the condition of water activity. Addition of the oils of orange, mandarin, and lemon promoted the growth of fungi, causing deterioration of bakery products at low water activity level (a_w), although citrus oils have been suggested to have antifungal activities (Guynot et al., 2003). A similar effect was reported in the addition of some citrus oils on *P. angolensis*, causing citrus leaf and fruit spot disease (Kuate et al., 2006). The potential properties of citrus oils have been researched and suggested as antimicrobial materials against various microorganisms causing foodborne diseases, human skin trouble, tinea pedis, and dandruff. Further, citrus essential oil was suggested as a preservative for animal feed against aflatoxin contamination (Nam et al., 2006). They detected aflatoxin in control and treated feed samples with citrus oil on days 16 and 21. Aflatoxin was not detected in feed samples treated with citrus oil. More over, citrus oil did not influence ruminal pH, or dry or organic matter digestibility over 8 h of incubation in rumen fluid. From this research, it was proposed that citrus oil had bio-properties to enhance preservation of animal feed as well as antimicrobial activity (Nam et al., 2006).

Recently, the antimicrobial activities of essential oils and aroma compounds have been examined not only in vitro but also in vivo. However, it has been reported that the activities of essential oils and aroma compounds were different between in vitro and in vivo. Usually, the inhibitory effect was lower in vivo than in vitro. One reason for the minor activity in vivo could be that the active aroma components of essential oils, known to be lipophilic, interact with food components such as proteins and lipids (Guynot et al., 2003).

Several studies have been conducted to understand the mechanism of action of essential oils (Chang et al., 2001); however, it is still unclear. Some studies suggest that compounds penetrate inside the cell, where they interfere with cellular metabolism (Marino et al., 2001). Other studies suggest that they disturb the cellular membrane and react with active sites of enzymes or act as a H^+ carrier, depleting the adenosine triphosphate pool (Farag et al., 1989; Chang et al., 2001; Ultee et al., 2002).

6.3.4 Orange (*Citrus sinensis*)

Orange oils have been tested to discover their antimicrobial possibilities against various fungi and bacteria as shown Table 6.11. However, orange oils seem to be not as powerful on antimicrobial action as other citrus oils. Subba et al. (1967) reported that 2,000 ppm of orange oil had an effect similar to 10 ppm of tylosin as an antibiotic compound, on all the gram-positive cultures tested. At the concentration, yeasts and molds were suppressed but not bacteria. The possibility of using orange oil as a preservative in food is indicated.

Although orange oil does not show powerful activity against bacteria, it seems to have potential effects on fungi. Sharma and Tripathi (2006) supported the fungitoxicity of orange oil. In their report, orange oil was extremely fungitoxic for spore germination on 10 postharvest pathogens. And orange oil of 300–500 ppm was sufficient to check the inhibition effect of spore germination (Sharma and Tripathi, 2006; Table 6.13). Fungitoxicity of orange oil is most effective especially against *A. niger* (Sharma and Tripathi, 2006, 2008; Viuda-Martos et al., 2008). It was observed that treatment with orange oil induced irreversible deleterious morphological modifications in germination of *A. niger* (Sharma and

TABLE 6.13. Inhibition effect of orange (*Citrus sinensis*) oil on spore germination of 12 postharvest pathogens at 25°C

Spore Germination (%)	Concentration of Oil (ppm)							
	Control	25	50	100	200	300	400	500
A. alternate	100	71.2	58.3	43.2	19.6	8.2	0.0	0.0
A. mali	100	70.6	43.6	19.1	5.6	0.0	0.0	0.0
A. niger	100	74.3	46.2	21.0	10.2	4.5	0.0	0.0
B. cinerea	100	66.1	32.4	15.6	9.6	0.0	0.0	0.0
B. theobromae	100	88.9	68.3	59.6	44.2	31.6	24.2	12.6
C. cladosporidiodies	100	73.6	44.8	31.3	19.4	12.6	0.0	0.0
C. fulvum	100	78.8	58.3	49.6	35.2	21.3	11.2	0.0
M. roridum	100	100	98.6	79.8	61.9	48.6	35.3	21.6
P. chrysogenym	100	86.2	65.6	53.4	38.6	25.2	11.8	0.0
P. expansum	100	89.3	69.8	54.8	37.6	28.3	13.6	0.0

Tripathi, 2006, 2008; Table 6.14). The main morphological changes were loss of cytoplasm in fungal hyphae, and budding of the hyphal tip, which resulted in cell wall disruption. The fungitoxicity of orange oil against *A. niger* did not change even at exposure to 100°C and autoclaving (Sharma and Tripathi, 2008).

The oils of *Citrus sinensis* inhibited and delayed microbial growth such as molds and bacteria in bread (Rehman et al., 2007; Table 6.15). The essential oil of *C. sinensis* was added in the dough and sprayed on the whole loaf, on all slices of bread, and on wrapping material for in vivo testing. Though the maximum inhibitory effect was achieved against molds and bacteria by spraying on all slices of bread, the effect of spraying citrus oil on wrapping material was much higher than that of the other samples treated with the same citrus oil. Rehman et al. (2007) indicated an important problem related to the quality of the food product, when it is treated with the citrus oil in vivo. In their research, the application of citrus essential oil significantly affected the sensory characteristics of bread, such as symmetry of form, character, and color of crust, and taste, texture, aroma, and grain of bread. The anti-viability effect of orange peel oils (terpeneless oil, normal oil, and aqueous aroma) against *Salmonella* was assayed, and terpeneless oil showed the strongest effect (Parish et al., 2003). Orange peel oil was also effective on the inhibition of ethanol production by *Zymomonas mobilis* at 30° and 37°C until 72 h (Wilkins, 2007).

6.3.5 Bergamot and Lime (*Citrus aurantifolia*)

Bergamot essential oil is widely used in the pharmaceutical industry because of its antibacterial and antiseptic activity (Verzera et al., 2003). Three types of bergamot oils (the natural essence and furocoumarin-free and distilled extracts) were suggested as having a potential role in the topical treatment of dermatophytoses such as *Candida* infections (Romano et al., 2005; Sanguinetti et al.,

TABLE 6.14. Effect of different concentrations of *Citus sinensis* epicarp oil against *Aspergillus niger*

Concentration of oil (μg/mL)	Radial Growth Inhibition (%)	Spore Germination (%)	Mophorogical Change
Control	—	100.0	• Magnification of a single hyphal tip • Mycelium showing conidial heads on conidiophore
0.1	5.9	74.3	No examination
0.5	31.4	21.0	• Mycelium distorted • Squashed and flattened conidiophore bearing damaged conidial head
1.0	63.1	4.5	• Highly budded apical tip of hyphae • Flattened hyphae clearly visible • Presence of punctured hyphae
2.0	87.1	0.0	• Cell wall disruption • Squashed and degrading hyphae clearly visible
2.5	92.9	0.0	
3.0	100.0	0.0	
3.5	100.0	0.0	

Morphological change was observed by using scanning electron microscopy.

TABLE 6.15. Inhibitory effect of *Citrus sinensis* oil against bacteria and mold in bread at different storage intervals

Treatments	0 h	24 h	48 h	72 h	96 h	Means
			Bacteria/g			
Control	60	90	160	210	270	158
Addition in the dough	50	80	150	200	250	146
Spraying on the whole loaf	—	80	140	190	220	126
Spraying on all slices	—	—	—	50	80	26
Spraying on wrapping material	—	—	60	90	120	54
			Mold/g			
Control	—	210	240	270	290	202
Addition in the dough	—	120	160	230	260	154
Spraying on the whole loaf	—	80	140	180	240	128
Spraying on all slices	—	—	—	100	150	50
Spraying on wrapping material	—	—	90	160	200	90

Colony-forming count unit is based on one gram of bread.

TABLE 6.16. In vitro susceptibility of *Candida spp.* isolates to three bergamot oils

Strain	MIC_{90}		
	Natural Essence	Furanocoumarin-Free Oil	Distilled Oil
C. albicans			
24 h	5	5	1.25
48 h	5	2.5	2.5
C. glabrata			
24 h	5	1.25	0.63
48 h	>10	5	1.25

MIC_{90} means the minimum concentration (% v/v) of substance that inhibited 90% of the isolates.

2007). As shown in Table 6.16 (Romano et al., 2005), the highest activity was observed with distilled extract, which was absolutely devoid of nonvolatile residues including the phototoxic bergaptene, followed by furocoumarin-free extract. This result seems to be important in preparing the best bergamot oil with antimycotic action (Pizzimenti F Tulino et al., 1998; Romano et al., 2005; Sanguinetti et al., 2007). Bergamot oil was more susceptible in bactericidal activity against common foodborne pathogens including *C. jejuni*, *E. coli* O157, and *A. butzleri* strains than lemon and sweet orange oils. The effect of bergamot oil was similar to that of citral and linalool among citrus components (Fisher and Phillips, 2006; Fisher et al., 2007). Bergamot ethanolic fraction and flavonoids extracted from peel also showed also good inhibition effects on gram-negative bacteria; therefore bergamot peel was suggested as a potential source of natural antimicrobials (Mandalari et al., 2007).

Lime extract showed inhibition effects on the growth of upper respiratory tract bacterial pathogens (Adeleye and Opiah, 2003). Lime (*Citrus aurantifolia*) oil has the potential for antimicrobial activity against fungi, yeast, and various bacteria strains (Smith-Palmer et al., 1998; Hammer et al., 1999; Adeleye and Opiah, 2003; Aibinu et al., 2007).

6.3.6 Lemon (*Citrus limon*)

Lemon peel oil showed fungitoxicity against *Epidermophyton floccosum*, *Microsporum gypseum*, and *Trichophyton mentagrophytes*, which activity was not affected by autoclaving and storage (Misra et al., 1988). Concentrated lemon juice and essential oils inhibited *Vibrio cholerae* O1 completely at all studied dilutions (at concentrations of 10^2~10^8 colony-forming units/mL) and exposure times (5~30 min). From the results, lemon fruit and oil were suggested as a biocide against *V. cholerae* O1; these are natural and harmless to humans as an efficient decontaminant (De Castillo et al., 2000). Lemon oil showed synergistic activity against *S. aureus* in preservative concentration for use in health-care hand rub (Shintre et al., 2006). Viuda-Martos et al. (2008) examined the antifungal activities of citrus essential oils such as orange, lemon, mandarin, and grape-

TABLE 6.17. Reduction effect of orange, lemon, mandarin, and grapefruit essential oils upon the growth of fungi

	% Growth Reduction (mean and SD $n = 3$)				
	Concentration (%)	*A. niger*	*A. flavus*	*P. verrucosum*	*P. chrysogenum*
Orange	0.27	29.5^{aA}	15.4^{bA}	26.1^{cA}	25.3^{dA}
	0.47	36.4^{aF}	25.2^{bF}	39.9^{cF}	39.7^{dF}
	0.71	48.1^{aJ}	32.0^{bJ}	47.7^{cJ}	48.8^{dJ}
	0.94	100.0^{a}	100.0^{a}	100.0^{a}	100.0^{a}
Lemon	0.27	21.6^{aB}	51.1^{bB}	20.5^{cB}	22.3^{dB}
	0.47	26.0^{aG}	52.9^{bG}	38.0^{cG}	38.4^{dG}
	0.71	40.0^{aK}	57.2^{bK}	47.2^{cK}	47.7^{dK}
	0.94	100.0^{a}	100.0^{a}	100.0^{a}	100.0^{a}
Mandarin	0.27	5.1^{aC}	55.5^{bC}	17.2^{cC}	19.2^{dC}
	0.47	14.7^{aH}	62.8^{bH}	31.2^{cH}	35.7^{dH}
	0.71	31.9^{aL}	64.8^{bL}	42.6^{cL}	46.3^{dL}
	0.94	100.0^{a}	100.0^{a}	100.0^{a}	100.0^{a}
Grapefruit	0.27	6.7^{aD}	48.6^{bD}	34.5^{cD}	35.5^{dD}
	0.47	25.7^{aI}	54.4^{bI}	43.5^{cI}	41.2^{dI}
	0.71	35.0^{aM}	57.4^{bM}	48.3^{cM}	48.1^{dM}
	0.94	100.0^{a}	100.0	100.0^{a}	100.0^{a}

1. The same small letters within the same line are not significantly different ($p > 0.05$) according to Tukey's multiple-range test.
2. The same letters (A–D) within the same column are not significantly different ($p > 0.05$) at the same concentration according to Tukey's multiple-range test.
3. The same letters (F–I) within the same column are not significantly different ($p > 0.05$) at the same concentration according to Tukey's multiple-range test.
4. The same letters (J–M) within the same column are not significantly different ($p > 0.05$) at the same concentration according to Tukey's multiple-range test.
5. The fungi were tested by agar dilution method.

fruit against the fungi *A. niger*, *A. flavus*, *P. chrysogenum*, and *P. verrucosum*. They reported the best inhibitor citrus oil against each fungus. According to their report, lemon oil was not the best inhibitor on all fungi tested. However, it was suggested that lemon oil had good antifungal activities to apply for inhibition of various food spoilages because it was the second–best inhibitor against each fungus tested (Viuda-Martos et al., 2008; Table 6.17).

6.3.7 Mandarin (*Citrus unshiu*)

Antibacterial and antifungal activities of mandarin oil were examined against general human skin–resident microflora and specific disease-related microorganisms causing tinea pedis and dandruff, for its use as a functional material for food and cosmetic composition (Jo et al., 2004). Mandarin oil significantly reduced the

TABLE 6.18. Growth inhibition of mandarin essential oil on the microorganisms related to human skin disease

Related Disease	Strain	Control	Treatment
Human skin problem	*Bacillus subtilis*	7.40	5.17
	Staphylococcus aureus	9.41	7.09
	Escherichia coli	9.02	7.50
	Candida ablicans	7.47	Not growth
	Aspergillus niger	0.43	0.09
Athlete's foot (tinea pedis)	*Trichophyton rubrum*	0.77	0.07
	Trichophyton mentagrophytes	0.60	0.11
Dardruff	*Pityrosporum ovale*	2.58	Not growth

1. The growth of *B. subtilis*, *S. aureus*, *E. coli*, *C. abicans*, and *P. ovlae* was counted by plate-count method (Log CFU/g) and that of *A. niger* and *T. spp* was counted by dried weight method (g).
2. Control did not contain mandarin oil in a broth; treatment contained 0.1% mandarin oil in a broth.

*Significant difference between control and treatment.

growth of *C. albicans*, which causes human skin problems, and *A. niger*, one of the skin-resident fungi, and its inhibition effect was strong on the microorganisms relating to both tinea pedis and dandruff (Jo et al., 2004; Table 6.18). However, against the fungus *A. niger*, the activity of mandarin oil was not as strong as that of orange oil (Viuda-Martos et al., 2008; Table 6.17). Mandarin oil was suggested as the best inhibitor of *A. flavus*, which causes food spoilage (Viuda-Martos et al., 2008; Table 6.17). Different kinds of microbial properties were examined in mandarin by Mizuki et al. (1990). They observed a significant inhibition effect of methane fermentation in anaerobic digestion of *Citrus unshu* peel, which was mainly due to peel oil (Mizuki et al., 1990).

6.3.8 Grapefruit (*Citrus paradisi*) and Other Citrus

The oils from pummelo (*Citrus maxima*) and from grapefruits were most active in reducing radial growth and sporulation in the same conditions against the same fungus, *P. angolensis* (Kuate et al., 2006). Grapefruit essential oil significantly reduced the growth of fungi causing food spoilage, especially *P. chrysogenum* and *P. verrucosum* (Viuda-Martos et al., 2008). It was reported that the ethyl acetate extract of Buntan (*C. grandis*) flavedo and the methanol extract from its albedo tissue showed strong antibacterial activity against gram-positive and -negative bacteria, although Buntan oil was not used (Mokbel et al., 2006; Mokbel and Suganuma, 2006). Citrange (*Citrus* sinensis × *P. trifoliate*) oils such as "Troyer" and "Carrizo" seem to have powerful activity against *P. italicum* and *P. digitatum*, which was higher than that of orange, lemon, and grapefruit (Caccioni et al., 1998). *P. italicum* was found to be especially, resistant to the antifungal activity of citrus oils; however, citrange oils had only the equivalent effect on this fungus as on *P. digitatum* among citrus oils.

6.3.9 Volatile Aroma Component (Terpene Component)

The relationship between the abundance of chemical classes or volatile compounds in citrus oils and antimicrobial efficacy has been examined (Caccioni et al., 1998). It had seemed difficult to prove the correlation between the antimicrobial activity and the amount of single volatile compounds or chemical classes. However, antibiotic action of volatile components, especially terpene components, has been investigated, and some volatile compounds of citrus oils have been suggested as significant active sources in the inhibition of microorganisms.

Terpenes or terpenoids seem to be active against bacteria, fungi, viruses, and protozoa (Cowan, 1999). Among industrial citrus essences used in a soft-dink factory, some terpenes such as citral, β-pinene, and *p*-cymene strongly inhibited the growth of *S. cerevisiae*, a foodborne pathogen (Belletti et al., 2004).

Caccioni et al. (1998) reported that the content of oxygenated monoterpenes affected antimicrobial activity. Oxygenated monoterpenes were more abundant in the lemon oil from the winter harvest, and this lemon oil showed higher activity than that from the summer harvest against *P. digitatum* and *P. italicum.*

Thymol, carvacrol, eugenol, and perillaldehyde among 23 oil compounds were the most active against four species of bacteria control: *C. jejuni*, *E. coli*, *S. enterica*, and *L. monocytogenes* (Friedman et al., 2002). Citral was found to be the fungitoxic factor of lemon peel oil (Misra et al., 1988). Citral also showed the most effective antimicrobial activity among some components of orange and lemon oils (Caccioni and Deans, 1993; Caccioni et al., 1995). Carvacrol was more effective in suppressing *Staphylococcus aureus* than allyisothiocyanate, having antimicrobial activity (Ogawa and Isshiki, 1996). Antibacterial activities of thymol and carvacrol were strong against *Pseudomonas aeruginosa* and *Staphylococcus aureus*. Such inhibition effect is due to damage in membrane integrity, which further affects pH homeostasis and equilibrium of inorganic ions. Thymol and carvacrol render bacterial cell membranes permeable (Lambert et al., 2001). There was research related to the application of citrus essential oils and natural aroma compounds such as hexenal, 2-(*E*)-hexenal, and hexyl acetate to improve the shelf-life and safety of minimally processed fruits (Lanciotti et al., 2004).

The aroma compounds with phenolic structures, such as carvacrol, thymol, and eugenol, are suggested to be highly active against bacteria and fungi (Dorman and Deans, 2000; Table 6.19; Figure 6.10). Members of this class are known to be either bactericidal or bacteriostatic agents, depending on the concentration used (Pelczar et al., 1988). It is reported that the strong antimicrobial activity of these compounds is not affected by their relatively low capacity to dissolve in water (Mahmoud, 1994; Kim et al., 1995; Hili et al., 1997; Dorman and Deans, 2000). The activities of these aroma compounds with phenolic ring seem to be influenced by the relative position of the hydroxyl group and alkyl substitution (Pelczar et al., 1988; Dorman and Deans, 2000).

Shin and Lim (2004) suggested that monoterpene alcohols such as geraniol and citronellol could be clinically practical antifungal agents because of their

TABLE 6.19. Antibacterial activity of volatile terpenes

Bacterial Strain	Carvacrol	Thymol	Eugenol	Nerol	Geraniol	Geranyl Acetate	Limonene	α-Pinene	β-Pinene
A. calcoacetica	45.3	29.8	15.4	11.4	6.1	10.3	NI	NI	11.2
A. hydrophila	37.7	26.8	17.0	7.7	6.4	9.0	NI	NI	7.1
A. feacalis	21.8	32.5	12.3	7.1	7.0	10.5	NI	NI	7.8
B. subtilis	39.5	39.2	21.8	12.4	6.4	10.8	NI	NI	NI
B. natriegens	14.1	50.1	20.8	11.3	6.2	10.8	NI	NI	6.5
B. linens	21.7	42.0	12.7	11.7	7.3	12.5	NI	NI	NI
B. thermosphacta	25.5	29.3	14.1	9.0	7.4	9.2	NI	NI	5.9
C. freundii	17.7	46.5	9.1	7.8	9.2	6.8	7.8	6.0	5.9
C. sporogenes	20.3	NI	9.7	NI	12.9	20.4	10.3	5.7	7.5
E. faecalis	21.2	26.3	10.0	NI	12.9	7.5	NI	9.2	7.8
E. aerogenes	18.5	30.5	9.9	7.2	6.4	7.6	7.1	NI	NI
E. carotovora	15.5	32.0	10.0	7.7	8.1	8.7	7.4	8.7	NI
E. coli	29.2	34.3	13.3	7.6	9.7	11.0	11.2	8.9	7.8
F. suaveolens	26.0	25.8	11.6	7.0	7.0	11.0	10.6	6.5	8.4
K. pneumoniae	23.6	40.0	10.9	NI	NI	7.8	7.0	8.1	7.9
L. plantarum	18.7	>90.0	21.5	19.1	6.2	12.9	NI	NI	NI
M. luteus	26.6	53.1	11.7	7.4	6.1	8.0	NI	7.6	6.3
Moraxella sp.	21.6	39.1	10.1	NI	6.1	9.0	7.9	6.2	4.8
P. vulgaris	26.5	33.5	8.3	NI	5.6	9.8	7.4	7.5	6.6
P. aeruginosa	26.0	13.4	15.5	13.6	5.7	6.5	NI	NI	6.5
S. pullorum	27.1	31.5	12.9	NI	6.3	8.7	11.2	7.9	6.0
S. marcescens	22.5	42.6	22.9	8.5	5.7	6.8	6.5	NI	5.4
S. aureus	20.2	31.6	11.5	9.4	5.2	6.6	NI	8.3	7.4
Y. enterocolitica	22.4	27.7	11.6	7.1	8.0	8.2	7.1	6.6	5.8

Values are zone of growth inhibition (mm); well diameter, 4.0 mm. NI: no inhibition.

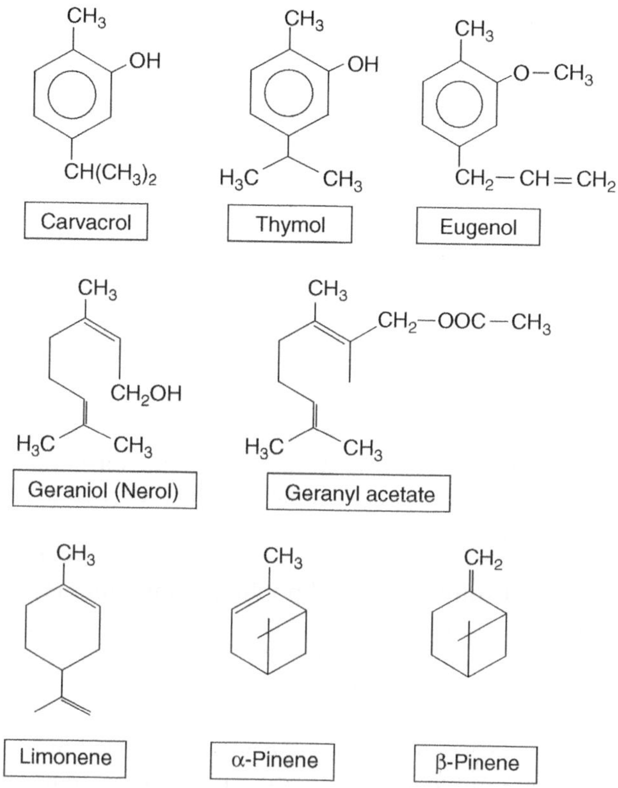

Figure 6.10. Chemical structures of terpene compound.

stability, especially in different pH conditions, although the clinical utility of phenolic compounds such as eugenol or thymol may be restricted in higher pH conditions.

Dorman and Deans (2000) reported that the antimicrobial activities of geraniol and borneol were higher than those of their acetate compounds such as geranyl acteate and bornyl acetate (Table 6.10; Figure 6.10). From this result, they proposed that the presence of an acetate moiety in the structure may increase the activity of the parent compound.

Aldehydes, especially formaldehyde and glutaraldehyde, are known to possess powerful antimicrobial activity. It has been suggested that an aldehyde group conjugated to a carbon-to-carbon double bond is a highly electronegative arrangement and the increase of electronegativity induces high antimicrobial activity (Kurita et al., 1979; Moleyar and Narasimham, 1986). The electronegativity of the aldehyde compound may interfere in biological processes involving electron transfer and react with vital nitrogen components and therefore induct the bactericidal and bacteriostatic effects (Dorman and Deans, 2000). About the ketone group, it has been proposed that the bacteriostatic and fungistatic action of terpenoids is increased when it is carbonylated by the presence of an oxygen function in the framework (Naiger et al., 1996).

An alkenyl substituent (1-methylethenyl) incorporated into a non-phenolic ring structure seem to increase antibacterial activity, compared to an alkyl substituent (1-methylethyl). Limonene, an alkenyl type, showed antibacterial activity; however, p-cymene with double bond only on the phenolic ring had no effect against the test bacteria (Dorman and Deans, 2000). An allylic side chain of aroma compound seems to enhance the inhibitory effects of a component and chiefly against gram-negative organisms (Pelczar et al., 1988; Dorman and Deans, 2000; Table 6.19; Figure 6.10).

The stereochemistry of a compound is an important factor in inhibiting the action of microorganisms. The majority of α-isomers and *cis*-isomers are inactive relative to β-isomers and *trans*-isomers (Hinou et al., 1989; Dorman and Deans, 2000; Table 6.19; Figure 6.10). It has been suggested that compounds with methyl-isopropyl cyclohexane rings, such as terpinolene and terpineol, have stronger effect, and unsaturation of the cyclohexane ring further increases the antibacterial activity (Hinou et al., 1989).

The mechanism of action of terpenes is not fully understood but is speculated to involve membrane disruption by the lipophilic compounds (Cowan, 1999). The lipophilic properties of the constituent terpenes have been suggested as a factor of their bioactivation. Their action appears to be at the phospholipid bilayer. Lipophilic compounds including terpenes affect biochemical mechanisms catalyzed by the phospholipid bilayers of the cell, that is, the inhibition of electron transport, protein translocation, phosphorylation steps, and other enzyme-dependent reactions (Knobloch et al., 1986). The antibioactivity of terpenoids in vivo have to be regarded not only in the structure of the terpenoids, but also the chemical composition of the cell membrane (Knobloch et al., 1988). Mendoza et al. (1997) also supported these mechanisms. They found that increasing the hydrophilicity of kaurene diterpenoids by addition of a methyl group drastically reduced their antimicrobial activity.

The balance of volatile composition in citrus oils was pointed out. Caccioni et al. (1998) suggested that antimicrobial activities of essential oils could be the result of a certain quantitative balance of various components. French (1985) proposed that the various components of any oil may act sinergically while several compounds may have a stimulating action on fungal spore germination. Although some volatile compounds show significantly distinctive activities according to their abundance, the synergic and additive effects of volatile compounds in citrus oils may prevail over contrasting effects of each single compound (Caccioni et al., 1998).

In conclusion, citrus essential oils could be considered suitable alternatives to chemical additives for use in various industrial areas such as food, cosmetics, pharmaceuticals, cleansers or detergents, and agricultural chemicals in order to satisfy the demand of consumers for safety and natural components. Citrus oils have an attractive and mild aroma that can to mask food smells from fish, meat, garlic, and onion, and can destroy mild toxicities. Therefore these seem to be positive functions for use as industrial antimicrobial agents such as natural preservatives, especially in the food industry. Further study is needed to investigate various citrus oils having potent activity against microorganisms. Sensory evaluation must be another research point when citrus oils are applied to food and beverages as a preservative. The relationships between the compositions of citrus oils and antimicrobial efficacy and potent components or factors resulting in antimicrobial effects of citrus oils are continuously researched together with the examination of the microbial mechanism for antimicrobial activities of citrus oils and volatile components.

REFERENCES

Achiwa, Y., Hibasami, H., Katsuzaki, H., Kada, T., Komiya, T. (1996). Inhibitory effects of plant constituents on the mutagenecity of C-nitro and C-nitroso compounds formed by reaction of sorbic acid with sodium nitrite. *Nippon Shokuhin Kagaku Kogaku Kaishi* **43**: 493–501.

Achiwa, Y., Hibasami, H., Kada, T., Komiya, T. (1997). Inhibitory effect of vegetable and fruit juices on formation of *N*-nitrosodimethylamine. *Nippon Shokuhin Kagaku Kogaku Kaishi* **44**: 50–54.

Adeleye, I.A., Opiah, L. (2003). Antimicrobial activity of extracts of local cough mixtures on upper respiratory tract bacterial pathogens. *West Indian Medical Journal* **52**: 188–190.

Aibinu, I., Adenipekun, T., Adelowotan, T., Ogunsanya, T., Odugbemi, T. (2007). Evaluation of the antimicrobial properties of different parts of *Citrus aurantifolia* (lime fruit) as used locally. *African Journal of Traditional, Complementary and Alternative Medicines* **4**:185–190.

Arldoğan, B.C., Baydar, H., Kaya, S., Demirci, M., Özbaşar, D., Mumcu, E. (2002). Antimicrobial activity and chemical composition of some essential oils. *Archives of Pharmacal Research* **25**: 860–864.

Awika, J.M., Rooney, L.W., Wu, X., Prior, R.L., Cisneros-Zevallos, L. (2003). Screening methods to measure antioxidant activity of sorghum (*Sorghum bicolor*) and sorghum products. *Journal of Agricultural and Food Chemistry* **51**: 6657–6662.

Bandoniene, D., Murkovic, M. (2002). On-line HPLC-DPPH screening method for evaluation of radical scavenging phenols extracted from apples (*Malus domestica* L.) *Journal of Agricultural and Food Chemistry* **50**: 2482–2487.

Baratta, M.T., Dorman, H.J.D., Deans, S.G., Figueiredo, A.C., Barroso, J.G., Ruberto, G. (1998). Antimicrobial and antioxidant properties of some commercial essential oil. *Flavour and Fragrance Journal* **13**: 235–244.

Belletti, N., Ndagijimana, M., Sisto, C., Guerzoni, M.E., Lanciotti, R., Gardini, F. (2004). Evaluation of the antimicrobial activity of citrus essences on *Saccharomyces cerevisiae*. *Journal of Agricultural and Food Chemistry* **52**: 6932–6938.

Brock, B.L., Ketchum, H.M. (1951). The antibacterial action of citrus peel oil on the *Tubercle Bacillus* in vitro. *Chest* **20**: 671–674.

Burke, Y.D., Stark, M.J., Roach, S.L., Sen, S.E., Crowell, P.L. (1997). Inhibition of pancreatic cancer growth by the dietary isoprenpids farnesol and geraniol. *Lipids* **32**: 151–156.

Burt, S. (2004). Essential oils: Their antibacterial properties and potential applications in foods—a review. *International Journal of Food Microbiology* **94**: 223–253.

Caccioni, D.R.L., Deans, S.G. (1993). Action of citrus fruit essential oil components on germination of *Penicillium digitatum* and *Penicillium italicum*. *International Symposium on Industial Crops and Products*, Pisa, Italy, pp. 22–24.

Caccioni, D.R.L., Deans, S.G., Ruberto, G. (1995). Inhibitory effect of citrus fruit essential oil components on *Penicillium digitatum* and *Penicillium italicum*. *Petria* **5**: 177–182.

Caccioni, D.R.L., Guizzardi, M., Biondi, D.M., Renda, A., Ruberto, G. (1998). Relationship between volatile components of citrus fruit essential oils and antimicrobial action on *Penicillium digitatum* and *Penicillium italicum*. *International Journal of Food Microbiology* **43**: 73–79.

Cao, G., Sofic, E., Prior, R.L. (1996). Antioxidant capacity of tea and common vegetables. *Journal of Agricultural and Food Chemistry* **44**: 3426–3431.

Cerutti, P.A. (1985). Prooxidant states and tumor promotion. *Science* **227**: 375–381.

Chang, S.T., Chen, P.F., Chang, S.C. (2001). Antibacterial activity of leaf essential oils and their constituents from *Cinnamomum osmophloeum*. *Journal of Ethnopharmacology* **77**: 123–127.

Choi, H.S., Song, H.S., Sawamura, M. (2000). Radical-scavenging activities of citrus essential oils and their components: Detection using 1,1-diphenyl-2-picrylhydrazyl. *Journal of Agricultural and Food Chemistry* **48**: 4156–4161.

Chung, M.J., Lee, S.H., Sung, N.J. (2002). Inhibitory effect of whole strawberries, garlic juice or kale juice on endogenous formation of *N*-nitrosodimethylamine in humans. *Cancer Letter* **182**: 1–10.

Cowan, M.M. (1999). Plant products as antimicrobial agents. *Clinical Microbiology reviews* **12**: 564–582.

Crowell, P.L. (1997). Monoterpenes in breast cancer chemoprevention. *Breast Cancer Research. Treatment* **46**: 191–197.

De Castillo, M.C., De Allori, C.G., De Gutierrez, R.C., De Saab, O.A., De Fernandez, N.P., De Ruiz, C.S., De Ruiz Holgado, A.P., De Nader, M. (2000). Bactericidal activity of lemon juice and lemon derivatives against *Vibrio cholerae*. *Biological and Pharmaceutical Bulletin* **23**: 1235–1238.

Dorman, H.J.D., Deans, S.G. (2000). Antimicrobial agents from plants: antibacterial activity of plant volatile oils. *Journal Applied Microbiology* **88**: 308–316.

Dorman, H.J.D., Figueiredo, A.C., Barroso, J.G., Deans, S.G. (2000). *In vitro* evaluation of antioxidant activity of essential oils and their components. *Flavour and Fragrance Journal* **15**: 12–16.

Dutta, B.K., Karmakar, S., Naglot, A., Aich, J.C., Begam, M. (2007). Anticandidial activity of some essential oils of mega biodiversity hotspot in India. *Mycoses* **50**: 121–124.

Farag, R.S., Daw, Z.Y., Abo-Raya, S.H. (1989). Influence of some spice essential oils on *Aspergillus parasiticus* growth and production of aflatoxins in a synthetic medium. *Journal of Food Science* **54**: 74–76.

Fiddler, W., Pensabene, J.W., Doerr, R.C., Wasserman, A.E. (1972). Formation of *N*-nitrosodimethylamine from naturally occurring quaternary ammonium compounds and tertiary amines. *Nature* **236**:307.

Fisher, K., Phillips, C.A. (2006). The effect of lemon, ornage and bergamot essential oils and their components on the survival of *Camplobacter jejuni*. *Journal of Applied Microbiology* **101**: 1232–1240.

Fisher, K., Rowe, C., Phillips, C.A. (2007). The survival of three strains of *Arcrobacter butzleri* in the presence of lemon, orange and bergamot essential oils and their components *in vitro* and on food. *Letters in Applied Microbiology* **44**: 495–499.

Fisher, K., Phillips, C. (2008). Potential antimicrobial uses of essential oils in food: Is citrus the answer? *Trends in Food Science & Technology* **19**: 156–164.

French, R.C. (1985). The bio-regulatory action of flavor compounds on fungal spores and other propagules. *Annual Review Phytopatology* **23**: 173–199.

Friedman, M., Henika, P.R., Mandrell, R.E. (2002). Bactericidal activities of plant essential oils and some of their isolated constituents against *Campylobacter jejuni, Escherichia coli, Listeria monocytogenes* and *Salmonella enterica. Journal of Food Protection* **65**: 1545–1560.

Fukuda, Y., Osawa, T., Namiki, M. (1981). Antioxidants in sesame seed. *Nippon Shokuhin Kogyo Gakkaishi* (in Japanese) **28**: 461–464.

Fukuda, Y., Osawa, T., Namiki, M., Ozaki, T. (1985). Studies on antioxidative substances in sesame. *Agriculture and Biological Chemistry* **49**: 301–306.

Gangolli, S.D., van den Brandt, P.A., Feron, V.J., Janzowsky, C., Koeman, J.H., Speijers, G.J.A., Spiegelhalder, B., Walker, R., Wishnok, J.S. (1994). Nitrate, nitrite and *N*-nitroso compounds. *European Journal of Pharmacology and Environment of Toxicology and Pharmacology* **292**: 1–38.

Gould, M.N. (1997). Cancer chemoprevention and therapy by monoterpenes. *Environmment Health Prospection* **105**: 977–979.

Guynot, M.E., Ramos, A.J., Setó, L., Purroy, P., Sanchis, V., Marín, S. (2003). Antifungal activity of volatile compounds generated by essential oils against fungi commonly causing deterioration of bakery products. *Journal of Applied Microbiology* **94**: 893–899.

Hammer, K.A., Carson, C.F., Riley, T.V. (1999). Antimicrobial activity of essential oils and other plant extracts. *Journal of Applied Microbiology* **86**: 985–990.

Hili, P., Evans, C.S., Veness, R.G. (1997). Antimicrobial action of essential oils: The effect of dimethylsulphoxide on the activity of cinnamon oil. *Letters in Applied Microbiology* **24**: 269–275.

Hinou, J.B., Harvala, C.E., Hinou, E.B. (1989). Antimicrobial activity screening of 32 common constituents of essential oils. *Pharmazie* **44**: H4.

Jeongmok, K., Marshall, M.R., Wei, C. (1995). Antibacterial activity of some essential oil components against five foodborne pathogens. *Journal of Agricultural and Food Chemistry* **43**: 2839–2845.

Jo, C., Park, B.J., Chung, G.H., Kim, C.B., Cha, B.S., Byun, M.W. (2004). Antibacterial and anti-fungal activity of Citrus (*Citrus unshiu*) essential oil extracted from peel byproducts. *Food science and Biotechnology* **13**: 384–386.

Johann, S., de Oliveria, V.L., Pizzolatti, M.G., Schripsema, J., Braz-Filho, R., Branco, A., Smânia, Jr., A. (2007). Antimicrobial activity of wax and hexane extracts from *Citrus spp.* peels. *Mem Inst Oswaldo Cruz, Rio de Janerio* **102**: 681–685.

Joint FAO/WHO Expert Committee on Food Additives (1995). Forty-fourth meeting, Rome, Italy.

Kawaii, S., Tomono, Y., Katase, E., Ogawa, K., Yano, M. (1999). Quantitation of flavonoid constituents in Citrus fruits. *Journal of Agricultural and Food Chemistry* **47**: 3565–3571.

Khanum, M.N., Yamaguchi, T., Hiroishi, S., Muraoka, F., Takamura, H., Matoba, T. (1999). Radical-scavenging activities of fish and fishery products. *Food Science and Technology Research* **5**: 193–199.

Kikugawa, K. (2003). Reduction of mutagenic and/or carcinogenic compounds in foods. *Foods and Food Ingredients Journal of Japan* **208**: 174–183.

Kim, J., Marshall, M.R., Wei, C. (1995). Antibacterial activity of some essential oil components against five foodborne pathogens. *Journal of Agricultural and Food Chemistry* **43**: 2839–2845.

Knobloch, K., Weigand, N., Weis, H.M., Vigenschow, H. (1986). In: Brunke, E.J. (ed.), *Progress in essential oil research*. Berlin: Walter de Gruyther, p. 429.

Knobloch, K., Pauli, A., Iberl, N., Weis, H.M., Weigand, N. (1988). Modes of action of essential oil components on whole cells of bacteria and fungi in plate tests. In: Schreier P. (ed.), *Bioflavour*. Berlin: Walter de Gruyther, pp. 287–299.

Kuate, J., Foko, J., Ndindeng, S.A., Jazet-Dongmo, P.M., Fouré, E., Damesse, F. O., Ducelier, D. (2006). Effect of essential oils from citrus varieties on *in vitro* growth and sporulation of *Phaeoramularia angolensis* causing citrus leaf and fruit spot disease. *European Journal of Plant Pathology* **114**: 151–161.

Kunugi, A., Komoda, Y., Kurechi, T. (1983). Determination of nitrite and nitrate by high performance liquid chromatography. *Journal of Food Hydgienics Society of Japan* **24**: 324–328.

Kurechi, T., Kikugawa, K., Fukuda, S. (1980). Nitrite-reacting substances in Japanese radish juice and their inhibition of nitrosamine formation. *Journal of Agricultural and Food Chemistry* **28**: 1265–1269.

Kurita, N., Miyaji, M., Kurane, R., Takahara, Y., Ichimura, K. (1979). Antifungal activity and molecular orbital eneries of aldehyde compounds from oils of higher plants. *Agriculture and Biological Chemistry* **43**: 2365–2371.

Lambert, R.J.W., Skandamis, P.N., Coote, P.J., Nychas, G.J.E. (2001). A study of the minimum inhibitory concentration and mode of action of oregano essential oil, thymol and carvacrol. *Journal of Applied Microbiology* **91**: 453–462.

Lanciotti, R., Gianotti, A., Patrignani, F., Belletti, N., Guerzoni, M.E., Gardini, F. (2004). Use of natural aroma compounds to improve shelf-life and safety of minimally processed fruits. *Trends in Food Science & Technology* **15**: 201–208.

Lee, O.H., Lee, B.Y., Kim, Y.C., Shetty, K., Kim, Y.C. (2008). Radical scavenging-linked antioxidant activity of ethanolic extracts of diverse types of extra virgin olive oils. *Journal of Food Science* **73**: 519–525.

Lijinsky, W. (1999). *N*-Nitroso compounds in the diet. *Mutant Research* **443**: 129–138.

Lindsay, R.C. (1996). Food additives. In: Fennema, O.R. (ed.), *Food chemistry*. NY: Marcel Dekker, Inc., pp. 780–782.

Mahmoud, A.L. (1994). Antifungal action and aflatoxigenic properties of some essential oil constituents. *Letters in Applied Microbiology* **19**: 110–113.

Mandalari, G., Bennett, R.N., Bisignano, G., Trombetta, D., Saija, A., Faulds, C.B., Gasson, M.J., Narbad, A. (2007). Antimicrobial activity of flavonoids extracted from bergamot (*Citrus bergamia* Risso) peel, a byproduct of the essential oil industry. *Journal of Applied Microbiology* **103**: 2056–2064.

Manthey, J.A. (2004). Fractionation of orange peel phenols in ultrafiltered malasses and mass balance studies of their antioxidant levels. *Journal of Agricultural and Food Chemistry* **52**: 7586–7592.

Marino, M., Bersani, C., Comi, G. (2001). Impedance measurements to study the antimicrobial activity of essential oils from *Lamiaceae* and *Compositae*. *International Journal of Food Microbiology* **67**: 185–187.

McCalley, D., Torres-Grifol, J.F. (1992). Analysis of volatiles in good and bad conditions by gas chromatography and gas chromatography-mass spectrometry. *Analyst* **117**: 721–725.

Mendoza, L., Wilkens, M., Urzua, A. (1997). Antimicrobial study of the resinous exudates and of diterpenoids and flavonoids isolated from some Chilean *Pseudognaphalium* (Asteraceae). *Journal of Ethnopharmacology* **58**: 85–88.

Mirvish, S.S. (1986). Effects of vitamin C and E on *N*-nitroso compound formation, carcinogenesis, and cancer. *Cancer* **58**: 1842–1850.

Misra, N., Batra, S., Mishra, D. (1988). Properties of the essential oil of *Citrus limon* (L.) burm: against a few dermatophytes. *Mycoses* **31**: 380–382.

Miyake, Y., Yamamoto, K., Osawa, T. (1997). Isolation of eriocitrin (eriodictyol 7-rutinoside) from lemon fruit (*Citrus limon* Burm. f.) and its antioxidative activity. *Food Science and Technology Industry Tokyo* **3**: 84–89.

Mizuki, E., Akao, T., Saruwatari, T. (1990). Inhibitory effect of *Citrus unshiu* peel on anaerobic digestion. *Biological Wastes* **33**: 161–168.

Mokbel, M.S., Watanabe, Y., Hashinaga, F., Suganuma, T. (2006). Purification of the antioxidant and antimicrobial substances of ethyl acetate extracts from Buntan (*Citrus grandis* Osbeck) fruit peel. *Pakistan Jouranl of Biologica Sciences* **9**: 145–150.

Mokbel, M.S., Suganuma, T. (2006). Antioxidant and antimicrobial activities of the methanol extracts from pummelo (*Citrus grandis* Osbeck) fruit albedo tissues. *European Food Research Technology* **224**: 39–47.

Moleyar, V., Narasimham, P. (1986). Antifungal activity of some essential oil components. *Food Microbiology* **3**: 331–336.

Molyneux, P. (2004). The use of the stable free radical diphenylpicryl-hydrazyl (DPPH) for estimating antioxidant activity. *Songklanakaric Journal of Science Technology* **26**: 211–219.

Morris, J.A., Khettry, A., Seitz, E.W. (1979). Antimicrobial activity of aroma chemicals and essential oils. *Journal of the American Oil Chemist's Society* **56**: 595–603.

Naiger, R., Kalck, P., Roques, C., Roux, I., Michel, G. (1996). Comparison of antimicrobial properties of monoterpenes and their carbonylated products. *Planta medica* **62**: 275–277.

Nakaizumi, A., Baba, M., Uehara, H., Iishi, H., Tatsuma, M. (1997). *d*-Limonene inhibits *N*-nitrosobis(2-oxopropyl) amine induced hamster pancreatic carcinogenesis. *Cancer Letter* **117**: 99–103.

Nakamura, Y., Tomita, I. (1992). Test for toxin. In: Itokawa Y. (ed.), *Food additives*. Tokyo: Chijinshokan, pp. 159–171.

Nam, I.S., Garnsworthy, P.C., Ahn, J.H. (2006). Supplementation of essential oil extracted from citrus peel to animal feeds decreases microbial activity and aflatoxin contamination without disrupting *in vitro* ruminal fermentation. *Asian-Australasian Journal of Animal Sciences* **19**: 1617–1622.

Nogata, Y., Yoza, K., Kusumoto, K., Kohyama, N., Sekiya, K., Ohta, H. (1996). Screening for inhibitory activity of citrus fruit extracts against platelet cyclooxigenase and lipoxigenase. *Journal of Agricultural and Food Chemistry* **44**: 725–729.

Norman, S., Craft, C.C., Davis, P.L. (1967). Volatiles from injured and uninjured Valencia oranges at different temperatures. *Journal of Food Science* **32**: 656–659.

Obame, L.C., Koudou, J., Kumulnngui, B.S., Massolè, E.P., Ouattara, A.S., Traorè, A.S. (2007). Antioxidant and antimicrobial activities of *Canarium schweinfurthii* Engl. essential oil from Centrafrican Republic. *African Journal of Biotechnology* **6**: 2319–2323.

Ogawa, T., Isshiki, K. (1996). Antimicrobial activity of volatiles from edible herbs. *Nippon Shokuhin Kagaku Kogaku Kaishi* **43**: 535–540.

Ohshima, H., Bartsch, H. (1981). The influence of vitamin C on the *in vivo* formation of nitrosoamines. In: Counsell, J.N., Hornig, D.H. (eds.), *Vitamin C*. London: Applied Science, pp. 215–222.

Osawa, T., Mamiki, M.A. (1981). Novel type of antioxidant isolated from leaf wax of eucalyptus leaves. *Agricultural and Biological Chemistry* **45**: 735–739.

Osuna-García, J.A., Wall, M.M., Waddell, C.A. (1998). Endogenous levels of tocopherols and ascorbic acid during fruit ripening of new Mexican-type chile (*Capsium annuum* L.) cultivars. *Journal of Agricultural and Food Chemistry* **46**: 5093–5096.

Parish, E.P., Baum, D., Kryger, R., Goodrich, R., Baum, R. (2003). Fate of *Salmonellae* in citrus oils and aqueous aroma. *Journal of Food Protection* **66**: 1704–1707.

Pelczar, M.J., Chan, E.C.S., Krieg, N.R. (1988). Control of microorganisms, the control of microorganisms by physical agents. In: *Microbiology*. New York: McGraw-Hill International, pp. 469–509.

Pizzimenti, F., Tulino, G., Marino, A. (1998). Antimicrobial and antifungal activity of bergamot oil. *Program and Abstracts of the International Congress: Bergamotto 98. Stato dell'arte*, Reggio Calabria, Italy, Abstract no. 38.

Rapisarda, P., Tomaino, A., Cascio, L., Monia, F., Pasquale, A., Saija, A. (1999). Antioxidant effectiveness as influenced by phenolic content on the formation of *N*-nitrosodimethylamine. *Journal of Agricultural and Food Chemistry* **47**: 4718–4723.

Rehman, S., Hussain, S., Nawaz, H. (2007). Inhibitory effect of citrus peel essential oils on the microbial growth of bread. *Pakistan Journal of Nutrition* **6**: 558–561.

Romano, L., Battaglia, F., Masucci, L., Sanguinetti, M., Posteraro, B., Plotti, G., Zanetti, S., Fadda, G. (2005). *In vitro* activity of bergamot natural essence and furocoumarin-free and distilled extracts, and their associations with boric acid, against clinical yeast isolates. *Journal of Antimicrobial Chemotherapy* **55**: 110–114.

Saller, R., Reichling, J., Hellenbrecht, D. (1995). In: Wildi, E., Wink, M. (ed.), *Trends in medicinal plant research*. Heidelberg, Germany: Haug-Verlag, p. 69.

Sanguinetti, M., Posteraro, B., Romano, L., Battaglia, F., Lopizzo, T., De Carolis, E., Fadda, G. (2007). *In vitro* activity of *Citrus bergamia* (bergamot) oil against clinical isolates of dermatophytes. *Journal of Antimicrobial Chemotherapy* **59**: 305–308.

Sawamura, M., Song, H.S., Ozaki, K., Ishikawa, J., Ukeda, H. (1999). Inhibitory effects of citrus essential oils and their components on the formation of *N*-nitrosodimethylamine. *Journal of Agricultural and Food Chemistry* **47**: 4868–4872.

Sawamura, M., Wu, Y., Fujiwara, C., Urushibata, M. (2005). Inhibitory effect of yuzu essential oil on the formation of *N*-nitrosodimethylamine in vegetables. *Journal of Agricultural and Food Chemistry* **53**: 4281–4287.

Sharma, N., Tripathi, A. (2006). Fungitoxicity of the essential oil of *Citrus sinensis* on post-harvest pathogens. *World Journal of Microbiology & Biotechnology* **22**: 587–593.

Sharma, N., Tripathi, A. (2008). Effects of *Citrus sinensis* (L>) Osbeck epicarp essential oil on growth and morphogenesis of *Aspergillus niger* (L.) van Tieghem. *Microbiological Research* **163**: 337–344.

Shin, S., Lim, S. (2004). Antifungal effects of herbal essential oils alone and in combination with ketoconazole against *Trichophyton* spp. *Journal of Applied Microbiology* **97**: 1289–1296.

Shintre, M.S., Gaonkar, T.A., Modak, S.M. (2006). Efficacy of an alcohol-based healthcare hand rub containing synergistic combination of farnesol and benzethonium chloride. *International Journal of Hygiene and Environmental Health* **209**: 477–487.

Sirendi, M., Gohtani, S., Yamano, Y. (1998). Effect of some polysaccharides on oxidative stability of methyl linoleate in emulsion. *Journal of Dispersion Science and Technology* **19**: 679–694.

Smânia, Jr, A. (2007). Antimicrobial activity of wax and hexane extracts from *Citrus spp.* peels. *Mem Inst Oswaldo Cruz, Rio de Janerio* **102**: 681–685.

Smith-Palmer, A., Stewart, J., Fyfe, L. (1998). Antimicrobial properties of plant essential oils and essences against five important food-borne pathogens. *Letters in Applied Microbiology* **26**: 118–122.

Sohn, S.M., Yoneyama, T. (1996). NO_3^- of vegetables: Physiology and accumulation of NO_3^- by vegetables for human. *Nogyo Oyobi Engei* **71**: 1179–1182.

Song, H.S., Ukeda, H., Sawamura, M. (2001). Antioxidative activities of citrus peel essential oils and their components against linoleic acid oxidation. *Food Science and Technology Research* **7**: 50–56.

Stephany, R.W., Schuller, P.L. (1980). Daily dietary intakes of nitrate, nitrite and volatile *N*-nitrosamines in the Netherlands using the duplicate portion sampling technique. *Oncology* **37**: 203–210.

Stiborova, M., Hansikova, H., Schemeiser, H.H., Frei, E. (1997). An investigation of the metabolism of *N*-nitrosodimethylamine and *N*-nitrosodimethylaniline by horseradish peroxidase in vitro. *General Physiology and Biophysics* **16**: 285–297.

Subba, M.S., Soumithri, T.C., Suryanarayana Rao, R. (1967). Antimicrobial action of citrus oils. *Journal of Food Science* **32**: 225–227.

Suja, K.P., Jayalekshmy, A., Arumughan, C. (2004). Free radical scavenging behavior of antioxidant compounds of sesame (*Sesamum indicum* L) in DPPH system. *Journal of Agricultural and Food Chemistry* **52**: 912–915.

Swingle, W.T. (1943). The botany of *Citrus* and its wild relatives of the orange subfamily (family *Rutaceae*, subfamily *aurantioideae*). In: Mebber, H.J., Batchelor, L.D. (ed.), *The citrus industry*. Berkeley, CA: University of California Press, pp. 190–430.

Talcott, S.T., Percival, S.S., Pitter-Moore, J., Celoris, C. (2003). Phytochemical composition and antioxidant stability of fortified yellow passion fruit (*Passiflora edulis*). *Journal of Agricultural and Food Chemistry* **51**: 935–941.

Tanimura, A. (1980). Recent research on nitrite and related compounds. *Shokuhin Eisei Kenkyu* **33**: 1105–1111.

Teow, C.C., Trong, V.D., McFeeters, R.F., Thompson, R.L., Pecota, K.V., Yencho, G.C. (2007). Antioxidant activities, phenolic and β-carotene contents of sweet potato genotypes with varying flesh colours. *Food Chemistry* **103**: 829–838.

Tokoro, K. (1997). Antioxidants in grapefruit oil. *Aromatopia* **24**: 42–44.

Tsushida, T., Suzuki, M., Kurogi, M. (1994). Evaluation of antioxidant activity of vegetable extracts and determination of some active compounds. *Nippon Shokuhin Kogyo Gakkaishi* **41**: 611–618.

Ultee, A., Bennik, M.H.J., Moezelaar, R. (2002). The phenolic hydroxyl group of carvacrol is essential for action against the food-borne pathogen *Bacillus cereus*. *Applied and Environmental Microbiology* **68**: 1561–1568.

Verzera, A., Trozzi, A., Gazea, F., Cicciarello, G., Cortroneo, A. (2003). Effects of rootstock on the composition of bergamot (*Citrus bergamia* Risso et Poiteau) essential oil. *Journal of Agricultural food and Chemistry* **51**: 206–210.

Viuda-Martos, M., Ruiz-Navajas, Y., Fernández-López, J., Pérez-Álvarez, J. (2008). Antifungal activity of lemon (*Citrus limon* L.), mandarin (*Citrus reticulata* L.), grapefruit (*Citrus paradise* L.) and orange (*Citrus sinensis* L.) essential oils. *Food Control* **19**: 1130–1138.

Vogtmann, H., Biedermann, R. (1985). The nitrate story: No end in sight. *Nutrition and Health* **3**: 217–239.

Walters, C.L. (1981). The influence of ascorbic acid on the formation of *N*-nitrosoamines in foods, drugs, cosmetics and tobacco. In: Counsell, J.N., Hornig, D.H. (eds.), *Vitamin C*. London: Applied Science, pp. 199–213.

Walters, C.L., Smith, P.L.R. (1981). The effect of water-borne nitrate on salivary nitrite. *Food Chemistry and Toxicology* **19**: 297–302.

Wang, H., Cao, G., Prior, R.L. (1996). Total antioxidant capacity of fruits. *Journal of Agricultural and Food Chemistry* **44**: 701–705.

Wilkins, M.R. (2007). Effect of limonene on ethanol production by *Zymomonas mobilis*. *2007 ASABE Annual International Meeting* **11**: 8.

Willet, W.C. (1994). Diet and health: What should we eat? *Science* **264**: 532–537.

Wu, Y.N., Wang, H.Z., Li, J.S., Han, C. (1993). The inhibitory effect of Chinese tea and its polyphenols on in vitro and in vivo *N*-nitrosation. *Biomedical and Environmental Science* **6**: 237–258.

Wuryatmo, E., Klieber, A., Eileen, S. (2003). Inhibition of citrus postharvest pathogens by vapor of citral and related compounds in culture. *Journal of Agricultural and Food Chemistry* **51**: 2637–2640.

Yagi, K.A. (1970). A rapid method for evaluation of autoxidation and antioxidants. *Agricultural and Biological Chemistry* **34**: 142–145.

Yano, M. (1998). Health-promoting compounds in citrus fruits. *Up-to Date Food Process* (in Japanese) **33**: 4–7.

Zheng, G., Kenney, P.M., Lam, L.K.T. (1992a). Effects of carvone compounds on glutathione *S*-tranferase activity in A/J mice. *Journal of Agricultural and Food Chemistry* **40**: 751–755.

Zheng, G., Kenney, P.M., Lam, L.K.T. (1992b). Anethofuran, carvone, and limonene: Potential cancer chemopreventive agents from dill weed oil and caraway oil. *Planta Medica* **58**: 338–341.

Zhu, S.Y., Yang, Y., Yu, H.D., Ying, Y., Zou, G.L. (2005). Chemical composition and antimicrobial activity of the essential oils of *Chrysanthemum indicum*. *Journal of Ethnopharmacology* **96**: 151–158.

7

AROMATHERAPY

Chizu Kumagai
Municipal Ida Hospital, City of Kawasaki
Kanagawa, Japan

Aromatherapy involves the use of essential oils for medical purposes, and for promoting and maintaining health and beauty. It is one of the traditional folk medicines practiced since ancient times in Europe, and is defined as "the art based on the use of essential oils for a therapeutic purpose" (Torii, 2002, pp. 8–10). Essential oils have been studied for their antioxidant, antimicrobial, and antidepressant properties (Chang, 2008; Inoue and Abe, 2006; Nakayama et al., 2004). Thousands of years ago, essential oils were used in traditional herbal medicine, which was practiced in countries such as Egypt and India. However, the word *aromatherapy* was initially used by the French chemist René Maurice Gattefossé, in a book first published in 1937 (Gattefossé, 1993). Essential oils in aromatherapy are used for massages, inhalation, aromatic baths, compresses, cosmetic preparations, and many other specific applications to ease aches and pains, and relieve depression and anxiety (Han et al., 2006; Kim et al., 2005; Soden et al., 2004; Yip and Tam, 2008). Aromatherapy can be effective against several symptoms and diseases (Table 7.1) (Imanishi, 2006, p. 3).

Citrus Essential Oils: Flavor and Fragrance, Edited by Masayoshi Sawamura

TABLE 7.1. Symptoms and disorders for which aromatherapy can be effective

Respiratory disorder	Common cold, influenza, asthma
Arrergie	Hay fever
Skin disorder	Atopic dermatitis, contact dermatitis
Pregnancy, childbirth	Dysmenorrhea, premenstrual tension, menopause
Psychophysiological disorder	
Mental disorder	Insomnia, panic
Life-habit disorder	Hypertension, diabetes, adiposis
Aches and pains	Stiff shoulder, low-back pain, arthralgia, myalgia
Dysrhythmia	Jet lag
Gastrointestinal disorder	Constipation, dysorexia

7.1 APPLICATION FOR THERAPEUTIC EFFECT

Chizu Kumagai

7.1.1 Basic Fields of Aromatherapy

Clinical Aromatherapy. Several basic studies and clinical trials have examined the effectiveness of aromatherapy. It is a prescription therapy in France. Essential oils are administered orally. These are commonly used by physicians trained in phytotherapy, which involves aromatherapy as a part of medicine to treat infectious diseases.

Holistic Aromatherapy. Holistic aromatherapy is a touch-care therapy that employs essential oils and massage to treat physical and mental disorders. This form of treatment is conducted by well-trained practitioners in a medical clinic or treatment salon. The first consultation should involve an assessment of medical history, diet, exercise, general life-style, and physical and mental condition.

Home-Care Aromatherapy. Essential oils are popularly used for family and self-care, for inhalation, mouthwash, and massage, and as bath additives.

Beauty (Aesthetic) Aromatherapy. Many beauty therapists use ready-blended aroma oils for relaxation, slimming, or minor skin problems. Treatment is given by beauticians at aesthetic salons.

7.1.2 History

Aromatherapy commenced in ancient Egypt. A medical book, *The Papyrus of Ebers*, was written around 1550 B.C. This book describes the many aromatic plants used in Egyptian medicine. Prescriptions of many aromatic blends were also engraved on the walls of Egyptian temples. “Kyphi,” which is a blend of 16 kinds of aromatic substances such as saffron, cassia, spikenard, cinnamon, juniper, and frankincense, was used as a perfume, incense, and medicine (Torii, 2002, pp. 10–14). When the tomb of Tut'ankhamun was unearthed, archaeologists discovered an ointment jar that had retained its frankincense aroma. Furthermore, Egyptians used fragrant substances, such as myrrh and cassia, as preservatives during mummification, by wrapping the body in linen that was soaked in fragrant substances, such as cedarwood oil. Oil was infused with fragrance and applied to the body.

In the Gospels of the New Testament, John wrote: "Mary took a pound of costly perfume made of pure Nardo, anointed Jesus' feet, and wiped them with her hair. The house was filled with the fragrance of the perfume." "Nardo" means *spikenard* (*Nardostachys jatamansi*); its root was used as an aromatic stomachic or incense. This act of Mary was similar to aromatherapy.

In ancient Greece, Hippocrates, the father of medicine, recorded the hypnotic effect of poppies, and the analgesic effect of the willow leaf. During the Roman Empire, Dioscorides documented over 900 kinds of medicines and 500 species of plants, such as cypress, juniper, marjoram, and myrrh, into the *De Materia Medica*. In particular, he described "Kyphi," which has a sedative effect and is also used to ease an asthmatic attack.

In medieval Europe, a bouquet of herbs was used to prevent illness; many herbalists appeared by the seventeenth century. Infectious diseases were prevalent and many lives were lost. The cause of the disease was believed to be airborne. When disease broke out, disinfection was performed by burning frankincense, rosemary, and other things. Perfumers did not fall ill during this time, and it was believed to be because they were surrounded by essential oils.

The science of chemistry developed rapidly from the second half of the eighteenth century to the nineteenth century. It became possible to isolate and extract individual chemical substances from natural materials. Furthermore, different substances were made to react with each other to produce new chemical substances. However, herbal medicine declined with the development of modern medicine. In 1937, the French cosmetic scientist René Maurice Gattefossé coined the term *aromatherapy*. He was tragically burned in an explosion in his laboratory, but he covered the wounds in lavender oil and completely recovered with no scars. Significant interest in the medicinal usage of essential oils developed from this experience, resulting in the publication of the 1937 book, *Aromatherapie* (Gattefossé, 1993). The French doctor Jean Valnet treated a wounded soldier during World War I with an essential oil, which demonstrated its bactericidal effect. He went on to build the Foundation for Medical Aromatherapy in France. In Austria, the biochemist Marguerite Maury developed a special massage technique, which involved applying essential oils that were diluted in vegetable oil as an aromatherapy, resulting in the prescription of essential oils for massage. She described her medical and aesthetic treatment experiences with essential oils in her book, *The Secret of Life and Youth* (Maury, 1964).

Robert Tisserand, a British aromatherapist, explained the importance of aromatherapy in stress, pathology, revival of naturalism, and the social principle (Tisserand, 1977). He summarized aromatherapy as a systematic science in the book, *The Art of Aromatherapy*, in 1977. In modern medicine, strong single-component antibiotics have provided excellent results and have saved many lives; however, the side effects of powerful modern medicines emerged, and the basis for many diseases shifted from infectious to stress and lifestyle-related diseases. Today, aromatherapy attracts attention all over the world as an alternative medicine that produces both pharmacological and sense-of-smell effects.

7.1.3 The Sense of Smell

Odorous molecules, such as those present in essential oils, are transmitted as follows:

Odorous molecule → Olfactory epithelium of nasal cavity → Electrical signal → Olfactory neuron → Limbic system → Hypothalamus

When applied during massage, aromatic molecules are absorbed not only from the skin, but also from the respiratory and olfactory organs. Once the sense of smell is stimulated, the impulses reach the limbic system, which supports several functions, including emotion and memories. The olfactory stimulation is transmitted through the limbic system to the hypothalamus, which is the center of the autonomic nervous system and controls most of the involuntary activities that maintain life, such as digestion, heartbeat, and breathing, and also controls body temperature and hunger. The pituitary gland, which regulates parts of the endocrine system, is also stimulated.

7.1.4 Pharmacological Effects of Essential Oils

Essential oils are included in the national pharmacopoeia of many countries; for example, there are 26 essential oils in the *European Pharmacopoeia* (2008). Several basic research studies and clinical trials have been published recently that describe the anti-inflammatory, antimicrobial, and antioxidant properties of essential oils (Chaieb et al., 2007; Inoue and Abe, 2006; Nakayama et al., 2004).

Anti-Inflammatory Activity. Chamazulene, found in German chamomile (*Matricaria chamomilla*) oil, has been shown to be anti-inflammatory in vivo (Safayhi et al., 1994). Aqueous preparations include azulene as an active ingredient for treating inflammation of the oral cavity and throat. Azulene has been packaged as a tablet, gargle, instillation, and ointment. It exerts its anti-inflammatory effect by inhibiting the production of leukotriene B4 in the neutrophils (Safayhi et al., 1994). Leukotriene B4 is one of the chemicals released at the site of inflammation, and it causes further inflammation.

Antimicrobial Activity. Essential oils and their volatile constituents have antimicrobial properties. A broad range of bacteria have been tested for their susceptibility to tea tree, rosemary, cinnamon, clove, and others (Carson et al., 2006; Prabuseenivasan et al., 2006). The essential constituents, linalool, geraniol, and menthol, are active against bacteria and fungi. Among these, linalool is most potent against bacteria, followed by cineole and geraniol. Citral and geraniol are the most effective against fungi, followed by linalool, cineole, and menthol (Pattnaik et al., 1997).

Pharmacological Properties of the Main Essential Oil Constituents. These properties are shown in Table 7.2 for pharmacological properties of essential oil constituents (Imanishi, 2006, pp. 18–19) and in Table 7.3 for citrus essential oil profiles (Mikami, 2006).

TABLE 7.2. Pharmacological properties of essential oil constituents

Functional Groups	Pharmacological Properties	Constituents	Essential Oils	Effectiveness
Monoterpenes	antibacterial antivirus diuretic immune stimulant	myrcene	Lemongrass (*Cymbopogon citratus*)	analgegic
		limonene	Dill seed (*Anethum graveolens*) Citrus	antitumor
		caryophylene	Ylang ylang (*Cananga odorata*)	sedative
			Lavender (*Lavandula angustifolia*)	analgegic
			Sweet marjoram (*Origanum majorana*)	antibacterial
			Rosemary (*Rosmarinus officinalis*)	
Sesquiterpenes	anti-inflammatory antibacterial antivirus	chamazulene	Chamomile german (*Matricaria chamomilla*)	anti-inflammatory antiallergic
	antiallergic decreased body temperature	farnesene	Ginger (*Zingiber officinale*)	
		bisabolene	Black pepper (*Piper nigrum*)	

TABLE 7.2. *Continued*

Functional Groups	Pharmacological Properties	Constituents	Essential Oils	Effectiveness
Alcohols	antibacterial antivirus mental stimulant	geraniol	Palmarosa (*Cymbopogon martini*)	
		linalool	Lavender (*Lavandula angustifolia*) Neroli (*Citrus aurantium*) Thyme (*Thymus vulgaris*)	
		menthol	Peppermint (*Mentha piperita*)	antibacterial
		farnesol	Chamomile german (*Matricaria chamomilla*) Rose (*Rosa damascena*) Palmarosa (*Cymbopogon martini*) Ylang ylang (*Cananga odorata*)	
		terpineol	Bergamot (*Citrus bergamia*) Neroli (*Citrus aurantium*) Geranium (*Pelargonium graveolens*) Sweet marjoram (*Origanum majorana*)	antibacterial
		terpinen-4-ol	Tea tree (*Melaleuca alternifolia*)	antibacterial
Phenols	antibacterial immune stimulant mental stimulant	thymol	Thyme (*Thymus vulgaris*)	antiparasitic
		eugenol	Clove (*Syzygium aromaticum*) Cinnamon (*Cinnamomum zeylanicum*)	anti-inflammatory antidiarrheic
		carvacrol	Oregano (*Origanum vulgare*)	

TABLE 7.2. *Continued*

Functional Groups	Pharmacological Properties	Constituents	Essential Oils	Effectiveness
Aldehydes	ataraxic sedative anti-inflammatory antifungal	citronellal	Lemongrass (*Cymbopogon citratus*) Geranium (*Pelargonium graveolens*) Lemonbalm (*Melissa officinalis*)	antifungal
		geranial neral		
Esters	antispasmodic sedative antifungal	linalyl acetate	Clary sage (*Salvia sclalea*) Bergamot (*Citrus bergamia*) Lavender (*Lavandula angustifolia*)	
		geranyl acetate	Sweet marjoram (*Origanum majorana*)	
Ketones	cicatrizant mucolytic	menthone	Geranium (*Pelargonium graveolens*) Peppermint (*Mentha piperita*)	
Oxides	immune stimulant expectorant	cineole	Eucalyptus (*Eucalyptus radiata*) Rosemary (*Rosmarinus officinalis*)	mental stimulant
Lactones	mental stimulant mucolytic	alantolactone	Elecampane (*Inula helenium*)	
Coumarins		bergaptene	Bergamot (*Citrus bergamia*)	
		furanocoumarine	Lemon (*Citrus limon*)	

TABLE 7.3. Citrus essential oil profiles

Essential Oil	Sweet Orange	Bitter Orange	Neroli
Botanical name	*Citrus sinensis L.*	*Citrus aurantium L.*	*Citrus aurantium L.*
Family name	*Rutaceae*	*Rutaceae*	*Rutaceae*
Extraction	Expressed from peel	Expressed from peel	Steam distillation from flower
Origin	USA, Brazil, Mexico	Italy, USA, Spain	Tunisia, France, Morocco
Main components	limonene *n*-octanal sabinen *n*-decanal	limonene myrcene β-pinene linalyl acetate	linalool limonene α-pinene *trans*-β-ocimene
Main properties	antibacterial air purifier anti-inflammatory insect repellent sedative etc.	antibacterial analgesic sedative air purifier increased vascular flow etc.	sedative and arousal antipruritic skin tonic antibacterial nerve tonic etc.
IFRA regulation	none	phototoxic	none
Maximum use level		1.4%	
RIFM toxicity			
LD50 (oral)	>5 g/kg in rat	>5 g/kg in rat	4.4–4.6 g/kg in rat
LD50 (dermal)	>5 g/kg in rabbit	>5 g/kg in rabbit	>5 g/kg in rabbit
Irritation	mouse: none rabbit: moderate	mouse: moderate	mouse and rabbit: none
Phototoxicity	none	yes	none

7.1.5 Therapeutic Uses of Essential Oils in Aromatherapy

There are a wide variety of methods to use essential oils in aromatherapy.

Inhalation. Inhalation has been used for many centuries to ease respiratory problems such as colds, catarrh, sinusitis, sore throats, coughs, and so on. The simplest method is to put two or three drops of essential oil in a bowl of near-boiling water, lean over the bowl with a large towel enveloping both the bowl and your head, and inhale the steam for five minutes or more.

Bergamot	Grapefruit	Lemon	Petitgrain Bigarade	Yuzu
Citrus bergamia	*Citrus paradisi*	*Citrus limon*	*Citrus aurantium*	*Citrus junos*
Rutaceae	*Rutaceae*	*Rutaceae*	*Rutaceae*	*Rutaceae*
Expressed from peel	Expressed from peel	Expressed from peel	Steam distillation from leaves and twigs	Expressed from peel
Italy, Ivory, Guinea	USA, Israel, Brazil	North America, Italy, Spain	France, Tunisia, Italy, Spain	Japan, Korea, China
limonene linalyl acetate linalool γ-terpinene	limonene myrcene *n*-octanal *n*-decanal	limonene β-pinene γ-terpinene sabinene	linalool limonene β-pinene *trans*-β-ocimene	limonene γ-terpinene β-phellandrene α-pinene
analgesic antibacterial antifungal antispasmodic digestant etc.	lipolysis killing air bacteria antibacterial vasodilator stomachic etc.	antibacterial antifungal antivirus digestant air purifier etc.	antibacterial antifungal antivirus antispasmodic cicatrisant etc.	cartinostatic antibacterial antifungal deodorant antioxidant etc.
phototoxic	phototoxic	phototoxic	none	citrus; bergapten 75 ppm
75 ppm	4%	4%		
>10 g/kg in rat	>5 g/kg in rat	5 g/kg in rat	>5 g/kg in rat	no data
>20 g/kg in rabibt	>5 g/kg in rabbit	>5 g/kg in rabbit	>2 g/kg in rabbit	no data
no data (mouse)	mouse: none rabbit: moderate	rabbit: moderate		no data
yes	yes	yes	no data	no data

Massage Oils. This application can be used to treat problems from muscular aches and pains to skin conditions, anxiety, insomnia, and tension. The essential oil is diluted in vegetable-based oil for this purpose.

Aromatic Baths. Aromatic baths can be relaxing or sedative, stimulating, warming and calming, or an aphrodisiac. About five drops of essential oil are sprinkled into a tub filled with hot water, just before getting into the bath. The water is stirred to disperse the oil, which spreads to form a very thin film on the surface of the water, some of which adheres to the skin.

Diffuser or Spray. A vaporizer, oil burner, or electric diffuser can be used to diffuse essential oils. Diffusing essential oils can be useful during a cold; antibacterial oils, such as tea tree oil, may kill airborne bacteria and help prevent the spread of infection.

Compresses. Compresses are an effective way to treat muscular pain, sprains, and bruises. Warm compresses are prepared by adding one or two drops of essential oil to a bowl of hot water containing a towel. The excess water is squeezed out and the area to be treated is covered by the towel. Warm compresses are used for muscular and menstrual pain, whereas cold compresses are used for recent injuries such as sprains, bruises, swelling, and headaches.

7.1.6 Autonomic Nerve Activity and Citrus Essential Oils

In aromatherapy, citrus essential oils are used to treat depression (Chang, 2008), induce euphoria, and stimulate mental health; some studies have supported these positive effects. For example, lemon oil vapor relieves stress in mice (Komiya et al., 2006); pain and depression in hospice patients with terminal cancer were relieved using an aromatic hand massage with a blended oil of bergamot, lavender, and frankincense in the ratio of 1:1:1 (Chang, 2008).

It is hypothesized that these effects result from sensory signals in the olfactory mucous membrane, which are transmitted through the olfactory nerve to the limbic system as well as to the autonomic center in the hypothalamus.

Yuzu. We found that olfactory stimulation with the scent of yuzu oil decreases sympathetic nerve activity in the interscapular brown adipose tissue (BAT) and epididymal white adipose tissue (WAT) (Kumagai et al., 2009). Since BAT is a thermogenic organ, it produces heat in the mitochondria via the activation of uncoupling protein-1. This heat is stored in the BAT and distributed throughout the body. Thermogenesis is activated by brown adipose tissue sympathetic nerve activity (BAT-SNA). Body temperature, a marker of thermogenesis, is affected as a result of olfactory stimulation with the scent of yuzu oil. This stimulation lowers body temperature and plasma free-fatty acid (FFA) levels in unanesthetized rats (Kumagai et al., 2009), thus suggesting that the activation of sympathetic nerves innervating the WAT promotes lipolysis. These findings also suggest that olfactory stimulation with the scent of yuzu oil suppresses both thermogenesis and lipolysis, through a decrease in sympathetic nerve activity.

Materials and Methods. Eight-week-old male Wistar rats were used in the study. Essential oil of yuzu (*Citrus junos*; cultivated in Kochi, Japan) was prepared from yuzu peel waste post-squeezing, using steam-distillation under reduced pressure (Sawamura, 2005b). Rats were anesthetized with an intraperitoneal injection of urethane (1 g/kg in distilled water) to determine the electrical activity of sympathetic nerves innervating the interscapular BAT and epididymal WAT. Yuzu oil was suspended in a 10-fold volume of water, and cotton tube gauze, which was soaked in the suspension, was placed at the bottom of a plastic beaker, and the nose of the rat was placed inside the plastic beaker for 10 min.

A telemetry system was used to measure body temperature. In a subset of rats, a capsule containing a temperature sensor, battery, and transmitter was placed subcutaneously, above the interscapular BAT. Yuzu oil was suspended in a 100-fold volume of water, and cotton gauze, which was soaked in either water or yuzu oil, was placed on top of the animal cage for the entire experimental period (60 min), and body temperature above the BAT was measured.

A catheter consisting of a silicone tube was inserted into the right external jugular vein to determine plasma FFA levels. Blood samples were collected from the jugular catheter for 2 h at 30-min intervals. In this case, cotton gauze was soaked in either water or yuzu oil (1:1000 in water) and placed on top of the animal cage for the entire 2-h experimental period.

All data are expressed as mean ± standard error of the mean. Due to inter-individual variability in the pre-stimulation state, the percent change from baseline was also calculated for BAT-SNA, WAT-SNA, body temperature, and plasma FFA levels. Repeated-measures analysis of variance (ANOVA) was performed to compare group responses, and the Mann-Whitney *U*-test was applied to compare basal levels. Values of $p < 0.05$ were considered statistically significant.

Effect of Olfactory Stimulation with the Scent of Yuzu on BAT-SNA. Raw recording data from the BAT-SNA, before and after olfactory stimulation with the scent of yuzu oil, in urethane-anesthetized rats are shown in Figure 7.1 (left panel). The scent of yuzu oil gradually and significantly ($p < 0.0005$, $F = 71.4$ by ANOVA) reduced BAT-SNA compared with the BAT-SNA level in rats stimulated with water (Figure 7.1, right panel). No significant difference was observed between these basal values.

Effect of Olfactory Stimulation with the Scent of Yuzu on WAT-SNA. Raw recording data from the WAT-SNA, before and after olfactory stimulation with the scent of yuzu oil, in urethane-anesthetized rats are shown in Figure 7.2 (left panel). Olfactory stimulation with water did not change WAT-SNA (at 0 min). However, olfactory stimulation with the scent of yuzu oil reduced WAT-SNA up to 40 min after the start of olfactory stimulation, and then slightly increased SNA until the end of the experiment (Figure 7.2, right panel). The scent of yuzu gradually and significantly reduced WAT-SNA compared with the WAT-SNA level in rats stimulated with water ($p < 0.0005$, $F = 87.7$ by ANOVA). No significant difference was observed between these basal values.

Effect of Olfactory Stimulation with the Scent of Yuzu Oil on Body Temperature. Since olfactory stimulation with lavender (*Lavandula angustifolia*) oil suppressed BAT-SNA in urethane-anesthetized rats and lowered body

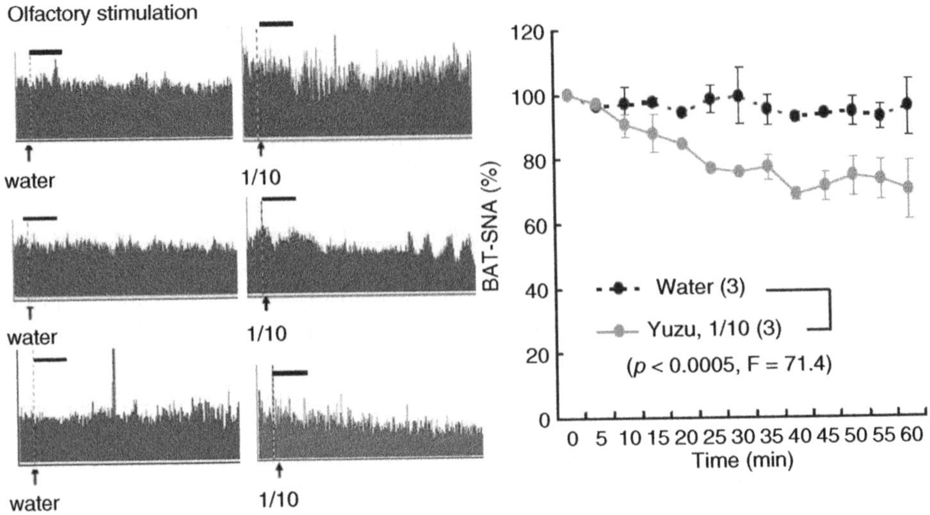

Figure 7.1. Effects of olfactory stimulation with scent of yuzu oil suspended in a 10-fold volume of water on BAT-SNA. *Left*: Raw recording data of BAT-SNA before and after olfactory stimulation with scent of yuzu oil and scent of water in urethane-anesthetized rats. Upper bars indicate a 10-min stimulation period. *Right*: Changes in BAT-SNA after 10 min of olfactory stimulation with scent of yuzu oil or water. Data are expressed as mean ± SEM of percentages of 0-min values. Differences between BAT-SNA values of water and scent of yuzu oil groups used are shown in parentheses. ANOVA was used to analyze differences in BAT-SNA at 5–60 min between water and yuzu groups.

temperature in conscious rats (Shen et al., 2005a), we examined whether olfactory stimulation with the scent of yuzu oil would elicit a decrease in body temperature, by monitoring the subcutaneous space above the interscapular BAT in conscious rats. Raw recording data for temperature are shown in Figure 7.3 (left panel). Olfactory stimulation with water initially induced a slight increase in body temperature, which subsequently fell to below the 0 min value (Figure 7.3, right panel). However, olfactory stimulation with the scent of yuzu oil gradually and significantly reduced body temperature to 99.2% of the 0 min value, 60 min after the start of olfactory stimulation (Figure 7.3, right panel). There was a significant difference between body temperatures in the water and scent-of-yuzu-oil groups for temperatures from 5 to 60 min ($p < 0.0005$, $F = 29.3$ by ANOVA). There were no significant differences between basal values.

Effect of Olfactory Stimulation with the Scent of Yuzu Oil on Plasma FFA Levels. Since the scent of yuzu oil inhibited WAT-SNA and the suppression of this nerve is known to reduce triglyceride hydrolysis, we examined the effect of olfactory stimulation with the scent of yuzu oil on lipolysis. Olfactory

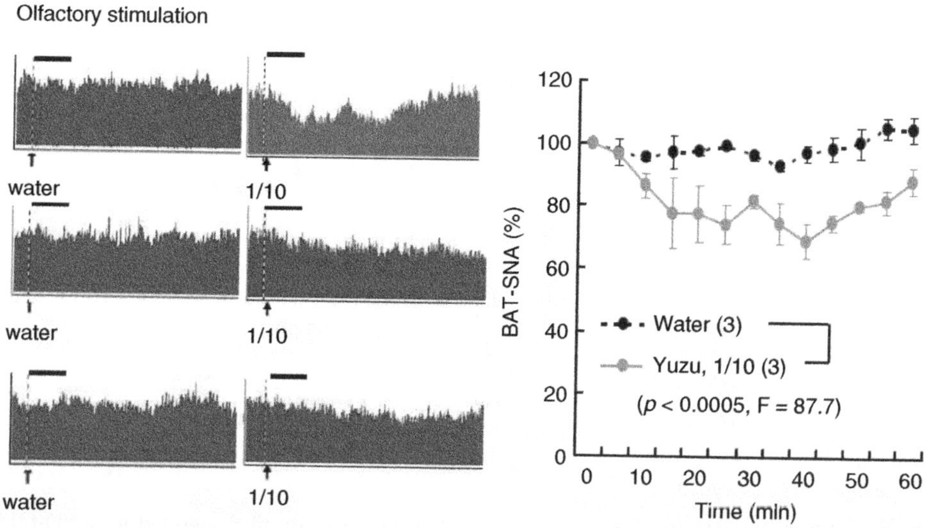

Figure 7.2. Effects of olfactory stimulation with scent of yuzu oil suspended in a 10-fold volume of water on WAT-SNA. *Left*: Raw recording data of WAT-SNA before and after olfactory stimulation with scent of yuzu oil and scent of water in urethane-anesthetized rats. Upper bars indicate a 10-min stimulation period. *Right*: Changes in WAT-SNA after 10 min of olfactory stimulation with scent of yuzu oil or water. Data are expressed as mean ± SEM of percentages of 0-min values. Differences between WAT-SNA values of water and scent of yuzu oil groups used are shown in parentheses. ANOVA was used to analyze differences in WAT-SNA at 5–60 min between water and yuzu groups.

stimulation with water caused a slight increase in plasma FFA levels (Figure 7.4), but olfactory stimulation with the scent of yuzu oil markedly and significantly ($p < 0.005$, F = 10.96 by ANOVA) decreased FFA levels compared with that of water (Figure 7.4). No significant difference was observed between the basal values. The results of the olfactory experiments indicate the following: (1) Olfactory stimulation with the scent of yuzu oil suspended in a 10-fold volume of water caused a reduction in BAT-SNA and WAT-SNA in urethane-anesthetized rats. (2) Olfactory stimulation with the scent of yuzu oil suspended in a 100-fold volume of water induced a significant decrease in body temperature in unanesthetized rats. (3) Olfactory stimulation with the scent of yuzu oil suspended in a 1000-fold volume of water resulted in a significant decrease in plasma FFA levels in unanesthetized rats (Kumagai et al., 2009).

Shen et al. (2005b) reported that olfactory stimulation with the scent of grapefruit oil increased the activity of sympathetic nerves innervating the BAT and WAT in urethane-anesthetized rats. Grapefruit oil contains 95% limonene, whereas yuzu oil contains about 70% limonene. Thus, the scent of yuzu oil was hypothesized to have similar effects to grapefruit oil on sympathetic nerves innervating the BAT and WAT. Indeed, olfactory stimulation with the scent of yuzu

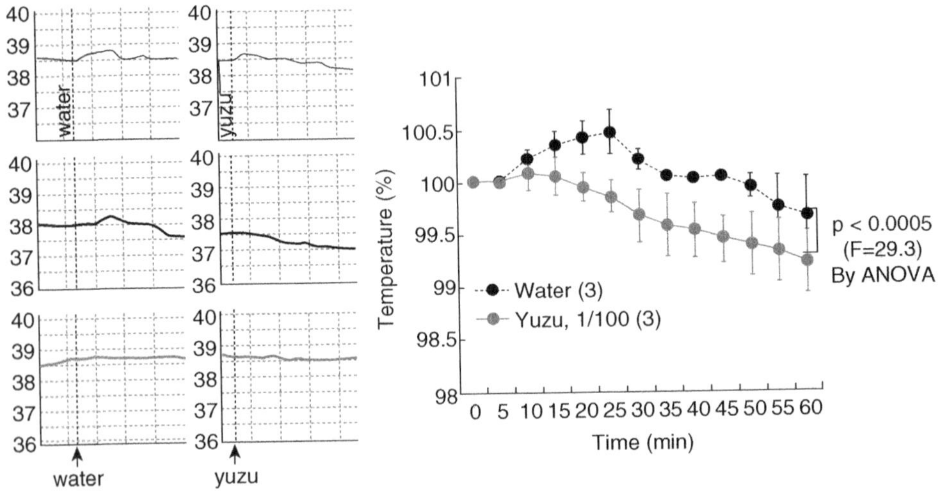

Figure 7.3. Effect of olfactory stimulation with scent of yuzu oil suspended in a 100-fold volume of water on body temperature. *Left*: Raw recording data for body temperature of rats stimulated with water or yuzu oil. *Right*: Changes in body temperature after olfactory stimulation with water or yuzu oil are expressed as mean ± SEM of percentages of 0-min values. Numbers of animals used are shown in parenthesis. ANOVA was used to analyze differences in body temperature at 5–60 min between water and yuzu groups.

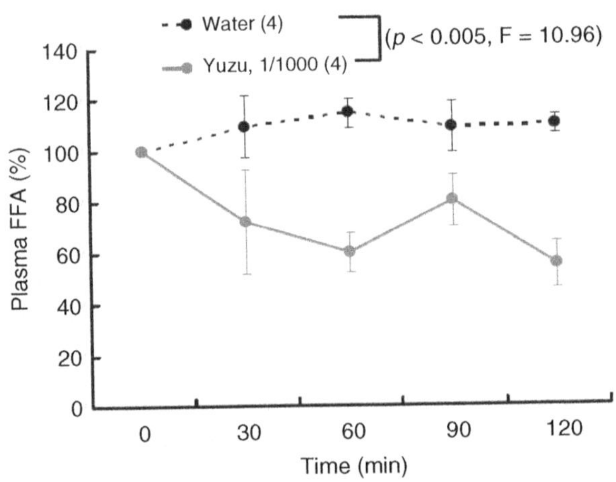

Figure 7.4. Effects of olfactory stimulation with scent of yuzu suspended in a 1000-fold volume of water on plasma FFA concentration. Data (mean ± SEM) are expressed as percentages relative to plasma FFA levels measured at 0 min. Differences between olfactory stimulation by water and yuzu oil at 0 min were not significant according to the Mann-Whitney *U*-test. Numbers of animals used are shown in parentheses. ANOVA was used to analyze differences between water and yuzu groups.

oil suspended in a 1000-fold volume of water increased BAT-SNA up to 380% (data not shown). Furthermore, olfactory stimulation with the scent of yuzu oil suspended in a 1000-fold volume of water increased the WAT-SNA (data not shown), that is, olfactory stimulation with yuzu oil suspended at a low concentration elicited a significant increase in BAT-SNA and WAT-SNA. However, a high concentration of yuzu oil showed the opposite effect, thus suggesting that the effects of linalool, another component of yuzu oil, elicit the opposite effect. Essential oil must be diluted 10 to 100-fold under anesthetized conditions to make the level of scent stimulation equal to the conscious state. Olfactory stimulation with the scent of yuzu oil suspended in a 100-fold volume of water reduced body temperature in conscious rats, and olfactory stimulation with the scent of yuzu oil suspended in a 1000-fold volume of water decreased plasma FFA levels, as a marker of lipolysis, in unanesthetized rats. Yuzu oils used in this study were composed of γ-terpinene (12.8%), β-phellandrene (4.4%), α-pinene (2.7%), myrcene (2.2%), and linalool (1.3%) at much higher levels than that found in grapefruit. This suggests that the concentrations of these components might have overcome any effects of limonene. However, future studies should examine this issue.

Olfactory stimulation with the scent of lavender oil reduces BAT-SNA and WAT-SNA, and suppresses body temperature and plasma glycerol levels. Linalool displays similar effects to lavender oil, that is, it reduces body temperature and plasma glycerol concentrations in unanesthetized rats. These findings indicate that linalool might be at least one of the essential components of yuzu oil causing the changes in BAT-SNA, WAT-SNA, body temperature, and lipolysis. However, further studies are required to clarify the effects of yuzu oil.

Grapefruit. Olfactory stimulation with the scent of grapefruit oil increases the activity of sympathetic nerves innervating the interscapular BAT and the epididymal WAT in urethane-anesthetized rats (Niijima and Nagai, 2003; Shen et al., 2005b; Tanida et al., 2005). Furthermore, grapefruit oil excites sympathetic nerves innervating the adrenal gland, suppresses gastric vagal (parasympathetic) nerve activity (Tanida et al., 2005), and increases plasma glycerol concentration and body temperature (Shen et al., 2005b). A 15-min exposure to the scent of grapefruit oil three times a week, reduced food intake and body weight, and limonene, the main component of grapefruit oil, induces a similar effect (Shen et al., 2005b). Olfactory stimulation with the scent of grapefruit oil, and particularly its main component, limonene, affects autonomic nerves, enhances lipolysis, and reduces appetite and body weight. Furthermore, a 10-min olfactory stimulation with the scent of grapefruit oil elevates renal sympathetic nerve activity and blood pressure (BP), and lowers gastric vagal nerve activity in urethane-anesthetized rats (Tanida et al., 2008). Olfactory stimulation with limonene also induces an increase in renal sympathetic nerve activity and BP in urethane-anesthetized rats (Tanida et al., 2008).

7.1.7 Essential Oil Safety

Bergapten. We have identified bergapten in 25 Japanese citrus essential oils and 27 other citrus essential oils (Table 7.4) (Sawamura et al., 2009). Bergapten

TABLE 7.4. Bergapten in citrus essential oils

Number	Citrus oil sample	Botanical name	Origin	Extraction	Bergapten (ppm)
1	Daidai	*Citrus aurantium* Linn. var. *Cyathifera* Y. Tanaka	Kochi	CP	660.0
2	Kabosu	*C. sphaerocarpa* Hort. ex Tanaka	Oita	CP	700.0
3	Kimikan	*C. flaviculpus* Hort. ex Tanaka	Kochi	CP	n.d.
4	Kiyomi	*C. unshiu* Marcov. × *C. sinensis* Osbeck	Kochi	CP	n.d.
5	Kiyookadaidai	*C. sp.*	Kochi	CP	280.0
6	Mochiyu	*C. inflata* Hort. ex Tanaka	Kochi	CP	n.d.
7	Naoshichi	*C. tagumasudachi* Hort. ex Y. Tanaka	Kochi	CP	250.0
8	Natsudaidai	*C. natsudaidai* Hayata	Kochi	CP	n.d.
9	Ponkan	*C. reticulata* Blanco	Kochi	CP	n.d.
10	Pummelo-1	*C. grandis* Osbeck forma *Tosa*	Kochi	CP	60.0
11	Pummelo-2	*C. grandis* Osbeck forma *Suisho*	Kochi	CP	n.d.
12	Satsuma mandarin	*C. unshiu* Marcov. var. *praecox* Tanaka cv. *Okitsu-wase*	Kochi	CP	n.d.
13	Yuko	*C. yuko* Hort. ex Tanaka	Kochi	CP	n.d.
14	Yuzu-1a	*C. junos* Sieb. ex Tanaka	Kochi	CP	0.5
15	Yuzu-1b	*C. junos* Sieb. ex Tanaka	Kochi (Purchase)	CP	n.d.
16	Yuzu-1c	*C. junos* Sieb. ex Tanaka	Kochi (Purchase)	SD	n.d.
17	Yuzu-2a	*C. junos* Sieb. ex Tanaka	Kochi	CP	n.d.
18	Yuzu-2b*	*C. junos* Sieb. ex Tanaka	Kochi	CP	n.d.
19	Yuzu-3	*C. junos* Sieb. ex Tanaka	Kochi (Purchase)	CP	3.8
20	Yuzu-4	*C. junos* Sieb. ex Tanaka	Kochi	CP	1.0
21	Yuzu-5	*C. junos* Sieb. ex Tanaka	Kochi	SSD	n.d.
22	Yuzu-6	*C. junos* Sieb. ex Tanaka	Ehime	CP	1.3
23	Yuzu-7*	*C. junos* Sieb. ex Tanaka	Kyoto	CP	11.5
24	Yuzu-8 (seedless)	*C. junos* Sieb. ex Tanaka	Kochi	CP	n.d.
25	Yuzu-9	*C. junos* Sieb. ex Tanaka	Korea	CP	18.4
26	Bergamot-1	*C. bergamia* Risso et Poit	Reggio Calabria, Italy	CP	4020.0
27	Bergamot-2	*C. bergamia* Risso et Poit	Purchase (R)	CP	2070.0
28	Bergamot-3	*C. bergamia* Risso et Poit	Purchase (N)	SD	n.d.

29	Bitter orange	C. *aurantium* Linn.	Kochi	CP	n.d.
30	Bitter orange	C. *aurantium* Linn. var. *Amara*	Purchase (M)	CP	4.3
31	Grapefruit-1	C. *paradisi* Maxima	Purchase (N)	CP	110.0
32	Grapefruit-2	C. *paradisi* Maxima	Purchase (S)	CP	33.0
33	Lemon-1	C. *limon* Burmann forma *Eureka*	Kochi	CP	n.d.
34	Lemon-2	C. *limon* Burmann forma *Monachello*	Sicily, Italy	CP	n.d.
35	Lemon-3	C. *limon* Burmann forma *Lisbon*	Kochi	CP	150.0
36	Lemon-4	C. *limon* Burmann	Purchase (N)	CP	110.0
37	Lemon-5	C. *limon* Burmann	Purchase (R)	CP	25.0
38	Lemon-6	C. *limon* Burmann	Purchase (T)	CP	100.0
39	Lime-1	C. *aurantifolia* Swingle	Ben Tre, Vietnam	CP	1200.0
40	Lime-2	C. *aurantifolia* Swingle	Hanoi, Vietnam	CP	210.0
41	Lime-3	C. *aurantifolia* Swingle	Vinh, Vietnam	CP	78.0
42	Lime-4	C. *aurantifolia* Swingle	Purchase (N)	SD	1.4
43	Lime-5	C. *aurantifolia* Swingle	Purchase (Q)	SD	5.0
44	Mandarin-1	C. *reticulata* Blanco	Purchase (B)	CP	n.d.
45	Mandarin-2	C. *reticulata* Blanco	Purchase (N)	CP	n.d.
46	Orange-1	C. *sinensis* Osbeck forma *Lima*	Kochi	CP	n.d.
47	Orange-2	C. *sinensis* Osbeck forma *Ogawa navel*	Kochi	CP	n.d.
48	Orange-3	C. *sinensis* Osbeck forma *Trovita*	Kochi	CP	n.d.
49	Orange-4	C. *sinensis* Osbeck forma *Valencia*	Kochi	CP	n.d.
50	Orange-5	C. *sinensis* Osbeck	Purchase (R)	CP	n.d.
51	Neroli	C. *aurantium* Linn.	Purchase (S)	SD	n.d.
52	Petitgrain	C. *aurantium* Linn. var. *Amara*	Purchase (N)	SD	n.d.

*seedling.
CP: Cold pressing.
SD: Steam distillation.
SSD: Supersonic distillation.
n.d.: Not detected.
Purchase: Commercial product.
B, M, N, Q, R, S, and T: Abbreviation of essential oil producer's name.

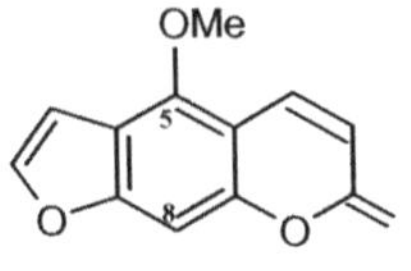

Figure 7.5. Chemical structure of bergapten.

was initially isolated from bergamot (Pomeranz, 1891). It is a furanocoumarin in which the furan ring is combined with the coumarin frame, that is, a psoralen derivative (Figure 7.5). 5-Methoxypsoralen, in which the methoxyl group is combined with carbon 5 of psoralen, is bergapten, and 8-methoxypsoralen has similar optical sensitization to, but lesser action than, bergapten (Schimmer, 1981). These are polycyclic molecules that possess the ability to absorb ultraviolet photons, store them, and release them in a burst onto the skin. This is the reason why itching, erythema, inflammation, and pigmentation are experienced on receiving ultraviolet rays with a high concentration of psoralens adhered to the skin (Tisserand and Balacs, 1995).

The International Fragrance Association (IFRA) has determined that the permissible limit for bergapten in essential oil is less than 15 ppm. Most furanocoumarins are found in *Rutaceae* and *Apiaceae*. In the *Citrus* group, bergapten is found in bergamot and lemon, whereas mandarin and the sweet orange include very little or no bergapten. Although bergapten has been found in many citrus essential oils (Dugo and McHale, 2002; Mondello et al., 1993), there are no reports of it in Japanese citrus, including yuzu. Nevertheless, it is possible that concentrations change with growing location, variety, or extraction method.

Bergapten was quantitatively determined in 25 Japanese citrus essential oils and 27 other citrus essential oils by means of a high-performance liquid chromatograph equipped with a photodiode array detector (SPD-M10Avp, Shimazu Corp.). Most of the essential oil samples were prepared by the cold-pressing method, so as to provide the native composition of the essential oils. The other citrus essential oil samples are extracted by supersonic steam distillation (Sawamura, 2005b), while commercial oils are extracted by steam distillation or cold-pressed methods. Among the Japanese citrus essential oils, the oils of kabosu, daidai, kiyookadaidai, and naoshichi contained bergapten in concentrations higher than 250 ppm (Sawamura et al., 2009). Bergapten was not detected in Satsuma mandarin, ponkan, natsudaidai, mochiyu, yuko, kimikan, or kiyomi essential oils. Twelve samples of yuzu oil were analyzed (Sawamura et al., 2009). Little or no bergapten was detected in the laboratory cold-pressed yuzu essential oils from Kochi, but more than 10 ppm of bergapten was found in those from Kyoto and Korea (Sawamura et al., 2009), thus suggesting that bergapten level may depend on the growing location. Bergapten, in concentrations greater than 100 ppm, was frequently detected in bergamot, grapefruit, lemon, and lime essential oils; however, no bergapten was detected in the *Eureka* and *Monachello* varieties of lemon (Sawamura et al., 2009).

7.2 AGEING OF ESSENTIAL OILS

Masayoshi Sawamura and U-Sun Son

Today, a great number of essential oil products for aromatherapy are commercially sold in new-age and other high-street shops, and the oil products are used in many situations requiring treatment with essential oils. In order to prevent oxidation, nitrogen is put in the bottle and antioxidants might be added to the essential oil products by some manufacturers. There is still little chemical information, however, on compositional changes during storage and/or usage (Choi and Sawamura, 2000; Njoroge et al., 1996). It is important for consumers and other parties concerned with aromatherapy to ensure the effectiveness and quality of essential oil products, in addition to guaranteeing their safety. The authors provide some information on the compositional change of commercial citrus essential oils for aromatherapy in consideration of practical applications.

7.2.1 Storage Conditions and Analysis

Commercial citrus essential oils, lemon (*Citrus limon* Burman), bergamot (*Citrus bergamia* Risso) and mandarin (*Citrus reticulata* Blanco), were provided from an international aroma-product company, Bay House Aromatics, England. The essential oils were of the highest quality on the market.

Two ml of the essential oil mixed with methyl myristate as internal standard in the ratio of 150:1 were placed in a 4-ml brown vial (Maruem Co., Osaka). The incubator used was a PIC-101 cool incubator (AS ONE Co., Tokyo). The samples were stored under four conditions as follows:

S-1: stored in an incubator set at 25°C with the vial being opened for 3 min every day

S-2: stored in an incubator set at 25°C with the vial opened for 3 min once a month

S-3: stored in a refrigerator set at 5°C with the vial opened for 3 min every day

S-4: stored in a refrigerator set at 5°C with the vial opened for 3 min once a month

The essential oil was analyzed using a Shimadzu gas chromatograph GC-14A with a DB-Wax column (60 m × 0.25 mm i.d., film thickness of 0.25 μm; J&W Scientific, Folsom, CA) equipped with a flame ionization detector. The column temperature was programmed from 70°C (2 min) to 230°C (20 min) at a rate of 2°C/min. Both injector and detector temperatures were 250°C. Nitrogen gas was used as a carrier gas at a flow rate of 2 ml/min. The split ratio was 1:50. The injection volume into GC was 0.2–0.5 μl depending on the peak separation. The measurement was performed in triplicate. A Shimadzu GC-17A coupled with a QP-5000 mass spectrometer was used for GC-MS. The GC condition was the same as that of the GC-14A. Ionization voltage was 70 eV and the ion source temperature was 250°C. The split ratio was 1:32 and the sample size was 0.2 μl.

7.2.2 Lemon Essential Oil

It is said that lemon was generated in India. From the eleventh to the sixteenth century, the lemon spread widely to Asia, Europe, Africa, and the Americas. In the modern age, lemon essential oil has been used commercially in food, beverages, cosmetics, and household products (Sinclair, 1984). Furthermore, lemon essential oil has been used in aromatherapy with refreshing effects. Lemon oil is one of the most important anti-bacterial oils used for infection or putrefaction. It is versatile in massage and bath oil blends, inhalations, and room fresheners. It blends well with many kinds of essential oils, and provides a top note to "lift" many fragrance blends (Susan, 1996).

Sixty-four volatile compounds of lemon essential oil were detected in the original oil, meaning the oil just before storage, and 60 were identified. As shown

TABLE 7.5. Compositionl changes in commercial lemon essential oil under four storage conditions (S-1 to S-4)

Functional Group Compound	Original	S-1					S-2				
	0	1[a]	3	6	9	12	1	3	6	9	12
Hydrocarbons	**97.1**	**87.6**				**30.7**	**93.9**	**85.3**	**87.0**	**74.1**	**72.2**
Aliphatic	*	**				**0.3**	**	**	**	**	**
Tetradecane	nd	nd	*	0.1	0.1	0.1	nd	nd	nd	nd	nd
Monoterpenes	**95.6**	**86.3**				**30.0**	**92.6**	**84.4**	**86.2**	**73.5**	**71.5**
α-Pinene	1.8	2.0	1.6	1.0	0.6	0.6	2.2	2.0	2.0	1.8	1.5
β-Pinene	12.2	11.1	9.4	5.8	3.9	4.0	12.3	10.9	11.2	11.1	9.0
Sabinene	2.0	1.8	1.3	0.7	0.4	0.4	1.9	1.7	1.7	1.6	1.3
Myrcene	1.4	1.2	0.8	0.3	0.1	0.1	1.4	1.2	1.2	1.1	0.9
α-Phellandrene	**	*	nd	nd	nd	nd	**	*	*	*	nd
α-Terpinene	0.1	**	nd	nd	nd	nd	0.1	**	**	**	nd
Limonene	68.5	61.9	52.6	32.8	24.0	20.1	65.1	60.5	61.9	50.2	51.7
β-Phellandrene	0.3	0.2	0.1	**	nd	nd	0.3	0.2	0.2	0.2	0.2
(*Z*)-β-Ocimene	0.1	**	**	*	**	nd	0.1	**	**	**	**
γ-Terpinene	7.2	4.0	0.4	*	**	**	7.0	5.5	4.9	3.7	2.7
p-Cymene	1.6	4.0	6.7	5.1	4.3	4.8	1.9	2.2	3.0	3.7	4.1
Terpinolene	0.3	0.1	**	nd	nd	nd	0.2	0.2	0.1	0.1	0.1
Sesquiterpenes	**1.5**	**1.3**				**0.4**	**1.3**	**0.9**	**0.8**	**0.6**	**0.7**
β-Caryophyllene	0.1	0.1	**	nd	nd	nd	0.1	0.1	**	**	*
(*Z*)-β-Farnesene	**	*	**	**	**	**	**	*	*	**	**
(*E*)-β-Farnesene	1.0	0.9	0.5	0.2	0.1	0.1	1.0	0.5	0.5	0.3	0.4

in Table 7.5, the oil was composed of terpene hydrocarbons (97.1%), aldehydes (1.7%), alcohols (0.6%), and esters (0.3%). Limonene was the most predominant component, accounting for 68.5%, which was similar to the results obtained in other research on lemon oil (Sawamura, 2000; Staroscik and Wilson, 1982). The proportions of β-pinene and γ-terpinene were 12.2 and 7.2%, respectively, which were at the same level as their reports. Sabinene, α-pinene, and myrcene were present in relatively high concentrations 2.0, 1.8, and 1.4%, respectively. The level of *p*-cymene is commonly as much as 0.03–0.2% on the basis of relative peak area in several varieties of fresh lemon oils, while it accounted for up to 1.6% (w/w) in the original sample (Njoroge et al., 1994; Sawamura, 2000; Staroscik and Wilson, 1982). Detailed information on the manufacture of current essential oil products has not been available until now. It has been reported that *p*-cymene in citrus essential oils increased during storage (Sinclair, 1984; Njoroge et al., 1996; Choi and Sawamura, 2000). It is therefore supposed that this lemon oil product might be blended with aged oils. Citral (neral and geranial) is the most character-impacting odor aldehyde of lemon, and its level has been used as an index for the assessment of lemon oil quality (Nursten, 1977; Ichimura and Uchiyama, 1989; Sawamura, 2000). The level was 1.4%, being comparable to that

S-3					S-4				
1	3	6	9	12	1	3	6	9	12
95.8	**83.7**	**80.9**	**75.3**	**64.9**	**89.3**	**86.5**	**93.5**	**94.8**	**93.8**
**	**	**	**	**	**	**	**	**	**
nd	nd	**	*	*	nd	nd	nd	nd	nd
94.5	**82.9**	**80.2**	**74.6**	**64.3**	**87.8**	**85.3**	**92.7**	**94.0**	**92.8**
2.3	1.9	1.7	1.4	1.1	2.2	1.9	2.2	2.3	2.1
12.0	10.5	10.0	8.7	7.2	12.4	11.1	12.0	12.5	12.3
2.0	1.7	1.6	1.3	1.1	2.0	1.7	1.9	2.0	1.9
1.4	1.2	1.2	1.5	0.8	1.4	1.2	1.4	1.4	1.3
**	**	*	nd	nd	**	**	**	*	*
0.1	0.1	**	**	nd	**	0.1	**	**	**
67.4	59.4	57.9	54.2	47.4	60.1	61.5	66.9	66.2	66.1
0.3	0.3	0.2	0.2	0.2	0.3	0.3	0.2	0.3	0.3
0.1	**	**	**	**	0.1	**	**	**	**
6.9	5.9	4.6	2.7	1.0	7.2	5.7	5.4	6.0	5.2
1.7	1.7	2.9	4.5	5.5	1.7	1.6	2.5	3.0	3.3
0.2	0.2	0.1	0.1	**	0.3	0.2	0.2	0.2	0.2
1.3	**0.8**	**0.7**	**0.7**	**0.6**	**1.5**	**1.2**	**0.8**	**0.8**	**1.0**
0.1	0.1	0.1	0.1	**	0.1	0.1	0.1	0.1	0.1
**	*	**	**	*	**	**	**	**	**
1.0	0.5	0.4	0.4	0.4	1.0	0.9	0.5	0.5	0.7

TABLE 7.5. *Continued*

Functional Group Compound	Original	S-1					S-2				
	0	1[a]	3	6	9	12	1	3	6	9	12
Aldehydes	**1.7**	**1.4**				**0.3**	**1.8**	**1.4**	**1.3**	**1.2**	**1.0**
Octanal	0.2	0.2	0.1	**	**	**	0.2	0.2	0.2	0.1	0.1
Neral	0.5	0.4	0.3	0.1	0.1	0.2	0.5	0.4	0.4	0.3	0.3
Geranial	0.9	0.7	0.4	0.1	0.1	**	0.9	0.7	0.6	0.6	0.5
Perillyl aldehyde	**	**	0.1	0.1	0.2	0.1	0.1	**	**	0.1	0.1
Alcohols	**0.6**	**0.7**				**4.8**	**0.6**	**0.5**	**0.7**	**1.2**	**1.1**
(*Z*)-β-Terpineol	*	nd	**	**	**	**	nd	nd	*	**	**
p-Mentha-1,8-dien-9-ol	*	0.1	0.1	0.2	0.3	0.3	**	**	0.1	0.1	0.1
2-Pentadecyn-1-ol	nd	nd	*	*	**	**	nd	*	*	*	**
Myrtenol	nd	nd	0.1	0.1	0.3	0.3	nd	nd	**	**	**
(*Z*)-Carveol	*	**	0.2	0.4	0.7	0.9	*	**	**	0.1	0.1
p-Cymene-8-ol	nd	nd	*	**	0.1	0.1	nd	nd	**	**	**
(*E*)-Carveol	*	**	0.1	0.2	0.3	0.4	*	**	**	**	0.1
Hydroxy linalool	**	**	0.1	0.1	0.2	0.3	**	**	**	**	**
1,2-Cyclohexanediol	0.2	0.2	0.5	0.6	1.0	1.3	0.1	0.1	0.2	0.3	0.3
Ketones	**	**				**1.6**	**	**	**	**0.2**	**0.2**
Carvone	**	**	0.2	0.4	0.7	1.0	**	**	**	0.1	0.1
Esters	**0.3**	**0.4**				**0.5**	**0.3**	**0.7**	**0.7**	**0.8**	**0.7**
Neryl acetate	0.1	0.1	0.4	0.2	0.2	0.2	0.1	0.4	0.4	0.5	0.4
Geranyl acetate	0.2	0.2	0.2	0.2	0.2	0.3	0.2	0.2	0.2	0.2	0.2
Oxides	**0.1**	**0.5**				**1.6**	**0.2**	**0.4**	**0.5**	**0.4**	**0.5**
(*Z*)-Limonene oxide	**	0.2	0.3	0.7	0.6	0.7	0.1	0.2	0.2	0.2	0.2
(*E*)-Limonene oxide	0.1	0.3	0.5	0.6	0.7	0.8	0.1	0.2	0.3	0.2	0.3
Acids	*	**				**0.2**	**nd**	**nd**	*	*	**nd**
Decanoic acid	nd	**	0.1	0.2	0.2	0.2	nd	nd	*	*	nd
Total volatiles (%)	**99.9**	**91.3**	**79.0**	**52.0**	**42.0**	**40.3**	**97.2**	**88.7**	**90.8**	**78.5**	**76.3**

[a]Period of storage (month).

*: Peak area detected less than 0.005%.

**: Peak area detected not less than 0.005% and less than 0.05%.

in previous reports (Ayedoun and Sossou, 1996; Njoroge et al., 1994; Sawamura, 2000; Shaw, 1979; Staroscik and Wilson, 1982; Vekiri et al., 2002). Eighteen alcohols were detected, but this group was detected in a proportion as low as 0.6%. Two esters, neryl and geranyl acetates, were detected in the original lemon oil in proportions of 0.08 and 0.24%, respectively. These esters are also characteristic compounds, in addition to neral and geranial. Njoroge et al. (1994) reported that

S-3					S-4				
1	3	6	9	12	1	3	6	9	12
1.8	**1.4**	**1.5**	**1.4**	**1.3**	**1.8**	**1.5**	**1.6**	**1.6**	**1.5**
0.2	0.2	0.2	0.2	0.2	0.2	0.2	0.2	0.2	0.2
0.5	0.4	0.4	0.3	0.3	0.5	0.4	0.4	0.4	0.4
0.9	0.7	0.7	0.6	0.5	0.9	0.7	0.8	0.8	0.7
0.1	**	0.1	0.1	0.1	0.1	0.1	0.1	0.1	0.1
0.7	**0.6**	**0.7**	**0.9**	**0.8**	**0.6**	**0.5**	**0.5**	**0.6**	**0.9**
*	nd	*	**	**	*	*	*	**	**
**	**	**	0.1	0.1	**	**	**	**	0.1
*	**	nd	nd	nd	*	*	nd	nd	nd
nd	nd	**	**	**	nd	nd	*	*	*
**	**	**	**	0.1	**	*	**	**	**
nd	nd	nd	nd	nd	nd	nd	nd	nd	nd
*	**	0.1	**	**	*	**	**	**	**
**	**	**	**	**	**	**	**	**	**
0.1	0.1	0.1	0.2	0.3	0.1	0.1	0.1	0.1	0.2
**	**	**	**0.1**	**0.2**	**	**	**	**	**0.1**
**	**	**	0.1	0.1	**	**	**	**	0.1
0.3	**0.7**	**0.6**	**0.8**	**0.7**	**0.3**	**0.3**	**0.7**	**0.8**	**0.8**
0.1	0.5	0.4	0.5	0.4	0.1	0.1	0.5	0.5	0.5
0.2	0.2	0.2	0.2	0.2	0.2	0.2	0.2	0.2	0.2
0.2	**0.2**	**0.2**	**0.4**	**0.5**	**0.2**	**0.2**	**0.2**	**0.4**	**0.3**
0.1	0.1	0.1	0.2	0.2	0.1	0.1	0.1	0.1	0.1
0.1	0.1	0.1	0.2	0.3	0.1	0.1	0.1	0.2	0.2
nd	**nd**	**	**0.1**	**0.1**	**nd**	**nd**	*	**	**
nd	nd	**	0.1	0.1	nd	nd	*	**	**
98.8	**86.9**	**84.6**	**79.1**	**69.0**	**92.4**	**89.2**	**97.1**	**98.6**	**98.1**

their respective proportions in fresh *Lisbon* cold-pressed oil were 0.31 and 0.23% on the basis of relative peak area, whereas neryl acetate was not detected in several varieties of lemon oils. (*Z*)- and (*E*)-Limonene oxides were quantified to be 0.05 and 0.07% in the original sample, respectively, although they are usually detectable in trace amounts in fresh lemon oils (Sawamura, 2000). Ketones were detected in trace amounts as well.

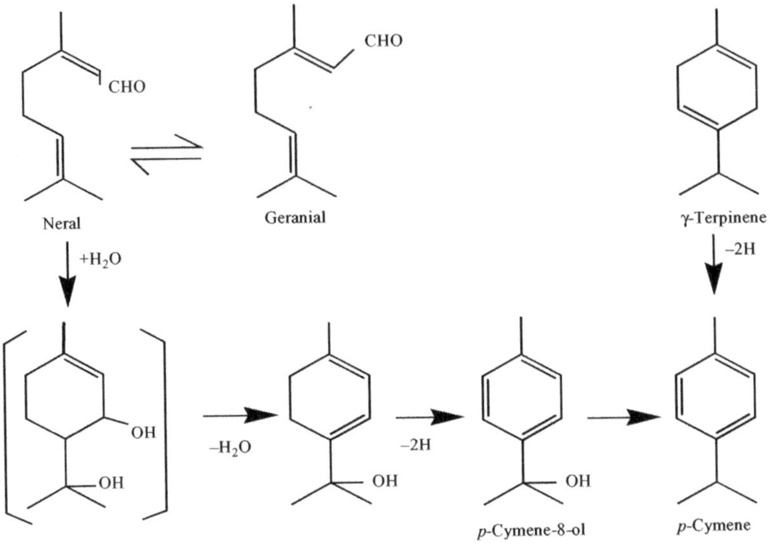

Figure 7.6. Postulated oxidative conversion mechanism of γ-terpinene and citral into *p*-cymene.

S-1. The relative compositional changes in commercial lemon essential oil stored in an incubator set at 25°C with the cap opened at given intervals are presented in Table 7.5. It focuses on the compositional changes of the commercial lemon essential oil under conditions S-1, S-2, S-3, and S-4 over a 1-, 3-, 6-, 9-, and 12-month period. Some compounds changed drastically and others changed slightly. The behavior of these components during storage showed the same tendency as in the previous experiment, in which cold-pressed yuzu (*Citrus junos* Tanaka) oil was stored at 20°C over one year (Njoroge et al., 1996; Sawamura, 2005a). The percentages of monoterpene hydrocarbons decreased remarkably from 95.5 to 30.0%. Limonene, a monoterpene hydrocarbon, which is usually the most abundant compound in lemon oil as well as in other citrus oils (Staroscik and Wilson, 1982; Njoroge et al., 1994; Ayedoun and Sossou, 1996; Sawamura, 2000; Vekiri et al., 2002), decreased remarkably from 68.5 to 20.1% over 12 months. *p*-Cymene, which is known as the main substance causing off-flavor in citrus oil, can be converted from γ-terpinene by oxidation (Sinclair, 1984). This conversion may have occurred here, because *p*-cymene increased from 1.6 to 7.1% during 6 months, and instead γ-terpinene decreased from 7.2 to 0.01%. It is also suggested that the formation of *p*-cymene-8-ol after 3 months is a proof of the existence of this mechanism. These oxidative conversion mechanisms are shown in Figure 7.6. α-Pinene and β-pinene are oxidized to their hydroperoxides with migration of the double bond in the presence of a photosensitizer via (*E*)-pino-carveol and myrtenol, respectively (Whittaker, 1972; Tomas, 1973). Actually, (*E*)-pino-carveol increased after 5 months and myrtenol appeared after 2 months, thereafter increasing gradually during storage. However, the levels of both compounds varied to a small extent, because they could be further converted into hydroperoxides. In addition, other monoterpene hydrocarbons such as sabinene and myrcene decreased considerably over one year, from 2.0 to 0.4% and 1.4 to 0.1%, respectively. α-Phellandrene and α-terpinene disappeared after 2 months of storage, while β-phellandrene and terpinolene were not detected after 9 and 4 months, respectively. The level of sesquiterpene hydrocarbons decreased, but not as much as that of monoterpene hydrocarbons. (*E*)-β-Farnesene decreased to 0.5% for 3 months. α-Bergamotene decreased from 0.4 to 0.2% over one year. The total level of aldehydes decreased from 1.7 to 0.3% over a one-year period, and the level of citral (neral and geranial) decreased from 1.4 to 0.2%. Octanal, one of the three aliphatic aldehydes detected, was quantified as 0.2% in the original sample, but it was present only as a trace amount after 6 months of storage. The level of alcohols increased noticeably from 0.6 to 4.8%. *p*-Cymene-8-ol, a characteristic compound of grapefruit (Ichimura and Uchiyama, 1989; Sawamura, 2000), occurred after 3 months of storage. Its conversion into *p*-cymene has been already described above. 1,2-Cyclohexanediol showed a considerable increase, from 0.2 to 0.6% in 6 months, and to 1.3% in 12 months. The levels of three carveol isomers increased noticeably: (*E*)-pino-carveol, from 0.1 to 0.4%; (*Z*)-carveol, up to 0.9%; and (*E*)-carveol up to 0.4% in one year. As for ketones, *p*-menth-8-one and carvone increased continuously up to 0.6 and 1.0%, respectively. 6-Methyl-5-hepten-2-one changed little. The total level of esters increased from 0.3 to 0.5%: Neryl acetate increased to 0.4% in 3 months and decreased to 0.2% over a 6-month period; geranyl acetate was almost stable at 0.2% over 9 months, increasing to 0.3% in 12 months. (*Z*)- and (*E*)-Limonene oxides increased from 0.05 to 0.7% and 0.1 to 0.8% in 5 months, and then maintained at levels between 0.7 and 0.8% up to the twelfth month. Decanoic acid, one of the newly formed compounds, increased gradually during storage, reaching 0.2% after 12 months. Decanal does not seem to be involved as a precursor of decanoic acid, because its level was low and varied little. Ten artifacts that had not been detected in the original lemon oil were formed during storage: (*Z*)-linalool oxide, 2,6-octadien-1-ol, 2-pentadecyn-1-ol, myrtenol, *p*-cymene-8-ol, tetradecane, 2-propyl heptanol, decanoic acid, and two unidentified compounds.

S-2. As shown in Table 5, the hydrocarbons in the S-2 sample decreased from 97.1 to 72.2% in one year. Monoterpenes diminished from 95.6 to 71.5%, where β-pinene and myrcene reduced from 12.2 to 9.0% and from 1.4 to 0.9%, respectively. α-Phellandrene and α-terpinene were detected until 9 months, but they were not detected thereafter. Limonene and γ-terpinene decreased from 68.5 to 51.7% and 7.2%, respectively. *p*-Cymene, on the other hand, increased from 1.9 to 4.1%. The relationship between γ-terpinene and *p*-cymene was examined in the S-1 experiment. Sesquiterpene hydrocarbons did not change as much as the monoterpenes, whereas (*E*)-β-farnesene decreased largely from 1.0 to 0.5% in 3 months. The total level of aldehydes decreased from 1.7 to 1.0% in one year. Neral and geranial decreased from 0.5 to 0.3% and from 0.9 to 0.5%, respectively. The alcohols were almost stable for 4 months, and then their levels increased to a small extent. (*Z*)-β-Terpineol, myrtenol, and *p*-cymene-8-ol were also detected during storage. The ketones, such as *p*-menth-8-one, 6-methyl-5-hepten-2-one, *d*-camphor, and carvone, increased to 0.1%. Neryl acetate increased from 0.1 to 0.4% in a year. The total levels of ketones, esters, and oxides were increased by 2 times over the levels in the original oil.

S-3. The concentration of hydrocarbons decreased predominantly from 97.1 to 64.9% in one year. In particular, the proportion of monoterpene hydrocarbons decreased remarkably as much as in the S-1 sample. The decrease in individual compounds in one year was as follows: β-pinene, 12.2–7.2%; sabinene, 2.0–1.1%; and γ-terpinene, 7.2–1.0%. The level of limonene diminished considerably from 68.5 to 47.4%, while *p*-cymene increased from 1.6 to 5.5%. The level of aldehydes decreased from 1.7 to 1.3% and that of alcohols was almost stable throughout one year. The total level of ketones, esters, and oxides showed a similar behavior to that of the S-2 experiment. It was found that the total level of monoterpene hydrocarbons changed noticeably in the aerobic condition. These results will provide a suggestion as to how to care for the commercial essential oils in daily use.

S-4. The least compositional change was observed in the S-4 experiment. The proportion of hydrocarbons decreased from 97.1 to 93.8% over a one-year period. The proportion of limonene changed from 68.5 to 66.1%, and that of γ-terpinene from 7.2 to 5.2%. The proportion of *p*-cymene doubled in one year, even when the sample was stored at 5°C. Neral and geranial changed slightly, from 0.5 to 0.4% and from 0.9 to 0.7%, respectively. The total level of alcohols increased from 0.6 to 0.9%.

Comprehensive Change. The compositional change of lemon essential oil for aromatherapy was studied under the four different storage conditions similar to those in practical use where the oil would be often exposed to air at a certain temperature. S-1 and S-3 may be common conditions for users consuming the oil. The qualitative and quantitative changes in the monoterpene hydrocarbon content were greater in S-1 than in S-3. In both conditions limonene, β-pinene, γ-terpinene, and *p*-cymene changed remarkably during storage. The level of alcohols also changed. The proportion of hydrocarbons in the S-3 sample changed noticeably, but that of the other compounds changed as little as in the S-2 and S-4 samples. These results suggest that the changes in the composition of lemon essential oil are accelerated by temperature and contact with atmosphere.

The amount of the total volatiles may be another indicator of the quality change of essential oil in addition to the compositional change. As for the S-1 sample, the total volatile amount determined by weight percent using GC decreased to 91.3% in one month (Table 7.5). This suggests that about one-tenth of the volatile compounds in the original essential oil converted to nonvolatile compounds during a period of one month. The rate of decrease of the volatile amount was shown to be at a minimum between the second and the fifth month. After 6 months of storage, the volatile proportion was as high as 52.0%. After 9 months, the amount of nonvolatile materials overcame that of the volatile materials in the essential oil. As shown in Table 7.5, the changes in the volatile compounds in S-2 showed a similar tendency to those in S-3. However, the amount retained in S-2 was 90.8% as compared with 84.6% in S-3 over a 6-month period. After 12 months, the nonvolatile substances were likely to account for about 30% in both samples. Sample S-2 was stored under an anaerobic condition at 25°C, while S-3 was stored in an aerobic condition at 5°C. These results suggest that the aerobic factor had a larger effect on conversion than temperature. Sample S-4 retained more than 90% of its volatile compounds throughout a one-year period. The ratio of decrease was about 10% in three months, but the volatile compounds increased again to the level of the initial amount after 6 months. This suggests that there would be a reversible conversion between the volatile and the nonvolatile compounds in the anaerobic condition at 5°C. The results of this study will contribute to the predictive knowledge concerning the compositional change in commercial essential oils for aromatherapy in practical use, and also to the consideration of how to care for and store aromatherapy materials.

In conclusion, compositional changes in lemon essential oil occurred predominantly in S-1, where terpene hydrocarbons including limonene, β-pinene, γ-terpinene and myrcene decreased from 97.1 to 30.4% in one year. The increase of *p*-cymene was associated with the decrease of γ-terpinene and citral. The detection of *p*-cymene-8-ol confirmed the conversion mechanism of citral into *p*-cymene. The compositional change in S-4 was minimal, while the aerobic condition (S-3) caused some decrease of the constituents during storage even at 5°C.

7.2.3 Bergamot Essential Oil

Bergamot cultivated in Reggio Calabria, Italy, is of the highest quality in the world. The production of bergamot essential oil began 300 years ago in Italy, and the oil has been used mainly in perfumes and cosmetics due to its characteristic aroma (Hodgson, 1967; Susan, 1996). There are many reports on the essential oil of bergamot (Calvarano, 1965; Cotroneo et al., 1992; Dugo et al., 1987, 1991; Giacomo and Mincione, 1995; Kirbaslar et al., 2001; Regione Calabria Assessoato All'agricoltura Consorzio del Bergamotto, 1989; Sawamrua et al., 1999; Verzera et al. 2003). It is remarkable that the proportion of monoterpene hydrocarbons in bergamot oil is much lower than that in other citrus oils, whereas linalyl acetate and linalool are much more abundant: 34–38% and 6–14%, respectively.

In the original bergamot essential oil before storage, 70 compounds were detected by GC, among which 68 were identified by GC and GC-MS. The oil was composed of terpene hydrocarbons (47.2%), aldehydes (0.4%), alcohols (16.8%), and esters (25.7%), as shown in Table 7.6. The bergamot oil presented a different composition from that of other citrus fruits (Cotroneo et al., 1992; Giacomo and Mincione, 1995; Moufida and Marzouk, 2003; Sawamura, 2000; Sinclair, 1984). Linalyl acetate and linalool in addition to limonene were the major components in the bergamot essential oil. The total proportion of these

TABLE 7.6. Compositional changes in commercial bergamot oil under four storage conditions (S-1 to S-4)

Functional Group Compound	Original	S-1				
	0[a]	1	3	6	9	12
Hydrocarbons	**47.2**	**44.2**				**18.8**
Aliphatic	*	**				**0.4**
1-Acetyl-2-(2'-oxo-propyl)-Cyclopentane	*	**	0.1	0.1	0.1	0.4
Monoterpenes	**46.9**	**43.7**				**17.8**
α-Pinene	1.2	1.1	0.8	0.7	0.4	0.4
β-Pinene	3.9	3.6	2.8	2.3	1.5	1.3
Sabinene	0.6	0.6	0.4	0.3	0.2	0.2
Myrcene	0.8	0.7	0.5	0.3	0.1	0.1
Limonene	34.4	32.2	24.6	21.7	14.2	12.9
γ-Terpinene	3.7	2.8	0.7	nd	nd	nd
p-Cymene	1.6	2.2	3.3	3.8	2.9	2.9
Terpinolene	0.2	0.1	**	*	nd	nd
Sesquierpenes	**0.3**	**0.5**				**0.6**
α-Bergamotene	0.3	0.3	0.3	0.2	0.2	0.2
(*E*)-β-Farnesene	**	**	0.1	0.1	0.2	0.3
Aldehydes	**0.4**	**0.4**				**0.1**
Neral	0.2	0.2	0.1	0.1	**	0.1
Geranial	0.2	0.2	0.1	0.1	**	**
Alcohols	**16.8**	**15.2**				**11.1**
Linalool	15.9	14.9	12.5	11.0	8.3	8.0
Terpinen-4-ol	0.4	nq	0.1	0.1	*	*
α-Terpineol	0.3	0.4	0.4	0.3	0.2	0.2
(*Z*)-Carveol	**	**	**	0.2	0.3	0.5
(*E*)-Carveol	**	**	**	0.1	0.2	0.3
Dihydrocarveol	**	**	0.1	0.1	0.3	0.3
Ketones	**0.1**	**0.1**				**0.8**
Solanone	0.1	0.1	**	0.1	0.1	0.1
(*S*)-(+)-Carvone	**	**	0.1	0.3	0.4	0.7
Esters	**25.7**	**24.7**				**17.3**
Linalyl acetate	24.6	23.5	21.1	19.1	15.4	15.6
Bornyl acetate	**	**				0.1
Nonyl acetate	nq	0.1	**	nq	0.1	nq
Neryl acetate	0.6	0.6	0.5	0.4	0.3	0.3
Geranyl acetate	0.4	0.3	0.3	0.2	0.2	0.2
Methyl laurate	**	0.1	0.2	0.5	0.7	1.0
Oxides	**0.3**	**0.4**				**3.3**
(*Z*)-Linalool oxide	0.1	0.1	0.2	0.5	0.7	1.0
(*Z*)-Limonene oxide	0.1	0.1	0.2	0.4	0.3	0.3
(*E*)-Limonene oxide	**	**	*	**	**	*
(*E*)-Linalool oxide	0.1	0.1	0.3	0.5	0.7	1.0
Acids	**nd**	**nd**				**0.1**
9,12,15-Octadecatrienoic acid	nd	nd	*	0.1	0.1	0.1
Triacetin	0.5	0.4	0.4	0.4	0.4	0.4
Total volatiles (%)	**91.0**	**86.1**	**71.7**	**66.1**	**51.6**	**52.4**

[a]Period of storage (month).

*: Peak area detected less than 0.005%.

**: Peak area detected not less than 0.005% and less than 0.05%.

nd: Not detected.

nq: Not quantified.

S-2				S-3				S-4			
1	3	6	12	1	3	6	12	1	3	6	12
38.3	**39.7**	**40.4**	**38.0**	**44.5**	**37.2**	**38.3**	**35.2**	**43.2**	**38.2**	**41.2**	**42.1**
**	**	**	**0.1**	**	**	**	**	**	**	**	**
**	**	**	0.1	**	**	**	**	**	**	**	**
38.0	**39.1**	**39.7**	**37.2**	**44.2**	**36.9**	**37.8**	**35.0**	**42.8**	**37.6**	**40.6**	**41.6**
0.9	1.0	1.0	0.9	1.1	0.9	0.9	0.8	1.1	0.9	1.0	1.0
3.1	3.3	3.3	3.0	3.7	3.1	3.1	2.8	3.6	3.1	3.4	3.5
0.5	0.5	0.5	0.5	0.6	0.5	0.5	0.4	0.5	0.5	0.5	0.5
0.6	0.6	0.8	0.5	0.7	0.7	0.6	0.6	0.7	0.6	0.7	0.7
28.0	28.7	29.3	27.6	32.4	27.0	27.8	25.9	31.4	27.7	29.9	30.7
2.9	2.5	1.8	0.9	3.4	2.9	2.8	2.2	3.4	2.9	3.0	2.7
1.5	2.0	2.7	3.5	1.7	1.5	1.6	1.9	1.5	1.4	1.6	2.1
0.1	0.1	0.1	0.1	0.2	0.1	0.1	0.1	0.2	0.1	0.1	0.1
0.3	**0.6**	**0.6**	**0.6**	**0.3**	**0.3**	**0.5**	**0.5**	**0.3**	**0.6**	**0.5**	**0.5**
0.3	0.3	0.3	0.3	0.3	0.3	0.3	0.3	0.3	0.3	0.3	0.3
**	0.1	0.1	0.1	**	*	**	**	**	0.1	**	**
0.4	**0.2**	**0.2**	**0.2**	**0.4**	**0.4**	**0.4**	**0.3**	**0.4**	**0.3**	**0.4**	**0.4**
0.2	0.1	0.1	0.1	0.2	0.2	0.2	0.1	0.2	0.1	0.2	0.2
0.2	0.1	0.1	0.1	0.2	0.2	0.2	0.2	0.2	0.2	0.2	0.2
14.3	**14.2**	**14.7**	**14.9**	**16.2**	**13.9**	**14.9**	**14.6**	**15.8**	**14.1**	**15.0**	**15.4**
13.5	13.5	13.9	13.9	15.2	13.0	14.1	13.9	15.0	13.3	14.3	14.7
0.3	0.1	0.1	0.1	0.3	0.2	0.2	0.1	0.3	0.1	nq	0.1
0.3	0.4	0.4	0.4	0.5	0.5	0.4	0.4	0.4	0.4	0.4	0.4
**	**	**	0.1	**	**	**	**	**	**	**	**
**	**	**	**	**	**	**	*	*	**	*	**
**	**	**	0.1	**	**	**	*	**	**	**	**
0.1	**0.2**	**0.2**	**0.2**	**0.1**	**0.1**	**0.1**	**0.1**	**0.2**	**0.1**	**0.1**	**0.1**
0.1	0.1	0.1	0.1	0.1	0.1	0.1	0.1	0.1	0.1	0.1	0.1
**	0.1	0.1	0.1	**	**	**	**	0.1	**	**	**
23.3	**23.1**	**23.5**	**23.6**	**25.2**	**22.9**	**23.6**	**23.4**	**25.0**	**22.8**	**23.9**	**24.4**
22.2	22.1	22.5	22.6	24.1	22.1	22.7	22.4	24.0	22.0	23.0	23.4
0.1	**	**	**	**	**	**	**	**	**	nq	**
nq	**	nq	nq	nq	*	nq	nq	**	nq	**	nq
0.6	0.5	0.5	0.5	0.6	0.5	0.5	0.5	0.6	0.5	0.5	0.5
0.3	0.3	0.3	0.3	0.3	0.3	0.3	0.3	0.3	0.2	0.3	0.3
**	0.1	0.1	0.1	**	**	**	0.1	**	**	**	0.1
0.3	**0.4**	**0.5**	**0.8**	**0.3**	**0.2**	**0.2**	**0.4**	**0.3**	**0.2**	**0.2**	**0.3**
0.1	0.1	0.1	0.2	0.1	0.1	0.1	0.1	0.1	0.1	0.1	0.1
0.1	0.1	0.1	0.1	0.1	**	**	0.1	0.1	**	**	0.1
**	**	**	0.1	**	**	**	**	**	**	**	**
0.1	0.1	0.1	0.2	0.1	0.1	0.1	0.1	0.1	0.1	0.1	0.1
nd	**nd**	**nd**	**nd**	**nd**	**nd**	**nd**	**nd**	**nd**	**nd**	**nd**	**nd**
nd	nd	nd	nd	nd	nd	nd	nd	nd	nd	nd	nd
0.4	0.4	0.4	0.4	0.5	0.4	0.4	0.5	0.4	0.4	0.4	0.5
77.2	**78.2**	**79.4**	**78.1**	**87.4**	**75.2**	**77.9**	**74.5**	**85.3**	**76.1**	**81.2**	**83.2**

three compounds was as high as 74.9%. Limonene was a predominant compound accounting for 34.4%, although its proportion was lower than that of other citrus fruits. β-Pinene, γ-terpinene, and *p*-cymene were present in relatively high proportions, 3.9, 3.7, and 1.6%, respectively. Many other identified compounds were determined in amounts of less than 0.1%. Sabinene and myrcene accounted for 0.6 and 0.8%, respectively. The sesquiterpene hydrocarbons identified were α-bergamotene, β-elemene, β-caryophyllene, β-santalene, (*E*)-β-farnesene, germacrene D, and β-bisabolene, accounting for more than 0.3%. β-Bisabolene was not quantitated since it was overlapped, as was the case of nonyl acetate. Alcohols and esters were present in relatively high amounts in the original oil. Linalool was one of the 19 alcohols (16.8%) detected in the original oil, accounting for 15.9%. Terpinen-4-ol and α-terpineol accounted for 0.4 and 0.3%, respectively. Esters were the second major group, accounting for 25.7%. The level of the linalyl acetate, in addition to the ratio of linalyl acetate to linalool, is considered to be one of the most important indices of the commercial quality of bergamot oil (Sawamura, 2000). The level of linalyl acetate in the bergamot oil was as high as 24.6%, although it was lower than that found in previous studies (Giacomo and Mincione, 1995; Kirbaslar et al., 2001; Sawamura, 2000). The total level of neryl acetate and geranyl acetate was 1.0%. Other esters were detected at less than 0.1% each. Neral and geranial were determined to be 0.2% each, and other aldehydes, octanal and decanal, were present in amounts less than 0.1%. (*Z*)- and (*E*)-Linalool oxides were both detected at 0.1%. Triacetin, which is known as glycerol triacetate and used as a solvent for perfume, was detected as high as 0.5% in the original oil. Acetic acid and butanoic acid were detected in trace amounts in the original bergamot oil.

S-1. The relative compositional changes in commercial bergamot essential oil stored in an incubator set at 25°C with the cap opened at given intervals are presented in Table 7.6. The compositional changes in the S-1 condition were remarkable. The total proportion of monoterpenes decreased predominantly from 46.9 to 17.8% over a 12-month period, whereas limonene decreased from 34.4 to 12.9%. The change of limonene level was small in the first month, but it decreased considerably by as much as 6.1% in the next month, then decreased by a few percent per month until the sixth month, reaching 21.7%. Then, it decreased by as much as 7.5%, between the sixth and the ninth months. Sinclair reported previously that limonene could be oxidized into its peroxide in the presence of atmosphere at a given temperature (Sinclair, 1984). In this bergamot oil, the change of limonene was remarkable in the S-1 condition. α-Pinene and β-pinene decreased to one-third over a 12-month period: from 1.2 to 0.4% and from 3.9 to 1.3%, respectively. The level of α-pinene decreased to about 0.3% in 2 months, and the level of β-pinene reduced sharply from 3.9 to 3.0% during the first 2 months, and further decreased to 2.6% in the 4th month of storage. Both α- and β-pinenes increased once in the fifth month. Sabinene, myrcene, and γ-terpinene decreased extensively, from 0.6 to 0.2%, from 0.8 to 0.1%, and from 3.7% to an undetectable level, respectively. Among them, the levels of sabinene and myrcene were reduced at a rate of 0.1% per month for 3 months. γ-Terpinene decreased remarkably at a rate of about 1.0% per month for 3 months from the initial term of storage. This result suggests that a sensitive and rapid reaction occurred in γ-terpinene in the S-1 condition. *p*-Cymene, which is known as a product from the oxidation of γ-terpinene as shown in Figure 7.6 (Sinclair, 1984), increased to around twice the proportion of the original oil after 6 months, accounting for 3.8%. It started increasing gradually from the initial period of storage, reaching 3.7% in the fourth month. *p*-Cymene tended to decrease after reaching the highest level, 3.8%, in the sixth month. The changes of γ-terpinene and *p*-cymene showed the same tendency in both bergamot and lemon oils. Seven compounds among the monoterpene hydrocarbons disappeared during a 12-month period: 3-carene, α-phellandrene, α-terpinene, β-phellandrene, (*Z*)-β-ocimene, γ-terpinene, and terpinolene. 3-Carene and α-phellandrene were initially detected in trace amounts and were not detected after 9 months. α-Terpinene decreased noticeably from 0.2% to a trace amount during 4 months and then disappeared. β-Phellandrene and (*Z*)-β-ocimene were not detected after 9 and 6 months, respectively. The total proportion of alcohols decreased from 16.8 to 11.1% over a 12-month period. Linalool decreased continuously until 9 months of storage, as much as half the original proportion, that is, from 15.9 to 8.0%. The proportion of linalool decreased little by little after 4 months of storage. α-Terpineol was in the range of 0.2–0.4% over the whole storage period. (*Z*)- and (*E*)-Carveols increased from a trace amount to 0.5 and 0.3%, respectively. They were in the range of less than 0.1% for 3 months. The nine compounds formed during storage were as follows: α-pinene oxide, furan, epoxylinalool, myrtenol, (*R*)-(-)-carvone, isopinocampheol, 9,12,15-octadecatrienoic acid, and two unidentified compounds. Myrtenol, which is reported to be produced by the oxidation of some terpene hydrocarbons in dissolution with cobalt solvent (Da Silva et al., 2003), was first detected in the fifth month. Linalyl acetate (24.6%), which was the secondary dominant compound of original bergamot oil, decreased to 15.6% in 12 months. The decrease in linalyl acetate was predominant during the initial 2 months. Neryl and geranyl acetates also decreased from 0.6 to 0.3% and from 0.4 to 0.2% over a 12-month period, respectively. The level of methyl laurate was low in the initial period, but it increased at a rate of 0.1% per month after 2 months, reaching 1.0% after 12 months. As a whole, the aldehydes, such as neral, geranial, octanal, heptanal, and decanal, changed little over a 12-month period. Among the six oxides, both (*Z*)- and (*E*)-linalool oxides increased tenfold, from 0.1 to 1.0%, due to oxidation of linalool. Both (*Z*)-and (*E*)-limonene oxides, on the other hand, increased little, essentially maintaining their initial proportions. One interesting result in this condition is the change of carvone oxide, which increased gradually from less than 0.1 to 0.9% over a 12-month period. Carvone, known as a characteristic ketone of dill and caraway oils, was formed in the process of oxidation of limonene (Newman, 1972; Sinclair, 1984). In the bergamot oil, (*S*)-(+)-carvone increased steadily from less than 0.1 to 0.7% over a 12-month period, while (*R*)-(-)-carvone was detected in a trace amount after 9 months.

S-2. As shown in Table 7.6, the total proportion of hydrocarbons for 12 months decreased from 47.2 to 38.0%, where the monoterpene hydrocarbons mainly diminished from 46.9 to 37.2%. The level of limonene decreased to 28.0% in the first month, but it maintained at about 28% thereafter. γ-Terpinene decreased from 3.7 to 0.9% over a one-year period. *p*-Cymene increased to 3.5% by the ninth month of storage. It held its initial level for the first month, and then it increased by 3.5% over a 12-month storage period. The total level of sesquiterpenes was constant at 0.6% after 3 months. The alcohols decreased considerably, from 16.8 to 14.3% in the first month of storage. Ninety-five percent of the alcohols was accounted for by linalool. (*Z*)- and (*E*)-Carveols increased greatly in the S-1 sample, but not in the S-2 sample. The total proportion of esters decreased from 25.7 to 23.3% in the first month of storage. Linalyl acetate was a major constituent, at a level of about 22% during storage. Among the aldehydes, there was a minute change in neral and geranial during storage. The concentration of oxides changed from 0.3 to 0.8% during storage, but the changes of the individual oxides were small, ranging between 0.1 and 0.2%. The total volatiles in the S-2 sample decreased drastically in the first month, and then varied little, in the range of 79.4 and 78.2%, over a 12-month period.

S-3. The compositional changes of S-2, S-3, and S-4 showed a similar tendency over a 12-month period except for terpene hydrocarbons, whose level decreased from 47.2 to 35.2%. Limonene and γ-terpinene, major monoterpene hydrocarbons, had a large change, from 34.4 to 25.9% and from 3.7 to 2.2% in a 12-month period, respectively. Limonene decreased from 34.4 to 27.0% within 3 months of storage. The levels of α-pinene, β-pinene, and γ-terpinene also decreased from 1.2 to 0.8%, from 3.9 to 2.8%, and from 3.7 to 2.2% in a 12-month period, respectively. Thus the change of *p*-cymene derived from γ-terpinene was so large, as much as 0.3%. Myrcene seemed to be stable at 0.6 to 0.7%. The total level of sesquiterpenes did not vary during the initial 3 months, but it increased in the sixth month of storage to account for 0.5%. α-Bergamotene, which was one of the main sesquiterpenes, was stable over a 12-month period. Both neral and geranial were also stable for one year. Linalool changed considerably, from 15.9 to 13.0% in 3 months storage. Esters also decreased to 22.9% after 3 months. The change of linalyl acetate among the esters was predominant, decreasing from 24.6 to 22.1% during the initial 3 months. There was no appreciable change in the aldehydes and ketones. The oxides did not vary appreciably over a one-year period.

S-4. The least compositional change was observed in the S-4 experiment. The total proportion of hydrocarbons decreased from 47.2 to 42.1% over a one-year period. The levels of limonene and γ-terpinene decreased from 34.4 to 30.7% and from 3.7 to 2.7%, respectively. The total proportion of alcohols decreased greatly, from 16.8 to 14.1% during 3 months of storage. This stabilized at 15% after 3 months. The change of linalool was minute over a one-year period. Most of the aldehydes and ketones retained their initial proportions over one year. The change of linalyl acetate decreased from 24.6 to 22.0% during a 3-month storage period. This suggests that, even in the least affected condition (S-4), linalyl acetate may be variable over a small range. The oxides were not variable, and the acids were not detected in the S-4 condition over the whole period of storage.

Comprehensive Change. Among the monoterpene compounds, it is worthwhile to compare the interconversion of γ-terpinene and *p*-cymene in all the conditions. In the previous study about the compositional change of essential oil during storage, the increase of *p*-cymene was markedly associated with a decrease of γ-terpinene (Sinclair, 1984). The relationship between these two compounds is presented in Figure 7.6 as a ratio of γ-terpinene to *p*-cymene. This ratio could be one of the indices of deterioration of the essential oil. In the S-1 condition, the ratio decreased steadily until the 6th month of storage when γ-terpinene was not detected. The ratio of the S-2 condition also decreased noticeably, but its rate of decrease was relatively slower than that of the S-1 condition. The decrease in the S-3 and S-4 conditions was not significant. Their decrease ratios were almost the same over the storage period, except for the period between the first and the third month in the S-3 condition. This suggests that the formation of *p*-cymene by withdrawal of hydrogen from γ-terpinene would take place in more aerobic and warmer conditions (S-1 and S-2) (Sinclair, 1984). Linalool and linalyl acetate have been used as principal constituents in perfumery (Bor-Karlson et al., 1996; Letizia et al., 2003a,b). Bergamot oil contains a high proportion of these two compounds, and this would be one reason why, among the citrus oils, bergamot essential oil is popular for use in perfumery (Moufida and Marzouk, 2003). The percentage of linalool and linalyl acetate in bergamot essential oil is reported to be in the range of 2–20% and 15–40%, respectively (Dugo et al., 1987). It was also reported that the levels of linalool and linalyl acetate in bergamot essential oil could be influenced by several factors such as the production region and storage condition. Furthermore, the ratio of linalool to linalyl acetate is regarded as one of the most important indices of commercial quality of bergamot oil (Giacomo and Mincione, 1995). The initial ratio was 1.6 in the original oil used in this study. The ratio seems to be lower than those in fresh cold-pressed oil of *C. bergamia* Risso var. *Fantastico* and bergamot commercial oil product from the Bergamot Consortium, which were 6.4 and 3.4, respectively (Sawamura et al., 1999). The ratios varied little more or less than 1.6 in S-2, S-3, and S-4 conditions during the entire period of storage. In S-1, the ratio increased slightly until the 6th month, and during that time linalyl acetate and linalool decreased by similar proportions. However, the ratio increased up to 2.0 thereafter due to a reduction in the quantity of linalool. These results suggest that the S-1 condition, which is aerobic at room temperature, will effect a considerable change in the composition of essential oil under ordinary usage.

In conclusion, compositional changes of bergamot essential oil occurred predominantly in S-1, where terpene hydrocarbons including limonene, β-pinene, and γ-terpinene decreased from 47.2 to 18.8% in a one-year period. The ratio of γ-terpinene to *p*-cymene decreased rapidly in S-1, followed by S-2. Linalool and linalyl acetate, predominant and characteristic compounds in the bergamot essential oil, decreased from 15.9 to 8.0% and from 24.6 to 15.6%, respectively. The change of volatile compounds in S-2, S-3, and S-4 showed a similar tendency to some extent. The change of S-4 was the least over a one-year period. The decrease of the total volatiles was the greatest in S-1, which was from 91.0 to 52.4% over the storage period. In S-1, S-3, and S-4, the total volatile was 78.1, 74.5, and 83.2% in 12 months, respectively.

7.2.4 Mandarin Essential Oil

In the 19th century, mandarin was introduced from Southeast Asia to Europe and was mainly cultivated in Italy and Spain. Forty years later, the mandarin spread to the United States, where it was named *tangerine* (Hodgson, 1967; Okamura, 1983). According to Swingle, all cultivars of mandarin belong to *Citrus reticulata,* while Tanaka classified mandarin into more than 30 different species (Lota et al., 2000). Nowadays, many varieties of *C. reticulata* Blanco var. *Mandarin* are cultivated around the world. Mandarin has gained a large acceptance among consumers because of its ease of peeling and pleasant flavor with a good balance of sweetness and sourness (Sawamura, 2000). Its aroma also has an extremely sweet smell with floral undertone. Mandarin oil has been used in massage and bath oils and air fresheners, and sweet orange oil is used in aromatherapy (Susan, 1996). It is preferred for use on children because of its low-irritant nature. The oil is also effective in soothing people and controlling hyperactivity; it not only calms the mind but can also be used for medical treatment of stress, nervous tension, insomnia, and dyspepsia. In the area of psychological remedy, it is said that mandarin is also appropriate if you have a tendency to feel sorry for yourself (Susan, 1996). There are many studies previously reported on the chemical composition of mandarin oil (Choi and Sawamura, 2002; Lota et al., 2000; Mitiku et al., 2002; Sawamura, 2000; Verzera et al., 2000). Limonene is the most predominant constituent, accounting for over 90% in mandarin oil. It is suggested that limonene is comparatively stable when it is kept away from air and light (Guenther and Althausen, 1949). Therefore, it would be useful to investigate the stability of limonene and its interaction with the other compounds in mandarin essential oil for aromatherapy during storage.

Original Sample. Fifty-seven volatile compounds were detected in the original oil and identified by GC and GC-MS. The oil consisted almost entirely of terpene hydrocarbons (97.8%), with limonene as the major component (93.2%) followed by myrcene (1.8%). Aldehydes (0.5%), alcohols (0.6%), and ketones (0.1%) were present in small amounts, as shown in Table 7.7. This composition was similar to that found in previous studies (Susan, 1996; Mitiku et al., 2002). The proportion of limonene in the original oil was higher than that of cold-pressed oil of *C. reticulata* Blanco, accounting for 89.9% (Sawamura, 2000). The proportion of myrcene and sabinene was relatively rich, as high as 1.8 and 0.6%, respectively. α-and β-Pinenes accounted for 0.7 and 0.4%, respectively. Among the monoterpene hydrocarbons, γ-terpinene and sabinene were also detected in small quantities, as much as 0.5 and 0.6%, respectively. In the tangerine oil, the amount of limonene and γ-terpinene was 90.8 and 2.9%, respectively (Moshonas and Shaw, 1974). These levels are remarkably low compared with those of other citrus fruits. Other monoterpenes were also detected in low levels: δ-3-carene and β-phellandrene, 0.1 and 0.2%, respectively. The total amount of aldehydes, octanal, decanal, dodecanal, and α-sinensal, accounted for 0.5%. The total amount of alcohol was small, as low as 0.6%, where 1,2-cyclohexanediol and linalool were 0.1 and 0.2%, respectively. (*S*)-(+)-Carvone was a main ketone, accounting for 0.1%.

S-1. During storage, 12 compounds were newly identified. Several artifacts were as follows: hexanal (trace), acetic acid (trace), (*E*)-3(10)-caren-2-ol (trace), 7-nonanoic acid (trace), styrene (0.1%), (*Z*)-linalool oxide, (*E*)-linalool oxide (trace), *p*-menth-8-en-2-one (0.1%), *d*-limonene diepoxide (0.3%), and three unidentified compounds. Many compounds changed distinctly during storage in the S-1 condition. Limonene was the most prominent compound that changed significantly in quantity. Limonene decreased extensively from 93.2 to 26.6% over a 12-month period. In the first month, the decrease of limonene was not noticeable as it accounted for 92.6%, although it was stored in an aerobic condition. However, this level of limonene decreased by about 23.4% in the period from the 2nd to the 3rd month, that is, from 85.5 to 65.1%. Thereafter, it further decreased from 63.7 to 46.8%. From the 9th to the 12th month, limonene decreased slowly from 31.4 to 26.6%. Other momoterpenes also decreased steadily over a 12-month period, but the reduction rate was small: α-pinene, from 0.7 to 0.1%; β-pinene, from 0.4 to 0.1%; sabinene, from 0.6 to 0.1%; myrcene, from 1.8% to a trace amount; and γ-terpinene from 0.5% to a trace amount. Among these minor compounds, myrcene decreased from 1.8 to 0.6%, that is, by as much as two-thirds in the 3rd month, and its level reached 0.1% after 6 months of storage. Myrcene, a cyclic monoterpene, occurs naturally, but it readily changes to other compounds such as linalool, citral, geraniol, and nerol (Guenther and Althausen, 1949; Diekman and Palamand, 1974), as shown in Figure 7.7. Furthermore, the proportion of γ-terpinene decreased remarkably in the first month from 0.5 to 0.1% and it was present only as a trace amount from the 2nd month. *p*-Cymene is known as an oxidation product of γ-terpiene and its increase indicates that the oil loses its freshness (Usai et al., 1992). In this experiment, the change of *p*-cymene was in the range between 0.2 and 0.5% over the whole period.

Aliphatic aldehydes were composed of six compounds and decreased from 0.3% to trace amounts. Decanal, known as a contributing compound to the aroma of mandarin, decreased from 0.1% to a trace amount in the 5th month of storage, which might have affected the aroma quality of the oil. Neral increased from a trace amount to 0.4%. Alcohols (8.1%), ketones (3.1%), oxides (1.3%), and acids (0.4%) increased over the 12-month period, as shown in Table 7.7.

TABLE 7.7. Compositionl changes in commercial mandarin essential oil under four storage conditions (S-1 to S-4)

Functional Group Compound		S-1					S-2				
	0	1[a]	3	6	9	12	1	3	6	9	12
Hydrocarbons	**97.8**	**96.3**				**27.4**	**96.8**	**91.7**	**92.0**	**98.0**	**94.4**
Monoterpenes	**97.7**	**96.2**				**27.3**	**96.7**	**91.7**	**91.9**	**97.9**	**94.3**
α-Pinene	0.7	0.5	0.3	0.2	0.2	0.1	0.5	0.5	0.5	0.5	0.5
β-Pinene	0.4	0.3	0.2	0.1	0.1	0.1	0.3	0.3	0.3	0.3	0.3
Sabinene	0.6	0.5	0.3	0.1	0.1	0.1	0.6	0.5	0.5	0.5	0.5
Myrcene	1.8	1.5	0.6	0.1	**	*	1.7	1.4	1.3	1.2	1.1
Limonene	93.2	92.6	65.1	43.9	31.4	26.6	92.6	88.3	88.7	93.5	91.2
γ-terpinene	0.5	0.1	**	**	**	**	0.4	0.3	0.2	0.2	0.1
p-Cymene	0.2	0.4	0.4	0.3	0.3	0.3	0.2	0.2	0.3	0.4	0.4
Styrene	nd	nd	nd	**	0.1	0.1	nd	nd	nd	nd	nd
Sesquiterpenes	**0.1**	**0.1**				**0.1**	**0.1**	**	**0.1**	**0.1**	**0.1**
β-Elemene	*	*	*	*	*	*	**	*	*	*	*
Germacrene D	nq	**	*	**	*	**	0.1	**	*	**	nd
α-farnesene	**	**	nq	*	*	nq	**	nq	**	*	**
Aldehydes	**0.5**	**0.2**				**0.5**	**0.3**	**0.4**	**0.3**	**0.3**	**0.2**
Decanal	0.1	0.1	0.1	**	*	**	0.1	0.1	0.1	0.1	0.1
Dodecanal	0.1	**	*	*	**	**	nq	**	*	*	nd
Neral	**	**	0.1	0.2	0.3	0.4	**	**	**	0.1	0.1
Geranial	**	**	*	*	**	**	**	**	**	**	*
Perill aldehyde	**	**	0.1	0.1	0.1	0.1	**	**	**	**	**
α-Sinensal	0.1	**	nd	nd	nd	nd	0.1	0.1	0.1	0.1	**
Alcohols	**0.6**	**0.7**				**8.1**	**0.6**	**0.6**	**0.8**	**1.1**	**1.3**
Aliphatic	**0.3**	**0.2**				**3.6**	**0.2**	**0.2**	**0.3**	**0.3**	**0.4**
Heptanol	*	*	*	*	nq	nq	*	nd	*	*	*
Octanol	**	nq	0.2	0.3	0.4	0.4	*	**	**	nq	nq
2-Cyclohexen-1-ol	**	0.1	0.4	0.6	0.8	0.8	**	0.1	0.1	0.2	0.2
1,2-Cyclohexanediol	0.1	0.1	0.2	0.7	1.7	2.3	0.1	**	0.1	0.1	0.2
Monoterpenes	**0.3**	**0.5**				**4.5**	**0.4**	**0.4**	**0.5**	**0.7**	**0.8**
Linalool	0.2	0.3	0.1	0.1	0.1	**	0.2	0.2	0.1	0.1	0.1
trans-p-2,8-Menthadien-dienol	**	0.1				0.8	**	0.1	0.1	0.2	0.2
(*Z*)-Carveol	**	0.1	0.8	1.4	2.0	2.3	**	0.1	0.1	0.2	0.2
(*E*)-Carveol	**	0.1	0.5	0.6	0.6	0.6	**	**	0.1	0.1	0.2
Hydroxylinalool	**	**	**	0.1	0.4	0.7	**	**	**	**	**
Sesquiterpenes	**	**				*	**	**	**	**	**
Perill alcohol	**	**	*	*	*	*	**	**	**	**	**
Oxides	**	**0.3**				**1.3**	**0.1**	**0.1**	**0.2**	**0.4**	**0.4**
(*Z*)-Linalool oxide	nd	nd	*	*	*	**	nd	nd	nd	nd	nd
(*Z*)-Limonene oxide	**	0.2	1.1	1.1	0.5	0.3	**	0.1	0.1	0.2	0.2

S-3					S-4				
1	3	6	9	12	1	3	6	9	12
95.7	**82.6**	**78.2**	**72.7**	**63.2**	**94.7**	**92.0**	**98.2**	**95.4**	**96.8**
95.6	**82.5**	**78.1**	**72.6**	**63.1**	**94.5**	**91.9**	**98.0**	**95.2**	**96.7**
0.5	0.4	0.3	0.3	0.3	0.5	0.5	0.5	0.5	0.5
0.3	0.3	0.2	0.2	0.2	0.3	0.3	0.3	0.4	0.3
0.4	0.4	0.4	0.4	0.3	0.6	0.5	0.6	0.6	0.6
1.6	1.3	1.3	1.0	0.7	1.8	1.5	1.7	1.7	1.6
91.9	79.3	75.2	70.3	61.1	90.3	88.3	94.0	91.0	92.7
0.4	0.3	0.2	**	**	0.4	0.4	0.4	0.4	0.3
0.2	0.1	0.2	0.4	0.4	0.2	0.2	0.2	0.3	0.3
nd	nd	nd	nd	nd	nd	nd	nd	nd	nd
0.1	**0.1**	**0.1**	**0.1**	**0.1**	**0.1**	**	**0.1**	**0.1**	**0.1**
*	*	*	*	**	**	*	*	*	**
0.1	**	**	**	**	0.1	**	**	**	**
**	**	**	**	**	**	nq	**	**	**
0.4	**0.4**	**0.3**	**0.3**	**0.2**	**0.4**	**0.4**	**0.4**	**0.4**	**0.4**
0.1	0.1	0.1	0.1	0.1	**	0.1	0.1	0.1	**
*	**	**	**	nq	nq	**	nq	**	**
**	**	**	0.1	0.1	**	**	**	**	**
**	**	**	*	**	**	**	**	**	**
**	**	**	**	0.1	**	**	**	**	**
0.1	0.1	0.1	nd	*	0.1	0.1	0.1	0.1	0.1
0.4	**0.4**	**0.6**	**1.3**	**1.8**	**0.4**	**0.5**	**0.4**	**0.5**	**0.6**
0.1	**0.1**	**0.1**	**0.4**	**0.5**	**0.2**	**0.1**	**0.1**	**0.2**	**0.2**
*	nd	*	*	**	*	*	*	*	nd
*	*	nq	0.1	0.1	*	*	**	**	**
**	**	0.1	0.2	0.3	**	**	0.1	0.1	0.1
**	**	**	0.1	0.1	0.1	**	**	**	**
0.3	**0.3**	**0.5**	**0.9**	**1.3**	**0.3**	**0.4**	**0.3**	**0.4**	**0.5**
0.2	0.2	0.1	0.1	0.1	0.2	0.2	0.2	0.2	0.2
**	**	0.1	0.2	0.3	**	**	**	0.1	0.1
**	**	0.1	0.3	0.5	**	**	**	0.1	0.1
**	**	**	0.2	0.3	**	**	**	**	**
**	**	**	**	*	**	**	**	**	**
**	**	**	**	**	**	*	**	**	**
**	**	**	**	**	**	*	**	**	**
0.1	**	**0.1**	**0.5**	**1.1**	**	**	**	**0.1**	**0.1**
nd	nd	nd	nd	**	nd	nd	nd	nd	nd
**	**	**	0.3	0.6	**	*	**	**	**

TABLE 7.7. *Continued*

Functional Group Compound	0	S-1 1[a]	S-1 3	S-1 6	S-1 9	S-1 12	S-2 1	S-2 3	S-2 6	S-2 9	S-2 12
(*E*)-Limonene-oxide	**	0.1	0.7	1.1	0.9	0.6	**	**	0.1	0.2	0.2
(*E*)-Linalool oxide	nd	nd	*	*	*	nq	nd	nd	nd	nd	nd
Ketones	**0.1**	**0.2**				**3.1**	**0.1**	**0.1**	**0.2**	**0.2**	**0.3**
(*S*)-(+)-Carvone	0.1	0.2	0.9	1.6	2.3	2.7	0.1	0.1	0.2	0.2	0.3
(*R*)-(−)-Carvone	**	**	0.1	0.2	0.2	0.3	**	**	**	**	**
Acids	*	*				**0.4**	**	**	**	**	**0.1**
Decanoic acid	*	*	0.1	0.2	0.2	0.3	*	*	*	**	*
Palmitic acid	*	*	**	0.1	0.1	0.1	*	**	**	**	**
Esters	0.1	**				nq	0.1	**	**	**	**
Geranyl acetate	**	**	**	*	**	nq	**	**	**	**	**
Total volatiles (%)	**99.1**	**97.9**	**73.5**	**54.9**	**45.4**	**41.7**	**98.0**	**93.1**	**93.7**	**99.2**	**97.0**

[a]Period of storage (month).
*: Peak area detected less than 0.005%.
**: Peak area detected not less than 0.005% and less than 0.05%.
nd: Not detected.
nq: Not quantified.

Among the alcohols, (*Z*)- and (*E*)-carveols increased substantially, from a trace amount to 2.3% and to 0.6%, respectively. 1,2-Cyclohexanediol also increased remarkably from 0.1 to 2.3%. In ketones, the isomers of carvones, (*S*)-(+)-carvone and (*R*)-(-)-carvone, increased considerably, as much as from 0.1 to 2.7% and from a trace amount to 0.3%, respectively. Four isomers of limonene oxides were detected over a 12-month period, where (*Z*)- and (*E*)-linalool oxides were detected after 2 or 3 months, and (*Z*)- and (*E*)-limonene oxides increased constantly until the 4th month, from trace amounts to 1.4% and to 0.9%, respectively. The levels of these compounds reduced to 1.1% in the 6th month, and continued to decrease to 0.3 and 0.6%, respectively.

S-2. The total proportion of terpene hydrocarbons decreased from 97.7 to 94.3%, where the amount of sesquiterpenes was minor. Aldehydes (0.2%), alcohol (1.3%), oxides (0.4%), and ketones (0.3%) were present, respectively, after 12 months. Limonene decreased to below 90% after one month and then increased again, reaching 93.5% in the 9th month. The initial level of myrcene, 1.8%, decreased continuously to 1.1% by the 12-month period. Other monoterpene hydrocarbons such as α-pinene, β-pinene, and sabinene maintained their original levels in the oil. γ-Terpinene steadily decreased from 0.4 to 0.1% over the whole storage period. The change of γ-terpinene seemed to be linked to the increase of *p*-cymene from 0.2 to 0.4%. Most aldehydes in the S-2 condition were stable. The change in the total level of alcohols was from 0.6 to 1.3%, where 2-cyclohexen-1-ol, 1,2-cyclohexanediol, (*E*)-*p*-2,8-menthadien-1-ol, and (*Z*)- and

S-3					S-4				
1	3	6	9	12	1	3	6	9	12
**	**	**	0.2	0.4	**	**	**	**	**
nd	nd	nd	nd	nd	nd	nd	nd	nd	nd
0.1	**0.1**	**0.1**	**0.6**	**0.8**	**0.1**	**0.1**	**0.1**	**0.1**	**0.2**
0.1	0.1	0.1	0.5	0.7	0.1	0.1	0.1	0.1	0.1
**	*	**	0.1	0.1	**	*	*	**	*
**	**	**	**	**	*	**	**	**	**
**	*	**	**	**	*	**	*	**	*
nd	**	**	**	**	*	**	**	**	**
0.1	**	**	nq	nq	**	**	*	**	**
**	**	**	nq	nq	**	**	*	**	**
96.8	**83.6**	**79.3**	**75.7**	**67.7**	**95.7**	**93.1**	**99.3**	**96.9**	**98.2**

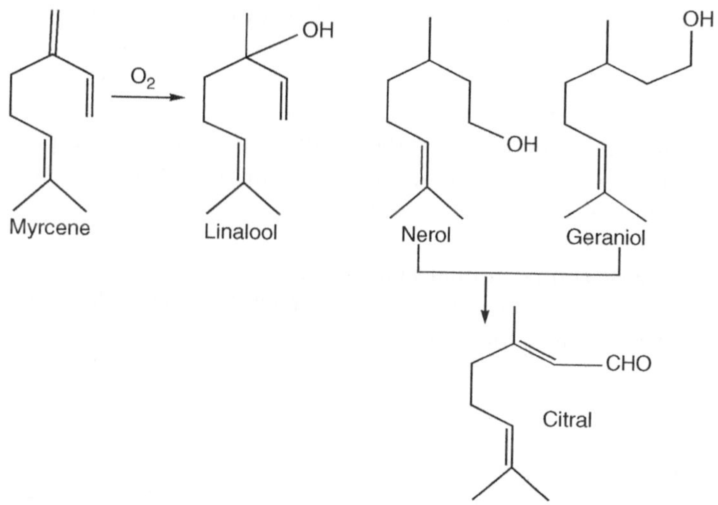

Figure 7.7. Change in myrcene in an aerobic condition.

(*E*)-carveols were detected. (*Z*)- and (*E*)-Limonene oxides increased to a small extent. (*Z*)- and (*E*)-Linalool oxides, which increased greatly in the S-1 condition, were not detected in this S-2 condition over the 12-month period. Limonene diepoxide was newly detected during the storage period in the S-2 condition. Concerning, the two main compounds of ketones, (*S*)-(+)-carvone increased from 0.1 to 0.3% and (*R*)-(−)-carvone remained constant in a trace amount.

S-3. The proportion of the compounds identified in the S-3 condition changed more noticeably than those in the S-2 and S-4 conditions: monoterpene hydrocarbons decreased to 63.1%, and alcohols, oxides, and ketones increased by 1.8, 1.1, and 0.8%, respectively. Several compounds were also detected in small amounts in the S-3 condition: (*E*)-3(10)-caren-2-ol (trace), acetic acid (trace), 7-nonanoic acid (trace), and (*E*)-linalool oxide (trace). The proportion of limonene decreased from 93.2 to 61.1% over the whole storage period. It diminished markedly to 79.3% in the initial 3 months, to 70.3% by the 9th month, and finally to 61.1% in the 12th month. Most monoterpenes decreased in relatively large amounts: α-pinene, β-pinene, sabinene, myrcene, and γ-terpinene decreased to roughly half of their initial proportions. The level of myrcene, particularly, decreased by as much as 1.1% in the 12-month storage period, reaching 0.7%, although the sample was stored in the refrigerator set at 5°C. The proportion of γ-terpinene decreased steadily from 0.5% to a trace amount. The proportion of *p*-cymene changed from 0.2 to 0.4% over the 12-month storage period. The variation of aldehydes, in spite of being noticeable in the S-1 condition, was not conspicuous in this condition. The alcohols and oxides, on the other hand, increased to a large extent, from more than 0.6% up to 1.8% and from a trace amount to 1.1%, respectively. (*E*)-*p*-2,8-Menthadien-1-ol, 2-cyclohexen-ol, and (*Z*)- and (*E*)-carveols showed a great increase after 6 months of storage. Despite a decrease in linalool, (*Z*)-and (*E*)-linalool oxides were not detected. (*Z*)-and (*E*)-Limonene oxides, which may have been derived from limonene, increased up to 0.6 and 0.4%, respectively, after 3 months. The extensive increase of the two compounds during the final period of storage was in contrast to the S-1 condition, where they increased in the early part of the storage period. It was noteworthy that (*S*)-(+)- and (*R*)-(-)-carvones increased from 0.1 to 0.7% and from a trace amount to 0.1%, respectively.

S-4. The least compositional change was observed in the S-4 experiment. The proportion of hydrocarbons decreased from 97.8 to 96.8% over a one-year period. The proportion of limonene ranged from 88.3 to 94.0% over a 12-month period. The proportion of myrcene was also less variable, from 1.8 to 1.6% during the storage period. γ-Terpinene and *p*-cymene also changed in a minor amount, in a narrow range around 0.1%. (*E*)-*p*-2,8-Menthadien-1-ol, 2-cyclohexen-1-ol, and (*Z*)-carveol increased to 0.1% each, and the total level of alcohols accounted for 0.6% in the 12th month. Limonene diepoxide was newly detected in a trace amount in the 12th month. Ketones were also stable in this condition.

Comprehensive Change. The total amount of volatiles may be another indicator of the qualitative change in essential oils accompanying the compositional change. As for the S-1 sample, the total volatile amount determined by weight percent analysis using GC decreased to 73.5% in three months. This suggests that about one-fourth of the volatile compounds in the original essential oil converted to nonvolatile compounds during a period of three months. This level was maintained for one month and then decreased again to 41.7% by the end of the 12th month. In the S-3 condition, the total volatiles decreased from 99.1 to 67.7%. In a practical condition of S-1 and S-3, under aerobic conditions, we can consider the possibility of the promotion of oxidation. Comparatively, in S-2 and S-4, the change in volatiles was not so noticeable, since its greatest decrease was only from 99.1 to 97.0% and to 98.2%, respectively. These results may provide predictive knowledge concerning the compositional changes in commercial essential oils for aromatherapy in practical use, and also for deliberations as to how to care for and store aromatherapy materials.

In conclusion, compositional changes of mandarin essential oil occurred predominantly in the S-1 condition followed by the S-3 condition during the storage period, where monoterpene hydrocarbons decreased from 97.7 to 27.3% and from 97.7 to 63.1%, respectively. The main compound, limonene, decreased remarkably in the S-1 and S-3 conditions, from 93.2 to 26.6% and from 93.2 to 61.6%, respectively. On the other hand, the changes of S-2 and S-4 were not significant. During a 12-month period, many compounds belonging to the alcohol, oxide, and ketone groups increased in concentration due to oxidation of terpene hydrocarbons.

7.2.5 Summary

Compositional changes in commercial essential oils for application in aromatherapy were investigated under four different conditions over a one-year period. Sample S-1 was stored in an incubator set at 25°C with the vial open for 3 min every day; sample S-2 was stored in an incubator set at 25°C with the vial open once a month for analysis; sample S-3 was stored in a refrigerator set at 5°C with the vial open for 3 min every day; and sample S-4 was stored in a refrigerator set at 5°C with the vial open once a month for analysis. The oil samples were analyzed quantitatively over a 12-month period using methyl myristate as an internal standard by GC and GC-MS. Finally, it is suggested that the S-1 and/or S-3 condition, which is aerobic or at room temperature, will effect a considerable change in the composition of essential oils under ordinary usage. These results may provide predictive knowledge concerning the compositional changes in commercial essential oils for aromatherapy in practical use, and also for deliberations as to how to care for and store aromatherapy materials.

REFERENCES

Ayedoun, A.M., Sossou, P.V. (1996). Volatile constituents of the peel and leaf oils of *Citrus limon*. Burm. f. from Benin. *Journal of Essential Oil Research* **8**: 441–444.

Bor-Karlson, A.K., Unelius, C.R., Valterova, L., Nilsson, L.A. (1996). Floral fragrance chemistry in the early flowering shrub Daphne Meserum. *Phytochemistry* **41**: 1477–1483.

Calvarano, M. (1965). La composizione di bergamotto. *Essenze Derivati Agrumari* **4**: 197–211.

Carson, C.F., Hammer, K.A., Riley, T.V. (2006). *Melaleuca alternifolia* (Tea tree) oil: A review of antimicrobial and other medicinal properties. *Clinical Microbiology Reviews* **19**: 50–62.

Chaieb, K., Hajlaoui, H., Zmantar, T., Kahla-Nakbi, A.B., Rouabhia, M., Mahdouani, K., Bakhrouf, A. (2007). The chemical composition and biological activity of clove essential oil, *Eugenia caryophyllata* (*Syzigium aromaticum* L. Myrtaceae): A short review. *Phytotherapy Research* **21**: 501–506.

Chang, S.Y. (2008). Effects of aroma hand massage on pain, state anxiety and depression in hospice patients with terminal cancer. *Taehan Kanho Hakhoe Chi* **38**: 493–502.

Choi, H.S., Sawamura, M. (2000). Effect of storage condition on the composition of *Citrus tamurana* Hort. ex Tanaka (Hyuganatsu) essential oil. *Bioscience, Biotechnology, and Biochemistry* **66**: 439–443.

Choi, H.S., Sawamura, M. (2002). Comparison of the cold-pressed oil composition between Korean and Japanese Satsuma mandarin (*Citrus unshiu* Macov. forma *Miyagawa-wase*) by GC, GC-MS and GC-O. *Journal of Food Science and Nutrition* **7**: 5–11.

Cotroneo, A., Stagno, I.A., Trozzi, A. (1992). On the Genuineness of citrus essential oils. Part XXXIV: Detection of added reconstituted bergamot oil in genuine bergamot essential oil by high resolution gas chromatography with chiral capillary columns. *Fravour and Fragrance Journal* **7**: 15–17.

Da Silva, M.J., Robles-Dutenhefner, P., Menini, L., Gusevskaya, E.V. (2003). Cobalt catalyzed autooxidation of monoterpenes in acetic acid and acetonitrile solutions. *Journal of Molecular Catalysis* **201**: 71–77.

Diekman, R.H., Palamand, S.R. (1974). Autioxidation of some constituents of hops: The monoterpene hydrocarbon, myrcene. *Journal of Agricultural and Food Chemistry* **23**: 498–503.

Dugo, G., Cotroneo, A., Verzera, A., Donato, M.G., Duce, R.D., Licandro, G., Crispo, F. (1991). Genuineness characters of Calabrian bergamot essential oil. *Flavour and Fragrance Journal* **6**: 39–56.

Dugo, G., Lamonia, G., Cotroneo, A., Trozzi, A., Crispo, F., Licandro, G., Gioffre, D. (1987). Sulla genuinita della frazione volatile dell'essenza di bergamotto calabrese. *Essenze Derivati Agrumari* **57**: 456–534.

Dugo, P., McHale, D. (2002). The oxygen heterocyclic compounds of citrus essential oils. In: Dugo, G., Giacomo, A.D., (eds.), *Citrus: The genus Citrus*. London: Taylor & Francis, CRC Press, pp. 355–390.

European Pharmacopoeia, 6th Edition. (2008). Supplement 6.2. Council of Europe, Strasburg, France.

Gattefossé, R.-M. (1993). *Aromatherapy*. Walden, UK: C. W. Daniel.

Giacomo, A.D., Mincione, B. (1995). *Olio essenzile di bergamotto*. Reggio Calabria: Laruffa Editore.

Guenther, E., Althausen, D. (1949). *The essential oils, vol. 2*. Toronto: D. Van Nostrand.

Han, S.H., Hur, M.H., Buckle, J., Choi, J., Lee, M.S. (2006). Effect of aromatherapy on symptoms of dysmenorrheal in college students: A randomized placebo-controlled clinical trial. *Journal of Alternative and Complementary Medicine* **12**: 535–541.

Hodgson, R.W. (1967). Sour or bitter oranges. In: Reuther, W., Webber, H.J., Batchelor, L.D. (eds.) *The citrus industry, vol. 1*. Berkley: University of California Press, pp. 489–496.

Ichimura, N., Uchiyama, T. (1989). Characteristic flavor components in citrus fruits. *Koryo* **164**: 73–80.

Imanishi, J. (2006). *Medical aromatherapy*. Tokyo: Kinpodo.

Inoue, S., Abe, S. (2006). A new development of anti-infectious aromatherapy. *Aroma Research* **26**: 121–131.

Kim, M.J., Nam, E.S., Paik, S.I. (2005). The effects of aromatherapy on pain, depression, and life satisfaction of arthritis patients. *Taehan Kanho Hakhoe Chi* **35**: 186–194.

Kirbaslar, F.G., Kirbaslar, S.I., Dramur, U. (2001). The compositions of Turkish bergamot oils produced by cold-pressing and steam distillation. *Journal of Essential Oil Research* **13**: 411–415.

Komiya, M., Takeuchi, T., Harada, E. (2006). Lemon oil vapor causes an anti-stress effect via modulating the 5-HT and DA activities in mice. *Behavioural Brain Research* **172**: 240–249.

Kumagai, C., Horii, Y., Shen, J., Tanida, M., Niijima, A., Okada, Y., Okuyama, T., Sawamura, M., Nagai, K. (2009). Effects of olfactory stimulation of Yuzu (*Citrus junos*) on autonomic nerves, lipolysis and body temperature. *Aroma Research* **10**: 156–161.

Letizia, C.S., Cocchiara, J., Api, A.M. (2003a). Fragrance material review on linalyl acetate. *Food and Chemical Toxicology* **41**: 943–964.

Letizia, C.S., Cocchiara, J., Api, A.M. (2003b). Fragrance material review on linalool. *Food and Chemical Toxicology* **41**: 965–976.

Lota, M.L., Serra, D.R., Tomi, F., Joseph, C. (2000). Chemical variability of peel and leaf essential oils of mandarins from *Citrus reticulata* Blanco. *Biochemical Systematics and Ecology* **28**: 61–78.

Maury, M., revised by Ryman, D. (1989). *The secret of life and youth*. Saffron, U. K.: C. W. Daniel.

Mikami, K. (2006). *Essential oils in Japan*. Tokyo: Fragrance Journal Ltd.

Mitiku, S.B., Njoroge, S.M., Sawamura, M., Koaze, H. (2002). Analytical discrimination of the cold-pressed oils of mandarins and their hybrids. *Journal of Essential Oil Research* **14**: 196–202.

Mondello, L., d'Alcontes, I.S., Duce, R.D., Crispo, F. (1993). On the genuineness of citrus essential oils. Part XL: The composition of the coumarins and psoralenes of Calabrian bergamot essential oil (*Citrus bergamia* Risso). *Flavour and Fragrance Journal* **8**: 17–24.

Moshonas, M., Shaw, P.E. (1974). Quantitative and qualitative analysis of tangerine peel oil. *Journal of Agricultural and Food Chemistry* **22**: 282–284.

Moufida, S., Marzouk, B. (2003). Biochemical characterization of blood orange, sweet orange, lemon, bergamot and bitter orange. *Phytochemistry* **62**: 1283–1289.

Nakayama, A., Shinohara, K., Nakao, S., Adachi, K., Hamazaki, H., Kubo, S., Sakurai, H. (2004). Reactive oxygen species-scavenging activity and biological response of herb essential oils. *Aroma Research* **18**: 123–128.

Niijima, A., Nagai, K. (2003). Effect of olfactory stimulation with flavor of grapefruit oil and lemon oil on the activity of sympathetic branch in the white adipose tissue of the epididymis. *Experimental Biology and Medicine* **228**: 1190–1192.

Njoroge, S.M., Ukeda, H., Kusunose, H., Sawamura, M. (1994). Volatile components of Japanese yuzu and lemon oils. *Flavour and Fragrance Journal* **9**: 159–166.

Njoroge, S.M., Ukeda, H., Sawamura, M. (1996). Changes in the volatile composition of yuzu (*Citrus junos* Tanaka) cold-pressed oil during storage. *Journal of Agricultural and Food Chemistry* **44**: 550–556.

Nursten, H.E. (1977). The important volatile flavour components of foods. In: Birch, G.G., Brennan, J.G., Parker, K.J. (eds), *Sensory properties of foods*. London: Applied Science Publishers, pp. 151–166.

Okamura, H. (1983). Mandarin oil. *Koryo* **138**: 53–57.

Pattnaik, S., Subramanyam, V.R., Bapaji, M., Kole, C.R. (1997). Antibacterial and antifungal activity of aromatic constituents of essential oils. *Microbios* **89**: 39–46.

Pomeranz, C. (1891). Über das Beergapten. *Monatsh Food Chemistry* **12**: 379–392.

Prabuseenivasan, S., Jayakumar, M., Ignacimuthu, S. (2006). *In vitro* antibacterial activity of some plant essential oils. *BMC Complementary Alternative Medicine* **6**: 39–46.

Regione Calabria Assessoato All'agricoltura Consorzio del Bergamotto. (1989). *Bergamotto Di Reggio Calabria*. Reggio Calabria: Laruffa Editore.

Safayhi, H., Sabieraj, J., Sailer, E.R., Ammon, H.P. (1994). Chamazulene: An antioxidant-type inhibitor of leukotriene B4 formation. *Planta Medica* **60**: 410–413.

Sawamura, M. (2000). Volatile components of essential oils of the *Citrus* genus. In: Pandalai, S.G. (ed.), *Recent research and development in agriculture and chemistry, vol. 4*. Trivandrum: Research Signpost, pp. 131–164.

Sawamura, M. (2005a). *Citrus junos* Sieb. ex Tanaka (Yuzu) fruit. In: Dris, R. (ed.) *Fruits: Growth, nutrition, and quality*. Finland: WFL, pp. 1–24.

Sawamura, M. (2005b). Essential oil extraction, Patent no. 3842794 (Japan).

Sawamura, M., Hasegawa, K., Kashiwagi, T., Nguyen Thi, L.P., Wada, M., Kumagai, C. (2009). Determination of bergapten in Japanese citrus essential oils. *Japanese Journal of Aromatherapy* **9**: 30–37.

Sawamura, M., Poiana, M., Kawamura, A., Itoh, T., Song, H.S., Ukeda, H., Mincione, B. (1999). Volatile components of peel oils of Italian and Japanese lemon and bergamot. *Italian Journal of Food Science* **11**: 121–130.

Schimmer, O. (1981). Vergaleich der photomutagenen wirkungen von 5-MOP (bergapten) und 8-MOP (xanthotoxin) in *Chlamydomonas reinhardii*. *Mutation Research Genetic Toxicology* **89**: 283–296.

Shaw, P.E. (1979). Review of quantitative analyses of citrus essential oils. *Journal of Agriculture and Food Chemistry* **27**: 246–257.

Shen, J., Niijima, A., Tanida, M., Horii, Y., Maeda, K., Nagai, K. (2005a). Olfactory stimulation with scent of lavender oil affects autonomic nerves, lipolysis and appetite in rats. *Neuroscience Letters* **383**: 188–193.

Shen, J., Niijima, A., Tanida, M., Horii, Y., Maeda, K., Nagai, K. (2005b). Olfactory stimulation with scent of grapefruits oil affects autonomic nerves, lipolysis and appetite in rats. *Neuroscience Letters* **380**: 289–294.

Sinclair, W.B. (1984). The essential oils. In: *The biochemistry and physiology of the lemon*. Berkeley, CA: Division of Agriculture and Natural Resources, University of California, pp. 218–309.

Soden, K., Vincent, K., Craske, S., Lucas, C., Ashlley, S. (2004). A randomized controlled trial of aromatherapy massage in a hospice setting. *Palliative Medicine* **18**: 87–92.

Staroscik, J.A., Wilson, A.A. (1982). Seasonal and regional variation on the quantitative composition of cold-pressed lemon oil from California and Arizona. *Journal of Agricultural and Food Chemistry* **30**: 835–837.

Susan, C. (1996). *Essential oils*. London: Aurum Press, pp. 10–25.

Tanida, M., Niijima, A., Shen, J., Nakamura, T., Nagai, K. (2005). Olfactory stimulation with scent of essential oil of grapefruit affects autonomic neurotransmission and blood pressure. *Brain Research* **1058**: 44–55.

Tanida, M., Shen, J., Niijima, A., Yamatodani, A., Oishi, K., Ishida, N., Nagai, K. (2008). Effects of olfactory stimulations with scents of grapefruit and lavender oils on renal sympathetic nerve and blood pressure in *Clock* mutant mice. *Autonomic Neurscience* **139**: 1–8.

Tisserand, R. (1977). *The art of aromatherapy*. Walden, U. K.: C. W. Daniel.

Tisserand, R., Balacs, T. (1995). *Essential oil safety*. Edinburgh: Churchill Livingstone, pp. 77–89.

Tomas, A.F. (1973). The synthesis of monoterpenes. In: ApSimon, J. (ed.), *The total synthesis of natural products*. New York: John Wiley & Sons, pp. 1–196.

Torii S (2002). *Science of aromatherapy*. Tokyo: Asakurashoten.

Usai, M., Arras, G., Fronteddu, F. (1992). Effects of cold storage on essential oils of peel of Thompson navel oranges. *Journal of Agricultural and Food Chemistry* **40**: 271–275.

Vekiri, S.A., Protopapadakis, E.E., Papadopoulou, P., Papanicolaou, D., Panou, C., Vamvakias, M. (2002). Composition and seasonal variation of the essential oil from leaves and peel of a Cretan lemon variety. *Journal of Agricultural and Food Chemistry* **50**: 147–153.

Verzera, A., Trozzi, A., Cotroneo, A., Lorenzo, D., Dellacassa, E. (2000). Uruguayan essential oil. Composition of Nova and Satsuma mandarin oils. *Journal of Agricultural and Food Chemistry* **48**: 2903–2909.

Verzera, A., Trozzi, A., Gazea, F., Cicciarello, G., Cotroneo, A. (2003). Effects of rootstock on the composition of bergamot (*Citrus bergamia* Risso et Poiteau) essential oil. *Journal of Agricultural and Food Chemistry* **51**: 206–210.

Whittaker, D. (1972). The monoterpenes. In: Newman, A.A. (ed.), *Chemistry of terpenes and terpenoids*. London: Academic Press, pp. 11–87.

Yip, Y.B., Tam, A.C. (2008). An experimental study on the effectiveness of massage with aromatic ginger and orange essential oil for moderate to severe knee pain among the elderly in Hong Kong. *Complementary Therapies in Medicine* **16**: 131–138.

8

INDUSTRIAL VIEW

Hisakatsu Iwabuchi

San-Ei Gen F.F.I., Inc.
Osaka, Japan

Down through the ages, people have been very interested in aromatic scents that give warmth and richness to the inner life. It is said that we have entered the age of aromatics, and aromatics receive great attention in our daily lives.

Aromatic materials used in creating flavors and fragrances for various applications are required to have not only a characteristic aroma with naturalness and strength that meets the tastes of consumers but also functional properties, such as heat and light resistance as well as aromatic and taste-enhancing effects. Among important aromatic materials are essential oils derived from a variety of plants. A pleasant aroma produced by a trace component in the essential oil imparts a distinctive character to flavors and fragrances.

The association between the aroma characteristics and the chemical structure (e.g., isomers, homologues, types of functional groups) of aroma compounds has long been studied. The advanced technology of analysis, particularly instrumental analysis, makes an important contribution to the study. Additionally, the progress of synthesis and extraction technologies has caused the advancement of formulation technology. The combination of these sophisticated technologies has enabled the identification of some of the key aroma components that had been hidden in a veil of mystery. The separation and determination of aroma components in

Citrus Essential Oils: Flavor and Fragrance, Edited by Masayoshi Sawamura

essential oils, fruits, and other foods are indispensable for developing flavors and fragrances with a natural aroma and the functional properties, and have long been studied by the flavor and fragrance industry.

Aromatic substances are used mainly to satisfy the diverse tastes of consumers in various products, such as foods, beverages, cosmetics, and household products. They are classified by application into two groups: flavors for foods and beverages, and fragrances for nonfood applications. They give warmth and richness to people's home, dietary, and fashion lifestyles as well as heighten the added-value of the abovementioned products.

Fragrances are used in perfumery and cosmetics (basic skin-care, makeup, and hair-care products, shampoo, soap, bath agents, etc.), household products (laundry detergents, kitchen detergents, bleaching agents, air fresheners, insecticides, etc.), and industrial products (paints, fuel oils, solvents, printing inks, fibers, etc.). They are required to appeal to the aesthetic sense of consumers.

Flavors are used mainly in confectionery, beverages, desserts and frozen desserts, soups, sauces and dressings, processed meat and seafood products, dairy products, fat and oil products, prepared foods, and processed agricultural products. Their aroma is a critical factor in producing delicious foods and beverages because it makes a certain contribution to the taste of final products.

Flavors are also used in nonfood products that are taken into the body, such as oral-care products, cigarettes, and pharmaceuticals. Some flavors are used in livestock feed to enhance the appetite of animals.

Aromatic substances have diverse functions that are not limited to imparting an aroma to the abovementioned products. Some of them act as antiseptics, antioxidants, attractants, repellents, pheromones, masking agents, and deodorants, as well as being used in aromatherapy.

The process of creating an objective aroma by blending various natural and synthetic aromatic materials is called *formulation*. Relying on olfaction, flavorists and perfumers select and blend aromatic materials in conformity with customer needs and product concepts, and record the final composition of flavors and fragrances, respectively. They are required to have not only extensive knowledge, such as of the aroma characteristics, the physical and chemical properties, the odor threshold, the optimal concentrations in various base materials, and the sensory properties depending on the concentration of each aromatic material, but also artistic sense and creativity. In addition, they are required to be familiar with scientific, safety, and regulatory knowledge of the final products, such as foods and cosmetics.

Aromatic materials were divided into natural and synthetic types. Citrus oils obtained from citrus fruits are among the most important aromatic materials. Citrus fruits are eaten by people all over the world, and their aroma and taste enjoy the greatest popularity. Among the world's fruit crops, grapes had long been in the first rank but were replaced by citrus in 1988. Citrus fruits on the global market are classified into five groups—orange, tangerine, lemon and lime, grapefruit and pummelo, and others—and their shares are about 52, 22, 4, 11, and 6%, respectively (Tsuchiya, 2008).

Citrus fruits are eaten raw, and processed into juice, canned foods, alcoholic beverages, confiture, dry peel, and so on. Large amounts of essential oils extracted from citrus fruits are used as materials for flavors and fragrances, and find wide application.

Citrus oils are used in fragrances mainly for perfumery, cosmetics, soap, bath agents, detergents, and air fresheners to impart a refreshing, light top note. Citrus flavors are among the most important ingredients in food processing, and are widely used mainly in fruit juice–containing beverages, soft drinks, desserts and frozen desserts, yogurt, confectionery, and bakery products. The production volume and price of citrus oils are critical factors in manufacturing flavors and fragrances, and largely depend on the weather. With rapid economic growth and environmental destruction from the twentieth century onward, the warming of the earth's atmosphere proceeds, bringing abnormal weather on a global scale. Floods, droughts, and cold waves as well as the increased scale of storms cause immense damage to plants and animals. Market prices of natural products fluctuate widely depending on the crops, and, in recent years, have been strongly affected by speculative dealing irrespective of the demands.

In squeezing juice from citrus fruits, a large amount of pomace is produced as industrial waste, and its effective utilization is an important issue. Pomace is rich in citrus oils, and the methods of efficiently extracting high-quality essential oils from pomace have been studied and put to practical use. Also, pomace is fermented and dried into compost. Essential oil recovery from waste was developed from the standpoint of the *eco-conscious system.*

In this chapter, the use of citrus oils in flavors and fragrances will be reviewed. Aroma formulations, the technology of making preparations of aroma formulations, and the effective utilization of citrus peel will be described in detail.

8.1 FORMULATION OF ESSENTIAL OILS FOR PROCESSED FOODS: PRODUCTION, TREND, AND MICROCAPSULATION

Chiyoki Yukawa and Masaki Shimada

8.1.1 Aroma Materials for Flavor/Fragrance Formulation

To prepare a flavor/fragrance formulation, natural and synthetic aroma materials are blended according to the intended use (Japan Patent Office, 1999). Natural aroma materials are generally divided into two types: plant derived and animal derived. Synthetic aroma materials consist of various organic compounds. For other aroma materials, there are Millard flavors, enzyme flavors, and so forth. Additionally, a single component isolated from aroma materials by physical methods, such as distillation and crystallization, is called "isolated aroma substances."

Plant-Derived Aroma Substances. Plant-derived aroma substances are produced from various parts of plants, such as flowers, leaves, seeds, fruits, peels, barks, roots, and resins. Depending on the production method, aroma substances derived from the same part of a plant may have different aroma components.

Natural aroma substances are classified by production method as follows:

1. Essential oils comprise volatile aroma components of the abovementioned plant tissues, and are obtained by steam distillation or pressing. Most citrus essential oils are produced by pressing. Essential oils produced by pressing at ordinary or low temperatures are called *cold-pressed* (CP) oils. The quality of essential oils depends on various factors, such as the production area and harvesting season of the plant, the weather in the growing season, and the oil production equipment. Essential oils are characterized by the harmonious balance of their aroma components.
2. *Oleoresin* is obtained by extracting aroma components from a ground plant aroma material with one or more volatile solvents and distilling off the solvents under reduced pressure. It contains both aroma and taste components, and has a distinctive aroma. Most spice extracts are of this type.
3. *Extract* is obtained by extracting aroma components from an aroma material with one or more solvents (except volatile solvents). Moisture ethanol is commonly used as an extraction solvent. The extract may be concentrated by distilling off part of the solvent. *Tincture*, included in this category, is an unconcentrated ethanol extract; that is, it contains the extraction solvent, ethanol. When liquid or supercritical carbon dioxide is used as an extraction solvent, the resultant product is called carbon dioxide extract.
4. There are other products obtained by extracting aroma components from an aroma material with one or more solvents and distilling off the solvents, such as *absolute*, *concrete*, and *resinoid*.
5. *Recovery essence* is obtained by recovering aroma components that distill simultaneously with water during the process of concentrating juice. The products are of two types—oil and concentrated aqueous solution—and will be described later in detail. Distilled water, the aroma component–containing aqueous distillate obtained during the process of producing essential oils by steam distillation, is also included in this category.

Animal-Derived Aroma Substances. Musk, civet, castoreum, and ambergris are animal-derived aroma substances. Today, only two of them, civet and castoreum, are in use. Although they are primarily used in fragrances for perfumery and cosmetics, they are sometimes used as food flavors as well.

Citrus Oils as an Aroma Material for Flavor/Fragrance Formulation. Among world fruit crops, grapes had long been in the first rank (Japan External Trade Organization, 2008). However, citrus fruit production increased and its production volume substantially matched that of grapes, around 64 million tons, in 1987. In the following year, 1988, citrus fruit production volume grew to 67 million tons, while grapes fell to less than 60 million tons. Consequently, citrus fruits ranked first, with the largest production volume in the world. The use of citrus flavors is particularly significant in food processing. Citrus flavors are widely used mainly in fruit juice–containing beverages, soft drinks, desserts and frozen desserts, yogurt, confectionery, and bakery products.

Although no accurate data concerning citrus oil production for recent years is available, the estimated production volumes of essential oils for 2007 are reported as follows (Lawrence, 2009): orange oil, 51,000 tons; lemon oil, 9,200 tons; lime distilled oil, 1,800 ton; mandarin oil, 460 tons.

Orange. Most orange crops are Valencia and Navel oranges. Blood orange is also produced in some quantities. Brazil is the world's largest producer of orange oil, and its total export is approximately 30,000 tons, roughly 30% of which is imported by the United States and Japan. The second largest producer is the United States, where 60% of the total volume is produced in Florida and 20–30% in California.

Orange production in the United States for the period from October 2006 to September 2007 was 6,684,741 tons (down by 15.9%, on a year-over-year basis). The significant drop in the volume of this period was attributed to bad weather; Florida's orange production areas were badly affected by hurricanes in 2004 and 2005, and California's orange production areas were severely hit by a great cold wave around the middle of January 2007.

In Brazil, orange production areas are concentrated in the state of São Paulo, with 80.4% of the total volume produced within this state. An increase in production is anticipated, as additional crop is expected from the new production areas. Brazil's orange production volume for the period from October 2007 to September 2008 is expected to grow significantly.

Lemon. Lemon (*Citrus limon* N. L. Burman) is believed to have originated in the eastern part of Himalayan Piedmont in India, or the regions ranging from southeastern China to the northern part of Myanmar. There are many different lemon varieties; the major varieties are *Lisbon*, *Eureka*, *Femminello ovale*, *Villafranka*, *Berna*, *Messero*, *Meyer lemon*, and so on. Argentina is the world's largest lemon producer, and the other major lemon-producing countries include the United States, Italy, Spain, and Brazil. Lemon production in the United States for the period from October 2006 to September 2007 was 637,762 tons (down by 28.3%, on a year-over-year basis). Lime (*Citrus aurantifolia* Swingle), a citrus fruit similar to lemon, belongs to Rutaceae family, and its birthplace is thought to have been in India. Today, the West Indies and Mexico are the major lime-producing regions.

Although lemon oil had been in steady supply for many years, its supply is now tight and the price has been soaring recently. Rising demand for fresh lemon in the world's three major lemon-producing areas seems to be behind these changes: It has led to the shortage of lemons for processing, consequently causing a significant decrease in the production of lemon oil as a byproduct of lemon juice processing. In the United States, central California was hit by a cold wave in January 2007 and the region's lemon crop for the 2007–2008 period decreased by more than 20%. Argentina was also badly damaged by cold summer weather in September 2007, resulting in more than a 20% drop in its lemon crop from the previous year. Global poor crops have boosted lemon prices, and brought a large portion of lemon crops to the fresh-fruits market where they are sold at higher prices, causing the shortage of lemons for processing. Moreover, a heat wave hit the southern part of Europe in June 2007, causing heavy damage to the fruits and flowers in Sicily. Consequently, the 2007–2008 crops plunged to a historically low level.

Grapefruit. Grapefruit (*Citrus paradisi* Macfadyen) belongs to the Rutaceae family, and is believed to have originated in the West Indies. Today, the United States (Florida and California), Israel, and South Africa are the major grapefruit-producing countries. Although Marsh Seedless, a white-pulp grapefruit, is the predominant variety, the red-pulp Ruby Red has been recently increasing in production.

Grapefruit production in the United States for the period from October 2006 to September 2007 was 1,430,654 tons (up by 28.0%, on a year-over-year basis). The United States is the top producer of grapefruit in the world, accounting for 40% of the total global production volume of a normal year. Florida supplies approximately 80% of the U.S. production.

In August 2004, Florida was struck by four devastating hurricanes, resulting in a more than 50% decrease in its grapefruit production. Florida was again hit by a hurricane in October 2005, suffering another significant drop in production. To make things worse, a citrus canker outbreak occurred when the citrus trees were becoming less resistant to diseases. Although production started to pick up again during the 2005–2006 period, the damage was so severe that a full recovery has not been brought about yet. In South Africa, grapefruit production volume for the period from February 2006 to January 2007 increased by 14.3% from the previous year to 414,948 tons (estimated).

Although white grapefruit is popular in Japan's markets as it suits Japanese tastes, sweet pink and Ruby Red grapefruits are predominant in Europe and the U.S. markets, where white grapefruit is not as well-received due to its somewhat bitter taste. White grapefruit CP oil and essence is mainly used in flavor formulations for beverages such as isotonic drinks. Other citrus aroma materials, such as lemon and lime, may be combined. Additionally, the recent increase in the production of NFC (Not From Concentrate) fruit juice is causing a continuous supply shortage of "recovery essence (oil and aroma)," a byproduct obtained during the fruit juice concentration process.

Citrus Recovery Essence. Citrus recovery essence, which is obtained by recovering aroma components that distill simultaneously with water during the process of concentrating juice, is differentiated from peel essential oil. The recovery essence is composed of a light oil phase (recovery essence oil) and a heavy aqueous phase (recovery aroma). The recovery essence oil contains higher quantities of components producing a juicy aroma characteristic of citrus than the peel oil, and is relatively stable.

When added to aqueous systems, such as fruit juice–containing beverages, the recovery essence oil is previously dissolved in a suitable solvent, for example, alcohol, or emulsified. In contrast, aroma components obtained by removing terpene hydrocarbons from the recovery essence oil by distillation or extraction are easily soluble and uniformly dispersible in concentrated and unconcentrated juices as well as beverages. Thus, use of neither the solvent nor emulsification is required.

Recovery aroma consisting mainly of water-soluble aroma components is miscible with beverages in all proportions, and imparts a mild aroma characteristic of citrus juice.

Processing Technologies of Natural Aroma Materials (Extraction/Refining). In this chapter, basic processing technologies of essential oils and formulation and preparation technologies of flavors will be explored in detail.

The processing method of citrus oil mainly consists of simple distillation, precision distillation, molecular distillation, and countercurrent extraction, fractionation, concentration, and extraction of specific components. Citrus oil is processed into various types of aroma materials with different levels of notes, flavor intensity, stability, and functionality depending on application, which provides characteristic aromas and specific functional properties to flavors.

As natural aroma substances are used for a wide variety of applications, various advanced technologies such as extraction and refinement are required to maximize the capabilities of natural aroma substances. Essential oils are generally extracted from plant materials through expression and steam distillation, and then directly used as aroma materials for flavors. Essential oils are also further refined into formulation materials for flavors because they are typically composed of many types of constituents (hydrocarbons and oxygenated components), and therefore are susceptible to oxidation, reduction, isomerization, decomposition, condensation, and polymerization during storage. Aroma of essential oils can be enhanced and maintained in such ways, including by removing depleted flavor components and polymeric substances, and by decolorizing colored essential oils. The method involves cutting of front and back fractions, steam distillation, absorption using porous absorbents, and filtration and washing treatments.

Synthetic Aroma Substances. Several thousand synthetic aroma substances have been developed over the years. They are obtained by chemical reactions and also synthesized from chemical compounds having defined chemical structures and flavor components.

Some synthetic aroma substances are chemically processed from isolated aroma substances originating in natural essential oils. Isolated aroma substances are prepared from plant-derived natural aroma materials (essential oils) by certain treatments such as distillation, extraction, and crystallization processes.

Synthetic aroma substances are classified into two types: nature-identical compounds and artificial flavors. Nature-identical compounds are produced synthetically from natural fruit peels, leaves, and branches but are chemically identical to their natural counterparts. Artificial substances are compounds that are artificially synthesized from entirely new aroma substances that have not yet been identified in natural plants. When classified by functional group, esters, alcohols, and aldehydes are the most important compounds and also are industrially produced in large quantities. Synthetic aroma substances can be stably supplied at reasonable prices and consistent quality.

Synthetic Citrus Aroma Substances. Citrus flavor materials are mainly composed of natural aroma materials (essential oils), but synthetic aroma materials are also frequently used. Synthetic aroma materials are mainly classified into two groups: The first group is substances that are chemically identical to their natural counterparts, which are found in essential oils of peels, leaves, and branches of citrus fruits, and the second group is substances that are not completely found in natural essential oils. Many of both types impart a fresh citrus note. Some of them exhibit a slightly unpleasantly strong citrus note at high concentrations, but exhibit a typical citrus note in a diluted form. Some synthetic aroma materials are used as a formulation material. Synthetic aroma substances imparting a citrus note and their unique aroma properties are briefly mentioned here, and their molecular structures are shown in Figure 8.1.

Aldehyde C-6 and aldehyde C-10. These are found in orange oil and lemon oil. Even small amounts of these components add dynamic impression to a citrus note.

***trans*-2-Dodecenal and *trans*-4-decenal.** These exibit an aldehydic note rather than a citrus note in a concentrated state, but give mandarin/orange notes in a diluted state.

Citral. This is found in lemon oil and other essential oils. It is widely used for the preparation of citrus notes. It should be used with care because it is susceptible to sunlight and alkali conditions.

Linalool and linalyl acetate. The combined use of these components and bergamot oil has been traditionally used to generate synergistic effects.

Nootkatone. This is found in lemon oil, orange oil, and grapefruit oil, and gives a grapefruit aroma and a long-lasting citrus note. Nootkatone is a useful flavor component to formulate a grapefruit note.

8,9-Didehydronootkatone. This is an important flavor component imparting a characteristically stronger grapefruit note than nootkatone.

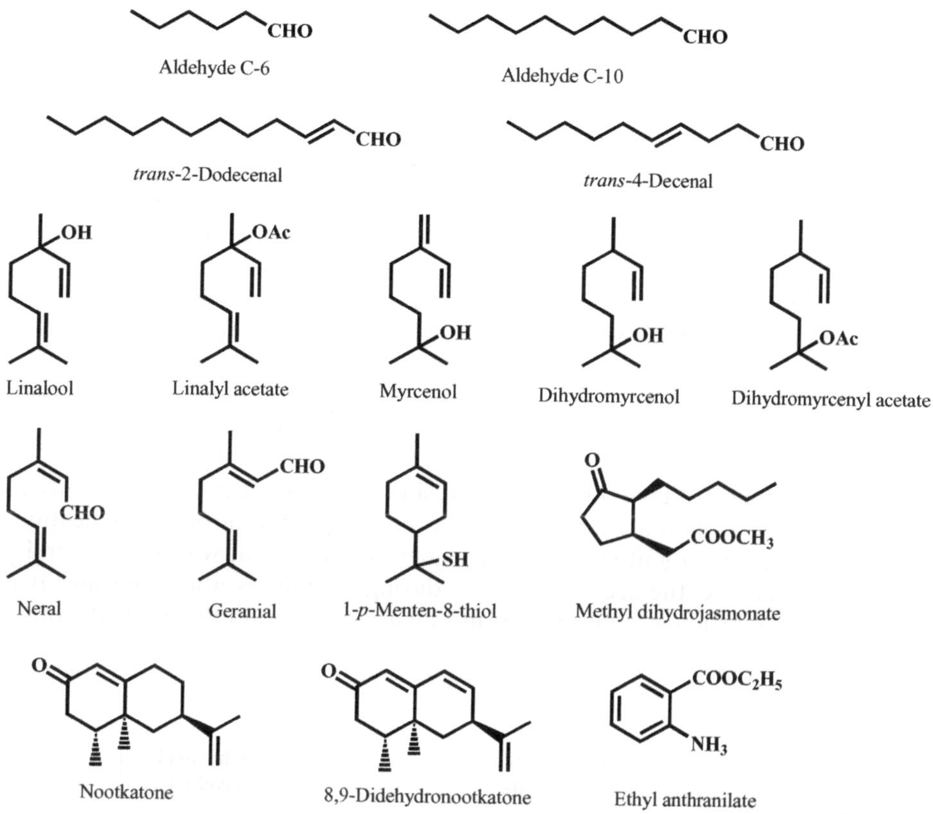

Figure 8.1. Molecular structures of citrus note compounds.

1-*p*-Menthen-8-thiol. This compound is originally found in natural grapefruits and belongs to the nature-identical type. It has the lowest odor threshold value and also exhibits the most powerful grapefruit note among flavors found in nature.

Dihydromyrcenol and dihydromyrcenyl acetate. Dihydromyrcenol has bergamot and lime notes. Dihydromyrcenyl acetate has a fresh lime note. Both of them are used as a citrus formulation material.

Methyl dihydrojasmonate. Combined use of this component with other citrus notes produces beneficial effects.

Ethyl anthranilate. This imparts a pleasant, neroli-like note in diluted form.

Other synthetic aroma substances including myrcenol (lime-like note), geranial (lemon note), *trans*-2-tridecenal, 2,6-docecadienal, citronellyl ethyl ether, and citral glyceryl acetal have their own characteristic aroma and are used to formulate a citrus note.

8.1.2 Fragrance Formulation

A fragrance formulation is prepared by blending aroma materials (Japan Patent Office, 2001). It is processed into various forms, such as oil, emulsion or water-soluble liquid, powder, or dispersion, according to the requirements of its intended application. New perfume and cosmetic products usually call for fragrances that match the current trend. For this reason, it is necessary to reflect the current trend and characteristics of perfumery and cosmetics in formulating a fragrance, in conformity with the properties of a new product. Additionally, flavor formulation techniques have been actively applied to fragrance formulations in recent years. The manufacturing process of flavor and fragrance formulations is outlined in Figure 8.2.

In general, perfumery and cosmetics require pleasant and mild fragrances because they are directly applied to human skin. However, as a fragrance naturally changes with time, its design should take this nature into consideration; it should be designed to give off a light, refreshing scent at an early stage followed by a soft, sweet scent at a later stage. However, fragrances for other applications such as laundry detergent should be designed in a different way. For a laundry detergent fragrance, the scent it releases during washing is not important. It is required to leave an agreeable, clean, and luxurious scent on the washed clothes

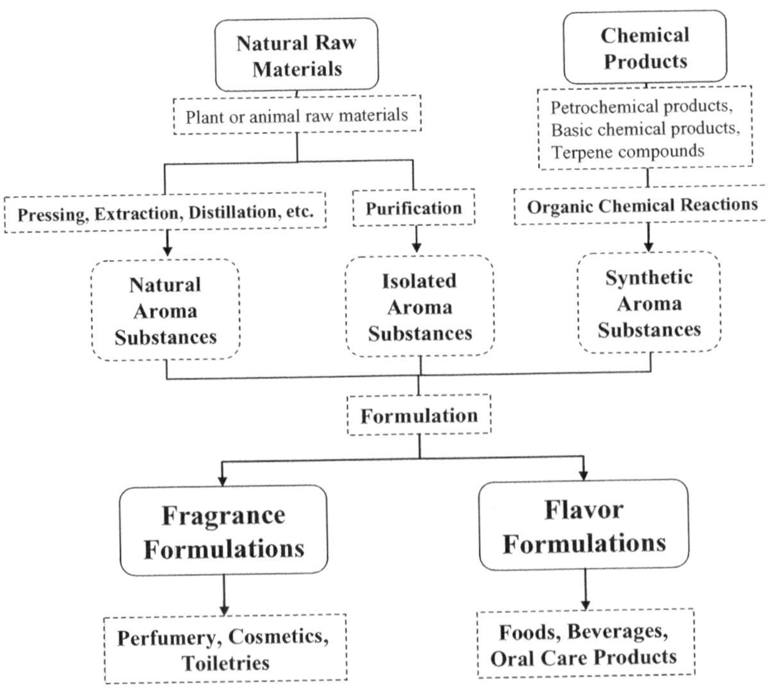

Figure 8.2. Outline of the manufacturing process of flavor and fragrance formulations.

after washing and drying. Fragrance formulation is the process of creating an objective fragrance for perfumery and cosmetics by blending various natural and synthetic aroma materials selected by perfumers in conformity with product planning, concepts, and fragrance trends in the market.

For fragrances, "citrus note" is an important top note. Citrus note is produced by blending an essential oil, such as lemon oil, orange oil, bergamot oil, lime oil, mandarin oil, or grapefruit oil, obtained by distillation or pressing of citrus peel, and synthetic substances with a citrus-fresh aroma. Compared to other notes, it is more prone to volatilize and does not last long. As a refreshing, light top note, citrus note is widely used in almost all types of fragrance formulations including floral bouquet, woody, aldehyde, and oriental.

"Orange" is the sweetest of all the citrus notes, and is widely used in a variety of cosmetics and soaps. "Lemon" is the most typical citrus note, and finds a broad range of applications. It is particularly employed in such applications as cologne, eau de toilette, kitchen detergent for washing dishes and vegetables, and room air freshener. "Lime" is rarely used as an independent top note. However, it well matches other citrus and spices, and is therefore suitable for a dry, lively masculine fragrance. "Grapefruit," in combination with spicy aromas, is employed in men's cologne applications. Refreshing "bergamot" is widely used in modern fancy perfumes including chypre and fougere. "Mandarin" adds mildness, and is therefore used in such applications as modern bouquet, neroli base, cologne, and chypre.

In manufacturing perfumery and cosmetics, liquid fragrance formulations are usually used without being processed into other dosage forms. Owing to their oiliness, fragrance formulations are mixed with the oily components of base materials of final products, and the mixture is emulsified and solubilized before dosing. When the base materials are in powder or granular form, spray dosing may be performed. In order to prevent volatilization and enhance the stability, aroma lifting, and lasting note of aroma components, fragrance formulations may be processed into cyclodextrin clathrates, capsules, and granules.

8.1.3 Formulation of Flavors

Developing a clear product concept is crucial for flavor creation (Japan Patent Office, 2000). Once a product concept has been determined, product developers design desirable flavors by considering application, product form, raw ingredients used, note and taste, price, and other factors. Flavor developers occasionally change flavor recipes for some areas to satisfy diverse consumer preferences, which greatly vary depending on region and country. They also have to consider all relevant regulatory requirements on food additives and prohibited religious practices.

Flavors are created by blending natural aroma substances and synthetic aroma substances at appropriate levels, and then applied to a wide variety of products such as beverages, confectionery, frozen deserts, dairy products, prepared foods, and toothpastes. Flavors play an important role in reconstructing aroma and taste of food products. They are added to foods to enhance aroma and consumer satisfaction and the value and appeal of food products. In this regard, flavors have completely different purposes from fragrances. Flavors are specially designed (custom-made) to satisfy customer-specific needs and requirements.

In developing flavors, flavorists are required to properly understand customer needs, desires, and product concepts, and also to grasp the overall image of a flavor held by customers. The flavor-creation process starts by first selecting appropriate aroma substances from hundreds of different types of aromas, and then deciding on the most appropriate compounding ratio of aroma substances (formula). Based on the formula recipe, flavorists accurately weigh each aroma material and mix them well. They subsequently evaluate the prepared samples in terms of aroma profiles and sensory perception, and decide whether the samples match the image of the aroma they are pursuing. If the samples do not fit the image, flavorists adjust the compounding ratio or use different aroma materials to reach the desired aroma. The trial-and-error process is repeated until the desired aroma is achieved.

Intended Use and Application of Flavors. Flavors play a major role in enhancing consumer acceptance and value of food products. They are among the most important and indispensable food additives for creating and developing new food products, responding to a changing distribution system, improving the quality of processed foods, and also satisfying consumer expectations.

Different aroma attributes are required depending on application and intended use. Flavors also have a major impact on the taste of food products. A harmonious combination of flavor and taste generates synergistic effects on food products.

Flavors are classified into three groups depending on the intended use:

1. Flavors that yield pleasant aromas that are attractive to consumers, to almost flavor-free food materials; flavors that enhance consumer satisfaction and expand the amplitude of aroma inherent in food materials
2. Flavors that enhance aroma intensity of food materials to prevent the aroma from being depleted, lost, or changed during the manufacturing process and distribution of food products
3. Flavors that suppress undesired odors that are inherent in food materials or that occur in the manufacturing process, and also enhance consumer acceptance

Flavors are designed into various types of formulations depending on applicational requirements. Water-soluble liquid flavors work well for clear carbonated beverages, whereas oily flavors are suitable for confectionery, where heat resistance is particularly required. Emulsified flavors are largely used for fruit juice drinks. Powdered flavors are used for chewing gums where aroma persistence is particularly needed.

Flavors are widely used not only for food products, such as confectionery, beverages, desserts and frozen desserts, soups, seasonings, processed meat and seafood products, dairy products, fat and oil products, prepared foods, and processed agricultural products, but also for nonfood products, including cigarettes, oral-care products, pharmaceuticals, feeds, and other industrial purposes.

Beverages. Flavors play a central role in enhancing the value and appeal of beverages. The main purposes of flavors in beverages are to provide and intensify aromas, and also to supply aromas that are likely disappear during the sterilization process and long-term storage.

Dairy products, milk beverages, *Lactobacillus* beverages. Flavors are used as a masking agent in combination with citrus, vanilla, and various fruit notes.

Desserts and frozen desserts. All types of sweet flavors are used. Liqueur flavors such as brandy and rummy notes are also frequently used.

Baked confectionery. Flavors such as milk, egg, and sugar are used. Spice flavors are sometimes used to give a characteristic impact. Oily flavor preparations and emulsified preparations are frequently used for baked confectionery in which flavors should be heat resistant. Reaction flavors are often used as a precursor imparting a roasted aroma.

Chewing gums. Mint, fruits, and coffee flavors are mainly used for chewing gums. Mint flavor particularly is considered the most important flavor. Oily flavors and powdered flavors are heavily used to release a long-lasting aroma.

Fat and oil products and chocolates. Oily flavor preparations are usually used to enhance a cacao aroma and impart a nut aroma to these food products.

Dressings. Various herb and spice flavors are used as hidden flavors and also to mask unpleasant odors of raw materials.

Seafood products. Crab flavor is used for fish-paste products. Various seafood flavors are used for fish delicacies. Dimethyl sulfide and other flavors imparting an ocean or a seaweed smell have been traditionally accepted in Japan. As fish-paste products become more popular globally as a healthy food, this type of flavor has gained widespread use.

Frozen and retort foods. Different types of herb and spice flavors are used to mask intrinsic odors of raw materials and also as hidden flavors. Reaction flavors are often used as a precursor imparting a roasted aroma.

Oral-care products. Mint flavor is predominantly used to give clean and fresh impressions.

Flavor Creation. The flavors of food products are reconstructed based on the composition and content of each flavor constituent in foods. Flavor constituents in foods consist of very small amounts of various elements. Using only a single flavor material cannot exactly recreate the flavor and aroma of foods. A wide variety of flavor materials, including natural aroma substances (essential oil, extract, oleoresin, isolated aroma substance, recovery essence oil, and others) and synthetic aroma substances (alcohols, esters, aldehydes, acetals, lactones, and others), are blended at an optimal ratio to create the desired flavor of foods.

The flavor-creation process involves selecting appropriate aroma materials, blending the selected aromas to create the body that is the key contributor to the desired aroma, and further adding the following four agents as necessary to create the fundamental form of flavors called "base":

1. *Blender.* This harmonizes various aromas and also adds richness and diversity to the body of the aroma.
2. *Modifier.* This imparts mellowness, richness, and breadth of aroma, and also harmonizes the overall aroma.
3. *Adjuvant.* This adds subtle nuances and makes an impressive impact on the aroma.
4. *Fixative.* This adjusts the volatility and aroma retention.

Other additives, such as colorants, antioxidants, and masking agents, are also added anywhere during the production of flavors.

Evaluation Method. Flavors generally consist of various components that differ in volatility. Flavors with a higher vapor pressure are more likely to volatilize, and therefore flavorists should effectively manage the flavor-creation process in a balanced manner.

Flavors consist of three different building blocks:

1. *Top note.* The top note of flavors is composed of aroma components that volatilize rapidly and have lower flavor retention. Top note is an important factor to define the first impression of the flavor.
2. *Middle note.* The middle note of flavors consists of aroma components that subsequently volatilize and have moderate flavor retention, and also forms the main body of the flavor.
3. *Base note.* The base note is a class of residual aroma components that volatilize very slowly and can linger for long periods of time. The base note contributes to determine aroma properties of the flavor.

A well-balanced combination of these three notes is the key to successful flavor creation. Unlike fragrances, flavors are used for products that are orally consumed. Not only the odor but the taste is a highly important factor in food development. Once flavor samples are fairly close to the desired level, they are incorporated into base materials such as water, syrup, starch syrup, and edible oils and fats to check the aroma created by flavorists, and sometimes are evaluated by sensory panelists. The finally selected flavor samples are incorporated into actual food products to examine their compatibility with base materials used and changes during processing. Further storage tests may be necessary to check the stability of flavors in the distribution process.

Aroma Component Analysis for Formulating Flavors. For developing flavors, thorough investigation of the aroma components of essential oils, fruits, and other foods is indispensable. For instance, there are wide variations in the aroma of apples, such as the aroma of the freshly picked apple, that of the ripe apple, and that of the green apple. In addition, how the aroma components of flavors change after food processing is a significant factor in producing delicious foods.

The aroma of a food is produced by many volatiles, whose contents are very low. Accordingly, techniques of collecting and concentrating the aroma components without degrading them as well as high-precision instrumental analyses are required for study of food aroma. In general, aroma components are separated from a food by steam distillation, extraction, or the head-space method, and analyzed by gas chromatograph–mass spectrometer (GC-MS). Owing to the improved precision of the analysis, key components that contribute to the aroma of each individual food have been gradually revealed.

The analysis results for the aroma components of a food are very useful to flavorists. If the aroma components are merely blended according to the results, however, it is impossible to accurately reproduce the original aroma of the food. For this purpose, the aesthetic sense and creativity of experienced flavorists are also required.

Flavors are formulated on the basis of the analysis data of aroma components, the knowhow of flavor manufacturers, and the accumulated knowledge of flavorists. First, a basic aroma is created. Next, by trial-and-error, the basic aroma is modified by using various aroma materials, and simple flavoring tests and sensory evaluations are repeated to find the optimum formulation. Finally, performance and stability tests on foods flavored with the resultant formulation are conducted. The concrete procedure is as follows:

1. Aroma materials are blended to prepare an aroma formulation.
2. If necessary, the formulation is kept standing for a certain period to mature the aroma.
3. The aroma of the formulation as well as the aroma and taste of foods flavored with the formulation are evaluated by a sensory panel.
4. If necessary, the volatility of the formulation is depressed by adding low-volatile substances to enhance the aroma retention.
5. If necessary, precipitates, sediment, water, colored substances, and so on produced during the manufacturing and storage of the formulation are removed by filtration and/or other methods. Filter aids, such as activated carbon, Celite, activated clay, sodium sulfate, and magnesium carbonate, may be used.

Manufacturing Process and Formulation of Citrus Flavors. Citrus fruits enjoy the greatest popularity, and the use of citrus flavors is particularly significant in food processing. Accordingly, there are various types of natural and synthetic citrus aroma materials.

In formulating citrus flavors, essential oils are generally employed as a body to reproduce the aroma of citrus fruits, but imitation flavors, combinations of synthetic flavors, may also be used. Then, selected aroma materials, for example, those with a character of freshness or ripeness, are added to the body.

Citrus flavors are widely used, for instance, in beverages (carbonated drinks, fruit juice–containing drinks, etc.), desserts and frozen desserts (yogurt, ice cream, ice-pops, etc.), confectionery (candy, chewing gum, etc.) and bakery products. As necessary, they are processed into water-soluble liquid, oil-soluble liquid, emulsion, and powder forms, which will be described later in detail.

Terpenes, including limonene, in citrus essential oils may undergo oxidation during storage. By the action of heat and enzymes, limonene is oxidized to carveol, 1,8-cineol, and so on, and γ-terpinene to *p*-cymene to emit so-called terpene odor. Low-temperature manufacturing, storage, and distribution as well as the use of antioxidants may be required to prevent oxidation.

There are various types of citrus fruits, and each type has a distinctive aroma. The differences in the aroma are attributed to those in the volatile composition. It is therefore very important to be familiar with the respective compositions of citrus essential oils.

Orange Flavors. Essential oils from orange fruits are generally blended with terpeneless oils or synthetic aroma substances. Oranges mainly used as raw materials of flavors are classified into three groups: sweet orange (*Citrus sinensis* Osbeck), sour orange (bitter orange) (*Citrus aurantium*), and mandarin (*Citrus reticulata* Blanco var. mandarin). The yield of orange peel oil ranges from 0.2 to 0.5%, depending on the variety, production area, and harvesting season of the fruit as well as the oil production method. The major components of the peel oil are terpene hydrocarbons, mainly *d*-limonene, and their content is more than 90%. The other main components are oxygen compounds, such as linalool, aldehydes, and esters. Linalool decreases with fruit ripening, but aldehydes and esters increase. The characteristic components of the peel oil are valencene, α-sinensal, aldol condensates (C_6–C_{10} alkyl acrorains), 2,4-decadienal, eudesm-11-en-ol, isoprene, and 3-methyl-1-butene. Its key aroma components are octanal, nonanal, linalool, decanal, neral, geranial, dodecanal, and α- and β-sinensals.

Orange flavors are required to have a refreshing and juicy character. It is preferable that orange flavors have a strong top note produced by aldehydes with a light aroma.

Lemon Flavors. The aroma components of lemon juice account for 0.001–0.005% of the total. Most aroma components are present in oil glands with a diameter of 1 mm in the peel. The cold-pressed oil is mainly employed, and the steam-distilled oil and the recovery essence are also used in formulating flavors.

The content of the essential oil in the peel is 0.5–0.6%. Terpenes account for more than 90% of the components of the essential oil, but their contribution to the aroma is small. The characteristic aroma components of the essential oil are citral, terpineol, octanal, citronellal, α- and β-pinenes, γ-terpinene, myrcene, β-bisabolene, caryophyllene, and α-bergamotene.

Lemon flavors may be used in combination with other citrus flavors, typically orange flavors. Sicily-type lemon oil with a high citral content and a sharp aroma is mainly used. California-type lemon oil may be used to enhance a character of sweet juice and pulp.

Lime Flavors. Limes are roughly divided into two groups: acid and sweet types. The acid type is called sour lime or Mexican lime (Key lime). The sweet type is considered to be a crossbreed of lemon and lime.

The following three types of lime oils are used in formulating flavors. Among them, the distilled oil is the most important ingredient.

1. *Distilled oil.* Lime juice obtained by pressing separates into three layers after being stored for two to four weeks. The intermediate layer is lime juice. Lime oil is obtained by steam distillation of the other two layers, and the yield ranges from 0.3 to 0.4%. The aroma of the oil depends on the production area of lime.
2. *Cold-pressed oil.* Obtained by pressing, as with lemon and orange oils. Contains citral, and has a lemon-like aroma.
3. *Recovery essence.* It has a fresh juicy character. Lime oil has similar components to lemon oil, but the contents of citral and esters are lower. It contains limonene in a smaller amount, and β-pinene and γ-terpinene in larger quantities than other citrus oils. Not only the abovementioned natural aroma substances, but also synthetic aroma substances, such as myrcenol and hydroxycitronellal, are used in formulating lime flavors.

Lime flavors are characterized by a refreshing fruity aroma as with lemon flavors, but their slightly heavier aroma sharpens the overall aroma of the resultant formulation. To enhance a character of sweeter pulp, orange flavors may be used in combination with lime flavors. Additionally, lime flavors have a distinctive oily odor, and should be carefully blended with other flavors. They are also used as adjuvants to impart an accent to mint and other citrus flavors.

Grapefruit Flavors. Grapefruits are classified by pulp color into three groups: white, red, and pink types. Their taste is an appropriate combination of sweetness and sourness, and has a refreshing character and bitterness. The bitterness is derived from a glycoside, naringin.

The main varieties are Duncan and Marsh (white type), Redblush and Hudson (red type), and Foster and Pink Marsh (pink type). Grapefruit oil is obtained by pressing the fruits in the process of manufacturing juice, and its yield ranges from 0.05 to 0.15%. It may be produced by steam distillation of the peel alone. The main components of the oil are *d*-limonene with a content of more than 90%, octanal, decanal, citral, geraniol, and geranyl acetate. Nootkatone, a sesquiterpenoid, contributes to the characteristic aroma of grapefruit. Grapefruit flavors used to impart a character of freshness or clearness are formulated on the basis of the essential oil. Nootkatone, styralyl isobutyrate, and so on, may be blended to enhance the flavoring effect.

When the natural and juicy characters of their aroma are too strong, however, grapefruit flavors are approximated to orange flavors. In addition, when the characters are weak, the flavoring effect is lost. Accordingly, the balance between the aroma characters and the flavoring effect should be carefully adjusted. For carbonated drinks, flavors with a refreshing aftertaste are preferable. Since nootkatone, a key aroma component, is difficult to extract with dilute alcohols, most grapefruit flavors have a slightly high alcohol content, and contain higher quantities of terpene hydrocarbons. Thus, when they are added to foods, food clouding due to the terpene hydrocarbons should be prevented.

When the essential oil is used in formulating grapefruit flavors, the resultant flavors may have a slight bitterness. In order to enhance a character of freshness or clearness, not the cold-pressed oil but the recovery essence may be employed.

Yuzu Flavors. Yuzu (*Citrus junos* Sieb. ex Tanaka) is a traditional citrus unique to Japan, and is said to originate from the upstream region of the Yangtze-Kiang in China. Owing to its distinctive aroma, the juice is used as vinegar, and the peel as condiments as well as in sauce (yuzu miso). Hence, yuzu flavors are used mostly in dressings and sauces.

For yuzu, the production volume is small and the production area is limited. Most yuzu products shipped are raw fruit and juice, but the peel oil is produced by steam distillation, solvent extraction, and pressing.

The analyses of the aroma components of the essential oil revealed that its characteristic components were oxygen compounds with a low boiling point and sesquiterpenoids with a high boiling point and that thymol and perillaldehyde were particularly important. In the peel oil, unsaturated aldehydes increase with fruit ripening. They have lower odor thresholds than saturated aldehydes, and significantly affect the characters of the peel oil. As key aroma components, 1-*p*-menthen-8-thiol (Yukawa and Iwabuchi, 1994) and 6,8,10-undecatrien-3-one (Miyazawa et al., 2008) were identified. They are contained in trace quantities, but have low odor thresholds, and contribute largely to the distinctive aroma. In other words, they are indispensable components in reproducing the aroma of yuzu.

Yuzu oil is used not only in formulating yuzu flavors but also as an adjuvant in lemon and grapefruit flavors.

A typical total ion chromatogram (TIC) obtained by GC-MS analysis of yuzu cold-pressed oil is shown in Figure 8.3, and the composition of the oil is listed

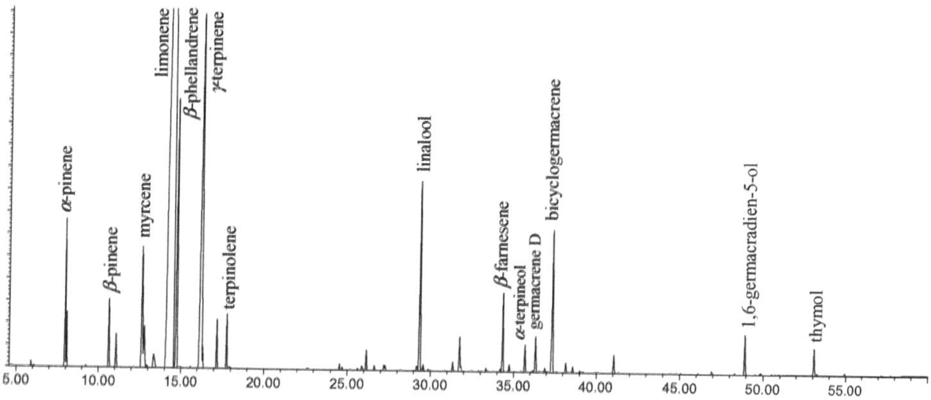

Figure 8.3. Typical total ion chromatogram of cold-pressed yuzu peel oil. GC/MS: Hewlett-Packard 5973 Mass Selective Detector; column: DB-Wax (J&W), 0.25 mm × 60 m; injection temperature: 250°C; column temperature: 50°C (2 min)–220°C, programmed at 3°C/min; split ratio: 70 : 1.

in Table 8.1. On the basis of these analysis data, various aroma materials are blended to prepare yuzu flavors. An example of yuzu flavor formulations is given in Table 8.2.

An essential oil may be used alone as a flavor or fragrance, but is usually blended with other aroma materials to prepare an aroma formulation. The aroma formulation is processed into liquid, emulsion, or powder form according to its intended use. The technology of processing aroma formulations is a significant factor in imparting aroma because different forms of an aroma formulation with the same composition have different aroma-lifting profiles and leave different impressions.

Classification of Flavors by Form. Since aroma sensitivity is high in the oral cavity and the flavor at a concentration higher than the appropriate value leaves an unpleasant impression, flavor processing technology is particularly significant for producing delicious foods. At present, flavors are available in several different forms appropriate to the form, properties, and manufacturing process of final food products. In fact, flavors are manufactured also considering various aspects that have no direct association with the aroma, such as user-friendliness, distribution and storage conditions, and effects on the environment.

Flavors are broadly classified by form into four groups: water-soluble liquid flavors, oil-soluble liquid flavors, emulsified flavors, and powdered flavors. Water-soluble liquid flavors are mainly used in transparent beverages, oil-soluble liquid flavors in oily cooked foods, and emulsified and powdered flavors in foods manufactured through a heating process during which the aroma retention and heat resistance of the flavor are required (Figure 8.4).

TABLE 8.1. Components identified in yuzu peel cold-pressed oil

Peak Number	Compound	Retention Index	%
1	α-Pinene	1023	2.37
2	α-Thujene	1026	0.75
3	Camphene	1066	0.02
4	β-Pinene	1110	1.30
5	Sabinene	1121	0.61
6	Myrcene	1162	3.05
7	α-Phellandrene	1165	1.17
8	α-Terpinene	1180	0.50
9	Limonene	1209	55.12
10	β-Phellandrene	1214	5.50
11	*cis*-Ocimene	1234	0.02
12	γ-Terpinene	1249	12.98
13	β-Ocimene	1250	0.32
14	*p*-Cymene	1270	0.85
15	Terpinolene	1283	0.96
16	Octanal	1287	0.02
17	Nonanal	1391	0.02
18	Dehydro-*p*-cymene	1435	0.10
19	α-Cubebene	1459	0.03
20	*trans*-Sabinene hydrate	1465	0.09
21	δ-Elemene	1471	0.37
22	α-Copaene	1494	0.10
23	Decanal	1496	0.08
24	β-Cubebene	1540	0.08
25	Linalool	1545	3.99
26	*cis*-Sabinene hydrate	1549	0.11
27	β-Elemene	1591	0.18
28	β-Caryophyllene	1600	0.71
29	Terpinen-4-ol	1602	0.08
30	γ-Elemene	1639	0.06
31	β-Farnesene	1664	1.56
32	α-Humulene	1673	0.14
33	α-Terpineol	1697	0.53
34	Germacrene D	1713	0.74
35	Bicyclogermacrene	1739	3.34
36	δ-Cadinene	1760	0.18
37	*p*-Mentha-1(7),2-dien-8-ol	1781	0.03
38	Germacrene B	1835	0.38
39	Isopiperitenone	1843	trace
40	Limonen-10-ol	1997	0.06
41	*trans*-Nerolidol	2037	0.02
42	12-Hydroxy-trans-9-dodecenoic acid lactone	2049	trace
43	1,6-Germacradien-5-ol	2055	0.83
44	Thymol	2180	0.55
45	1(10),5-Germacradien-4-ol	2186	0.04
46	β-Sinenesal	2231	trace
47	β-Eudesmol	2239	0.04

TABLE 8.2. Example of yuzu flavor formulations for beverages

Compounds	%
n-Octanal	0.1
cis-3-Hexenal	0.02
Perillaldehyde	0.01
Neryl acetate	0.03
Thymol	0.03
Linalool	0.05
Myrcene	0.1
Natural lemon oil	0.08
Lemon terpene	2.00
Tangerine cold-pressed oil	0.6
Yuzu flavor base	2.22
Lime oil	0.5
Yuzu oil	3.6
Methyl jasmonate	0.02
Triacetine	0.5
Glycerin	0.5
Ethanol	62.23
Ion exchange water	27.41
Total	100.0

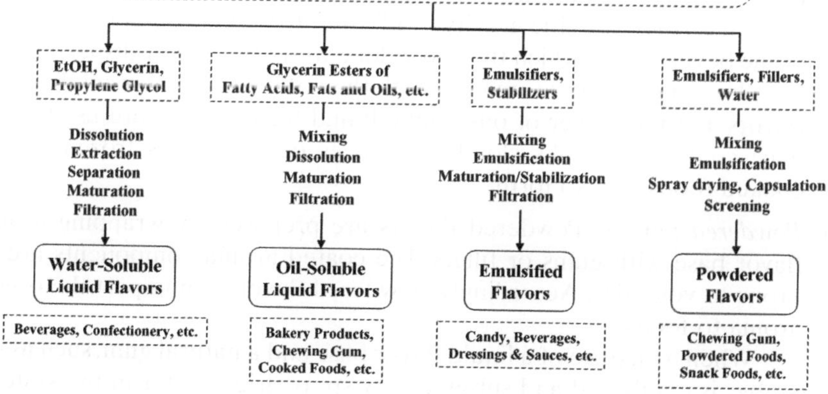

Figure 8.4. Different forms of flavors and their applications.

1. *Water-soluble liquid flavors.* One type of water-soluble liquid flavor is prepared by diluting a flavor base with moisture ethanol. Some components of the flavor base do not dissolve in moisture ethanol, and separate. Particularly for the flavor base containing essential oil, terpenic hydrocarbons usually separate. When the flavor base contains citrus essential oil, 1–2% of the aroma active components are extracted, and the remaining 98% is removed.

   The other type is prepared by adding one of the hydrophilic auxiliary materials, such as propylene glycol and glycerin, to the flavor base to enhance water solubility or dispersibility in aqueous food base materials. Water-soluble liquid flavors are employed in foods with a high water content, such as soft drinks, fermented milk, and desserts and frozen desserts.

2. *Oil-soluble liquid flavors.* Oil-soluble liquid flavors are prepared by adding lipophilic auxiliary materials, such as vegetable oils and glycerin esters of fatty acids, to a flavor base to enhance oil solubility. Seasoning oil flavors, which are obtained by heat extraction of aroma substances from spices, vegetables, meats, and so on with fats and oils without using the flavor base, are also included in this category.

   These are insoluble or semisoluble in water, have high aroma retention, and impart a powerful aroma to foods. Since their aroma components are less prone to volatilize at high temperatures, they are used in foods manufactured under relatively severe heating conditions, such as candy, bakery products, and cooked foods, as well as in foods whose base materials are compatible with fats and oils, such as chocolate, chewing gum, and margarine.

3. *Emulsified flavors.* These are uniform emulsions obtained by adding water and emulsifiers and stabilizers to a flavor base, followed by homogenization. When added to foods, they do not dissolve but disperse, and impart not only an aroma but also cloudiness. For emulsified flavors for beverages, their specific gravity is adjusted to a value comparable to that of the beverages to which they are added to stabilize their dispersion state for a long time. Their aroma has both the mildness of water-soluble liquid flavors and the power of oil-soluble liquid flavors. They are used in fruit juice–containing drinks, cloudy beverages, dessert jellies, frozen desserts, cooked foods, and so forth.

4. *Powdered flavors.* Powdered flavors are prepared by wrapping a liquid flavor base with gums or fillers. The coated aroma components are less prone to volatilize. Accordingly, powdered flavors can impart the original aroma to foods.

   When a mixture of a liquid flavor base and a natural gum, such as gum arabic, is emulsified and subsequently spray-dried, water in the system is removed, and powders in which the flavor base is coated with the gum are obtained. In this process, carbohydrates, such as dextrin, are used as fillers.

When cyclodextrin is used as a filler, powdered flavors with aroma retention enhanced by its molecular inclusion property are obtained.

In addition, there are powdered flavors prepared by adsorbing a flavor base onto one or more edible powders, such as lactose, starch, salt, anhydrous glucose, and microcrystalline cellulose.

Microcapsulization of Food Flavors. Retaining or enhancing and stabilizing food aroma, which is prone to be lost during food processing and distribution, is extremely important for food quality improvement (Hatano et al., 2000; Kondo, 1987; Tanaka, 2008). Particularly for processed foods manufactured through heating or drying, part of added flavors may be lost during these processes, leading to a weakened flavoring effect. Additionally, aroma degradation due to flavor oxidation during food processing and distribution should be prevented.

As a solution to these problems, coated flavors were developed. Locked-, spray-dried-, and double-coated-type powdered flavors are commonly used. Cyclodextrin clathrate flavors and microcapsulized flavors are also in practical use.

Microcapsulization is a method for preventing flavor degradation. Flavors in oil microdroplet, powder, crystal, and other forms are coated with a polymer film. They are protected from the surrounding environment, and their aroma is retained until they are used. The advantages of microcapsulization are summarized as follows:

- Converting the form of flavors from liquid to powder makes them easy to handle.
- The volatilization of aroma components is prevented for a long time.
- Protecting flavors from heat, moisture, and oxygen prevents their degradation.
- Controlled-release flavors can be manufactured.

Microcapsulization is mainly applied to flavors for foods manufactured through a heating process, such as powdered soup, instant lemon tea, gelatin desserts, and cake mix.

There are many methods of film formation in microcapsulization. Gelatin, gum arabic, sodium alginate, ethyl cellulose, methyl cellulose, dextrin, sodium caseinate, and so on are employed as film formers (shell materials). The methods are classified according to their processes into three groups: chemical, physicochemical, and physical methods.

1. *Chemical methods.* These are methods in which reaction products are used as shell materials. The interfacial polymerization method and the submerged hardening coating method are included in this category.
2. *Physicochemical methods.* These are methods in which shells are formed by using not chemical reactions but physicochemical phenomena, such as drying, precipitation, and coagulation. The phase separation method

(coacervation method), the submerged drying method, and the interfacial precipitation method are included in this category.

Phase separation method (coacervation method). Oil, aqueous solution, and solid can be employed as core materials.

3. *Physical methods.* These are methods in which microcapsules are produced by using physical force alone. The spray-drying method, the spray-chilling method, and the air suspension coating methods are included in this category.

   Spray-drying method. Along with fillers, emulsifiers, and stabilizers, a core material is dissolved or suspended in a solvent (mainly, water). The solution or suspension is sprayed through a nozzle or disk, and instantaneously dried by hot air blown simultaneously with spraying. The air temperature is high, 150–200°C, but the air instantaneously removes the heat of vaporization from the solvent, and relatively labile core materials can therefore be microcapsulized. Rapid vaporization of the solvent produces a porous film. Since continuous mass processing is feasible by this method, the processing cost is low. In addition, a broad variety of shell materials can be used. Accordingly, this method is widely applied to powdered flavors and fragrances, powdered detergents, milk powder, and so on. Representative microcapsulization methods utilized in the food industry are spray-drying, coacervation, emulsification, and drop hardening.

Yeast Capsules. The utilization of yeast capsules is a new unique method of encapsulating aroma substances (Matukura et al., 2008; San-Ei Gen, 2006). In recent years, yeast cell walls have been studied and are finding wide application in various industries. Yeast capsules are a powdered formulation produced through the following steps: First, generally available yeasts, such as beer yeasts, baker's yeasts, and torula yeasts, are cultivated. Next, active ingredients, such as aroma substances, are encapsulated with the yeast cell walls. Then, the outside surface of the yeast cell walls is coated with saccharides, and so on, and finally, the resultant solution is processed into powder form by spray drying, and so on. Yeast cell walls are known to be little affected by pressurization, heating, and freeze–thaw treatments. Owing to yeast cell walls having both toughness and flexibility, the storage stability of yeast capsules is higher than that of conventional powdered formulations.

Yeast capsules also have excellent aroma retention at high temperatures and high resistance to pressure, pH, friction, osmotic pressure, and enzymes. When they are in contact with water, the sugar coating dissolves and cracks open in the cell walls, leading to aroma release. The aroma released from yeast capsules feels stronger in the mouth and lasts longer.

Yeast capsules and a powdered flavor coated with a film of generally available gum arabic were prepared by using orange oil. After storage at 60°C for one week, the residual ratio of the orange oil and the aroma of 0.1% aqueous solution were evaluated. The residual ratio of the orange oil was higher for the yeast capsules than for the powdered flavor. In the sensory evaluation, an oxidized odor was detected in the powdered flavor solution, but little in the yeast capsule solution. In other words, the aroma of the yeast capsules underwent smaller changes and was more stable.

As described above, yeast capsules are a novel type of microcapsule, characterized by their excellent stability, aroma retention, and long-lasting flavor release, and suitable for foods manufactured through a heating process, such as bread, confectionery, and deep-fried foods.

8.2 ECO-CONSCIOUS SYSTEM OF OIL EXTRACTION FROM CITRUS PEEL WASTES

Takehiro Kashiwagi and Masayoshi Sawamura

Among Japanese citrus sour fruits, yuzu (*Citrus junos* Sieb. ex Tanaka) is the most popular in Japan. Yuzu is said to have originated in China. According to Swingle (1943), yuzu is considered to be a hybrid of sour mandarin (*C. reticulata* var. *Austera*) and Ichang papeda (*C. ichangensis*). Recently, it has been cultivated mainly in Japan and Korea. A photograph of a yuzu tree bearing mature fruit is shown in Figure 8.5.

Yuzu has an important commercial value in Japan and Korea. Annual production in both countries amounts to approximately 20,000 and 15,000 tons, respectively. In Japan, yuzu fruit with good appearance is used as a traditional dish called *Yuzu-gama*, literally meaning "yuzu bowl." Appetizer is stuffed into

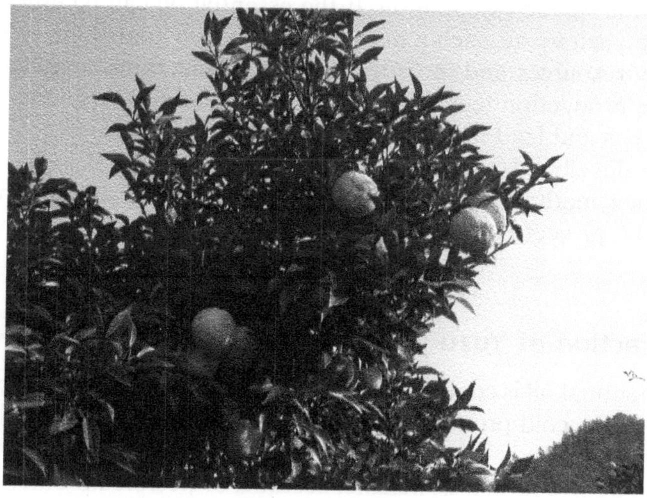

Figure 8.5. *Citrus junos* Sieb. ex Tanaka (yuzu).

the yuzu bowl, from which the flesh is scooped out. Yuzu juice is popularly utilized in a dressing called *ponzu* in Japanese, and as a flavoring for various dishes and foods. It is also used for soft drinks and some liquors. Yuzu outer peel is used to garnish some dishes as an aromatic zest: *Yuzu kosho* (literally "yuzu and pepper") is a hot-spicy Japanese sauce made from ground green or yellow yuzu peel and chili pepper. The peel is also used for marmalade and jam or as an ingredient in cakes. During the winter solstice, Japanese people enjoy taking a bath prepared with yuzu fruit to enhance good health. Breathing the volatiles from yuzu in the bath promotes relaxation.

"Yuzu tea," sliced yuzu fruit sweetened with honey or sugar (like marmalade), is very popular in Korea. A teaspoon of yuzu tea is put into a cup of hot water to make a sweet-and-sour beverage. The export of yuzu juice from Korea to Japan has been greatly increasing since 2004. The amount exported in 2008 reached 2500 tons, which is about 16 times as much as that in 1999.

During the squeezing process of yuzu fruit most of the flavedo, albedo, pulp segment, segment well, endocarp, and seed (see Figure 2.17) is wasted. The yield of yuzu juice is only about 20% of fruit weight and it is 20–50% lower than that of other citrus fruits. The whole waste is estimated to be 10,000 tons per year. Most of it has been incinerated by fossil fuels, although the peel waste is a sometimes utilized for cake and marmalade. Thus, there has been a big problem of post-squeezing yuzu waste as well as other citrus wastes such as orange and mandarin.

Yuzu has a fresh, pronounced, and strongly characteristic aroma in comparison with other citrus fruits. The antioxidant activity for yuzu peel is higher than that of the flesh (Yoo et al., 2004). It is known that the essential oil suppresses the formation of *N*-nitrosodimethylamine, a carcinogenic compound (Sawamura et al., 1999). Recently, the demand for yuzu essential oil for beverages, confectioneries, pharmaceuticals, cosmetics, and perfumes has been increasing, not only in Japan but also in Western countries. The post-squeezing yuzu waste still remains around 1% of aromatic essential oil. If the essential oil can be efficiently recovered from the yuzu waste, such a new technology will contribute to reduction in use of energy resources and in CO_2 emissions. Concerning regional economics, an innovative production technology for yuzu essential oil will encourage yuzu-cultivating areas and lead to further regional development.

We have developed a new technology for extraction of yuzu oil from the waste and a new method of wastewater treatment with the aim of environmental protection. The project is illustrated in Figure 8.6. The details will be described below.

8.2.1 Extraction of Yuzu Oil

Citrus peel essential oil is commercially produced by the following three methods: solvent extraction, cold pressing, and steam distillation.

Solvent extraction is a method of moving flavor components in citrus peel into an organic solvent, that is, hexane, acetone, or petroleum ether. The solvent is finally removed from the extract by steaming. Yuzu solvent-extracted oil is

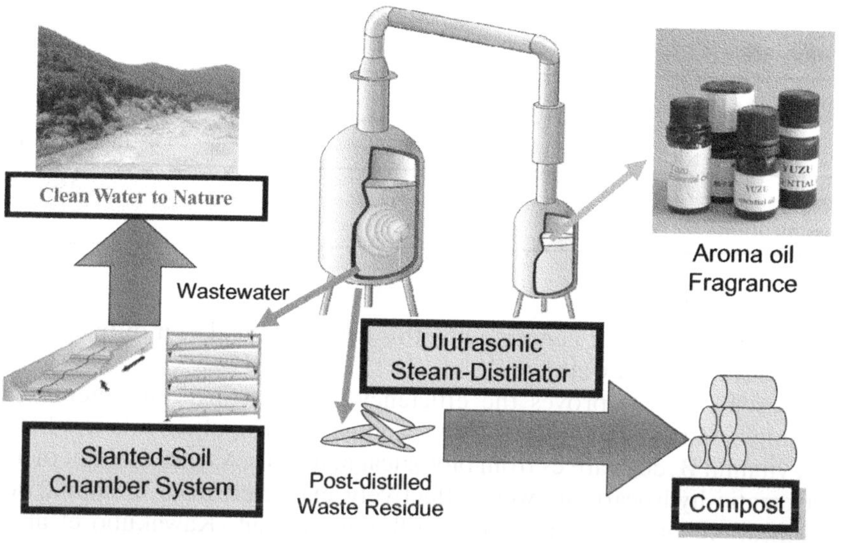

Figure 8.6. Concept of an eco-conscious system of oil extraction from citrus peel wastes.

widely used as a food flavor in Japan. There may be, however, some problems in the solvent-extracted oil. We should rigidly check for the absence of petrochemical residues in the oil. The solvent extraction may lose or denature its native chemical components in the steaming process to remove the organic solvent.

Citrus essential oil can be collected by mechanical pressing of flavedo, because the citrus fruit contains a lot of the oil in the oil gland. The essential oil is obtained under cool temperature by centrifuging a mixture of water and grated citrus flavedo or citrus juice after squeezing whole fruits. In the yuzu squeezing process, the cold-pressed oil is obtained as a by-product. The cold-pressed oil has an aroma close to the native yuzu fruit's, because this technique is done under lower temperature to minimize the decomposition and denaturing of constituents. The yield of cold-pressed oil is comparatively lower than solvent-extracted and distilled oil.

Steam distillation is the most popular method of extracting the oil from raw plant materials. As a mixture of material and water is warmed with steam, the essential oil is vaporized. The boiling points of the compounds are principally lowered in the presence of water or steam. Usually, citrus peel oil is extracted by distillation under reduced pressure at lower temperature, since the essential oil component is not so stable in heat and air. The steam-distilled oil has a lighter and fresher aroma than solvent-extracted oil and cold-pressed oil, because there is no nonvolatile constituent in the oil.

The yield of yuzu essential oil with steam distillation is lower than that of other citrus, because a lot of pectin and cellulose fiber in the peel interferes with releasing oil from the oil gland. Therefore, yuzu peel is preliminarily treated with either an acid or an enzyme to degrade pectin and cellulose. However, a variety

TABLE 8.3. Effect of ultrasonic distillation on the yield of yuzu essential oil at laboratory scale

Treatment	Yield	
	Essential Oil (%)	Distilled Water (mL)
Control	0.18	350
Ultrasonication	0.26	350

of soluble organic matter generated by this treatment makes it difficult to purify the post-distilled wastewater.

Ultrasonication improves the efficiency of extracting components from a solid sample. Hirose and Tsuge (1989) proposed to use ultrasonic irradiation to extract vitamin B_6 derivatives from biological materials. A trace amount of arsenic and aromatic hydrocarbons were effectively extracted from a sample soil by ultrasonication for determination of pollutants in soil (Kawakubo et al., 2007; Sun et al., 1998). Ultrasonic technique was also employed for soup processing from dried kelp and chicken bones instead of the conventional method (Kimura et al., 1996a,b, 1997).

Sawamura (2005) demonstrated at a laboratory scale that in the extraction of essential oil from wasted yuzu peel, distillation under ultrasonic irradiation was more effective than ordinary distillation. As shown in Table 8.3, the ultrasonic steam-distillation increased yuzu essential oil yield by 44% compared to the control. We have developed a new steam-distillation system equipped with an ultrasonic unit.

Yuzu whole fruits are squeezed by a specified caterpillar squeezer. The juice yield is usually about 20%. A highly squeezed juice gives a bitter taste due to flavonoids and terpenoids from the peel. The juice is processed into various products such as dressing, beverages and liquors. The post-squeezing waste is sliced to be separated into flavedo and other tissues such as albedo, segment well, seed, and so on. The flavedo is frozen at –20°C for storage until used. The minced flavedo is charged into a distillation still with an equal amount of water. An ultrasonic steam-distillation plant is shown in Figure 8.7. The plant is composed of a distillation still, a still receiver, a three-step condenser, and four ultrasonic oscillators. The ultrasonic generators are set on the bottom of the distillation still inside. There are four steam nozzles in front of each generator. The steam rushing out from these nozzles warms and strongly stirs the mixture. The still can load up to 400 kg of yuzu peel and its equal volume of water. The mixture of peel and water is heated under reduced pressure (7.3–15.3 kPa) by steam where the boiling point of the mixture is in the range of 52–57°C. The yield of the essential oil is 0.86% based on yuzu flavedo weight, which is about 15% more than that by nonultrasonic steam-distillation.

The chromatograms and weight percent of volatile components of ultrasonic steam-distilled oil (USDO) and conventional steam-distilled oil (CSDO) are

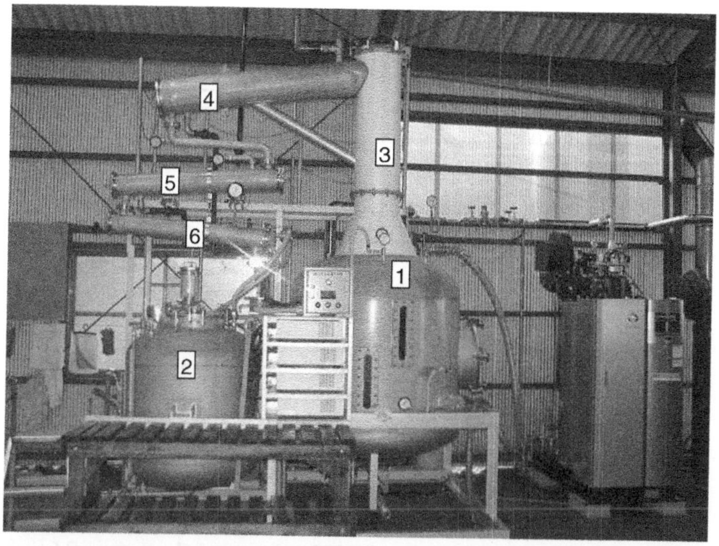

Figure 8.7. Ultrasonic steam-distillation plant under reduced pressure. (1) Distillation still; (2) still receiver; (3) distillation column; (4) first condenser; (5) second condenser; (6) third condenser; (7) ultrasonic generator; (8) vacuum control panel; (9) boiler.

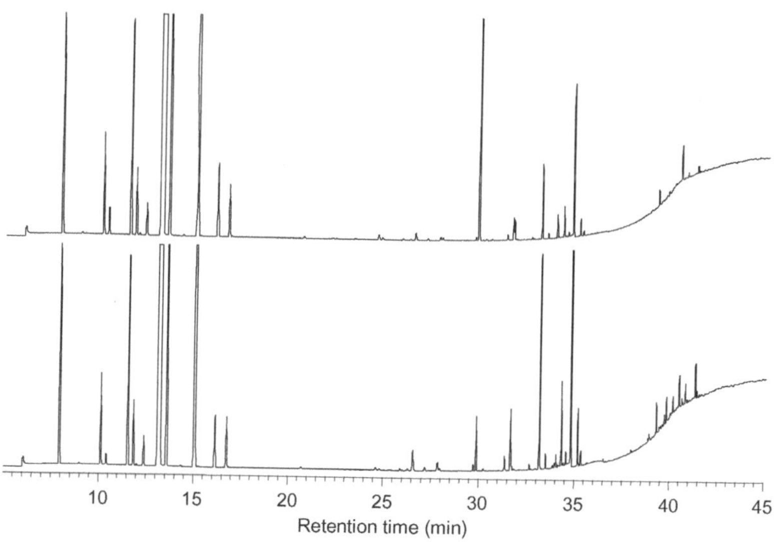

Figure 8.8. Total ion chromatograms of ultrasonic steam-distilled oil (*top*) and conventional steam-distilled oil (*bottom*).

shown in Figure 8.8 and Table 8.4, respectively. Forty-one volatile components were detected in the USDO, where 32 terpene hydrocarbons (96.7%) and 9 oxygenated compounds (3.2%) were determined. Monoterpene hydrocarbons representing 94.4% of the total concentration were the predominant volatile

TABLE 8.4. Volatile flavor components of USDO, CSDO, and CPO

Number	Compound	DB-Wax	Relatve Concentration (%)		
			CPO	USDO	CSDO
1	α-Pinene	1040	2.7	2.4	2.6
2	Camphene	1085	tr	tr	tr
3	β-Pinene	1126	1.1	1.0	0.9
4	Sabinene	1135	0.5	0.2	0.1
5	Myrcene	1171	3.2	2.1	2.1
6	α-Phellandrene	1179	0.9	0.7	0.7
7	Pseudolimonen	1184	tr	tr	tr
8	α-Terpinene	1193	0.3	0.3	0.3
9	Limonene	1222	63.1	69.6	68.2
10	β-Phellandrene	1229	5.4	4.3	4.1
11	β-Ocimene	1243	tr	tr	tr
12	γ-Terpinene	1262	12.5	12.3	12.2
13	*p*-Cymene	1282	0.6	0.8	0.6
14	Terpinolene	1295	0.7	0.6	0.6
15	Tetradecane	1397	tr	nd	nd
16	Nonanal	1399	tr	tr	tr
17	*p*-Isopropenylotluene	1445	tr	0.1	tr
18	1,3,8-Mentatriene	1449	tr	tr	tr
19	α-Cubebene	1467	tr	tr	tr
20	δ-Elemene	1479	0.2	0.1	0.3
21	Bicycloelemene	1489	tr	tr	tr
22	α-Copaene	1494	0.1	tr	0.1
23	Decanal	1504	0.1	tr	tr
24	β-Cubebene	1548	0.1	tr	0.1
25	Linalool	1555	2.8	2.6	0.5
26	(*E*)-α-Bergamotene	1564	tr	tr	tr
27	β-Elemene	1597	0.1	tr	0.1
28	β-Caryophyllene	1607	0.3	0.2	tr
29	4-Terpinenol	1612	0.1	0.1	tr

Tentatively identified; tr: Weight percent less than 0.05%; nd: Not detected.
USDO: Ultrasonic steam-distilled oil.
CSDO: Conventional steam-distilled oil.
CPO: Cold-pressed oil.

Number	Compound	DB-Wax	Relatve Concentration (%)		
			CPO	USDO	CSDO
30	Aromaderene	1626	tr	nd	nd
31	Caryophyllene	1644	tr	nd	nd
32	γ-Elemene	1646	tr	tr	tr
33	(*Z*)-β-Farnesene	1651	tr	nd	nd
34	(*E*)-β-Farnesene	1667	1.3	0.5	1.5
35	Humulene	1680	0.1	tr	0.1
36	α-Terpineol	1706	0.3	0.2	tr
37	Dodecanal	1716	tr	nd	nd
38	Germacrene D	1719	0.4	0.2	0.6
39	α-Muurolene	1734	tr	tr	0.1
40	Piperitone	1740	tr	nd	nd
41	Bicyclogermacrene	1746	2.0	1.0	2.5
42	δ-Cadinene	1766	0.1	0.1	0.4
43	Citronrllol	1770	tr	nd	nd
44	β-Sesquiphellandrene	1777	0.1	tr	0.1
45	Perillaldehyde	1790	tr	nd	nd
46	Nerol	1794	tr	nd	nd
47	Germacrene B	1841	0.2	nd	tr
48	β-Ionone	1953	tr	nd	nd
49	Perillyl alcohol	2007	tr	nd	tr
50	Nerolidol	2048	tr	nd	tr
51	(*Z*)-Oxacyclotridec-10-en-2-one	2051	nd	0.1	0.2
52	Germacrene D-4-Ol	2063	0.4	nd	0.1
53	Elemol	2091	tr	tr	0.1
54	Spathulenol	2119	tr	nd	0.1
55	Thymol	2193	0.3	0.2	0.2
56	α-Cadinol	2213	tr	nd	0.1
57	T-Cadinol	2248	tr	nd	0.2
	Monoterpens		91.1	94.4	92.4
	Sesquiterpens		4.5	2.3	5.9
	Alcohols		3.9	3.1	1.4
	Aldehydes		0.1	tr	tr
	Ketone		tr	tr	tr
	Esters and Ethers		tr	0.1	0.2
	Oxides		tr	tr	tr
	Total		99.5	99.9	99.7

group in yuzu oil, followed by sesquiterpenes (2.3%). Among the 16 monoterpene hydrocarbons identified in yuzu oil, limonene, which is well known to be a principal component of most citrus oils (Eskin, 1979), was the most prominent (69.6%). The relatively abundant monoterpene hydrocarbons in yuzu peel oil were γ-terpinene (12.3%), β-phellandrene (4.3%), α-pinene (2.4%), myrcene (2.1%), β-pinene (1.0%) and *p*-cymene (0.8%). Sixteen sesquiterpene hydrocarbons were identified in the yuzu peel oil. Among the sesquiterpene hydrocarbons, bicyclogermacrene was prominent, accounting for 1.0%, followed by (*E*)-β-farnesene (0.5%). The presence of these compounds was reported by Sawamura (2000), where germacrene D accounted for 0.2%. The sesquiterpenoids are often found in citrus oils (Lan-Phi et al., 2006; Sawamura, 2000). Other sesquiterpenes such as δ-elemene (0.1%), β-caryophyllene (0.2%), and δ-cadinene (0.1%) were also present in the essential oil. The yuzu peel oil contained six alcohols, accounting for 3.1% of the total content. Linalool was the most prominent (2.8%), followed by monoterpene alcohols such as thymol (0.2%), α-terpineol (0.2%), and 4-terpinenol (0.1%). Additionally, sesquiterpene alcohols such as germacrene D-4-ol, α-cadinol, and β-eudesmol was barely detected in the yuzu oil, along with two aldehydes and one ester. All aldehydes occurred at trace level. (*Z*)-Oxacyclotridec-10-en-2-one (0.1%), referred to as "yuzu lactone", initially isolated from and identified in *Medicago rugosa* leaves (Doss et al., 1989), was also detected in the yuzu USDO.

The composition of the yuzu USDO was compared with that of yuzu CSDO. The proportion of monoterpene hydrocarbons in the USDO (94.4%) was higher than that in the CSDO (92.4%). The USDO contained, on the other hand, sesquiterpene hydrocarbons (2.3%) whose content was approximately half that of the CSDO (5.9%). In addition, it is noted that the monoterpene alcohol content in USDO (3.1%) was about four times that in CSDO (0.8%). In particular, linalool in USDO (2.6%) was 5 times more than in CSDO (0.5%). Linalool is one of the characteristic constituents with a yuzu-like note (Lan-Phi et al., 2009). USDO also contained thymol (0.2%), α-terpineol (0.2%), and 4-terpinenol (0.1%), of which levels were higher than those of CSDO. These compounds are important, because they have a yuzu-like note (Song et al., 1999). The concentration of those monoterpene alcohols in USDO is similar to that in cold-pressed oil (CPO). Sesquiterpene alcohols were, on the contrary, detected at trace level. The sesquiterpene alcohols, such as spathulenol, elemol, α-cadinol, and T-cadinol, are off-flavor compounds, which increase during storage of yuzu essential oil at room temperature (Njoroge et al., 1996). Thus, the yuzu essential oil that was produced by our new technology is of the highest quality.

8.2.2 Treatment of Distillation Residue

Even after distillation of post-squeezing yuzu waste, there remain a lot of pasty solids containing pectic substances, fine fibers, and water. The residue of yuzu is much more troublesome in handling than that of other citrus fruits. Moreover, the yuzu wastewater has a high level of acidity (pH 3.8) and of both biological

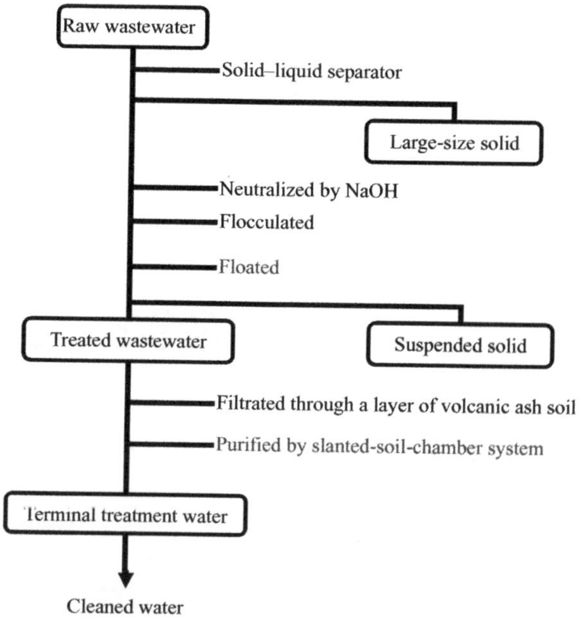

Figure 8.9. Flowsheet of treatment of post-distilled wastewater.

oxygen demand (BOD: 14,100 mg/mL) and chemical oxygen demand (COD: 87,300 mg/mL). In regard to environmental protection, however, we shall also solve these waste problems incidental to essential oil recovery processes.

Figure 8.9 shows the flowsheet for post-distilled yuzu wastewater treatment. At the first step, the wastewater is treated with a specified solid–liquid separator to remove large particles. The treated water still contains a large amount of suspended fine solid (SS). The density of SS is near to that of water. The resulting settling velocity is given by the following equation:

$$V_S = \frac{D_P^2(\rho_p - \rho_w)g}{18\eta}$$

where V_s is the particles' settling velocity (m/s); g is the gravitational acceleration (m/s^2), D_p is the radius of the particles (m), η is the wastewater's dynamic viscosity (Pa s), ρ_p is the mass density of the particles (kg/m^3), and ρ_w is the mass density of the wastewater (kg/m^3) (Lamb, 1993).

As indicated in the equation, the particles' settling velocity is directly proportional to the gravitational acceleration, to the difference between the mass density of the particles and that of wastewater, and to the square of the radius of the particles, and is inversely proportional to the wastewater's dynamic viscosity. Therefore, it is difficult to remove the suspended solid from highly viscous yuzu wastewater by sedimentation or centrifugation.

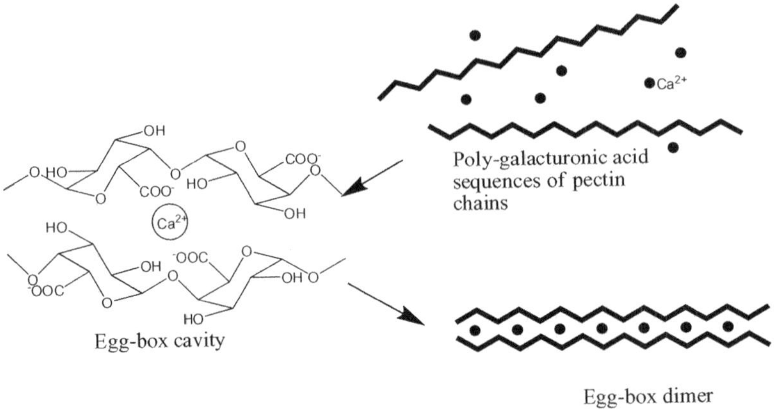

Figure 8.10. Schematic illustration of the egg-box model.

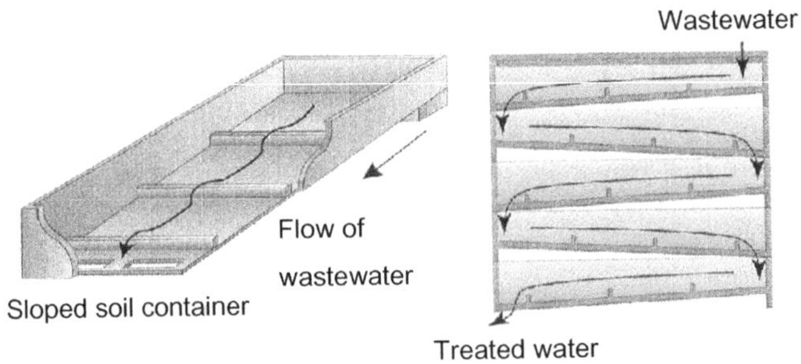

Figure 8.11. Slanted-soil-chamber system.

We developed a new treatment method for removing the suspended solid in yuzu wastewater. A typical feature of low-ester pectin is the ability to cross-link with divalent ions such as calcium ions. As illustrated in Figure 8.10, the cross-linking is considered to follow the so-called egg-box model (Grant et al., 1973; Morris et al., 1982; Powell et al., 1982; Tho et al., 2005). The pectin molecules in the suspended solid of wastewater will combine with a trace amount of calcium ion accompanied with sodium hydroxide chemical, as the acidic wastewater from which the large particles have been removed is neutralized with an aqueous solution of sodium hydroxide. The mixture is allowed to stand for several hours, and then carbon dioxide gas is generated by fermentation of bacteria to give buoyancy to the gel. As a result, the suspended solid can be coagulated together in the upper layer and separated easily from the lower water layer.

The treated wastewater is purified by the slanted-soil-chamber system developed by Yonden Consultants Inc., Japan. This water-cleaning system can be applied to a wide variety of wastewater. Filtration of suspended solid and biodegradation of organic matters are carried out while the wastewater runs slowly through a pile of volcanic ash soil or pumice stone, as shown in Figure 8.11. We

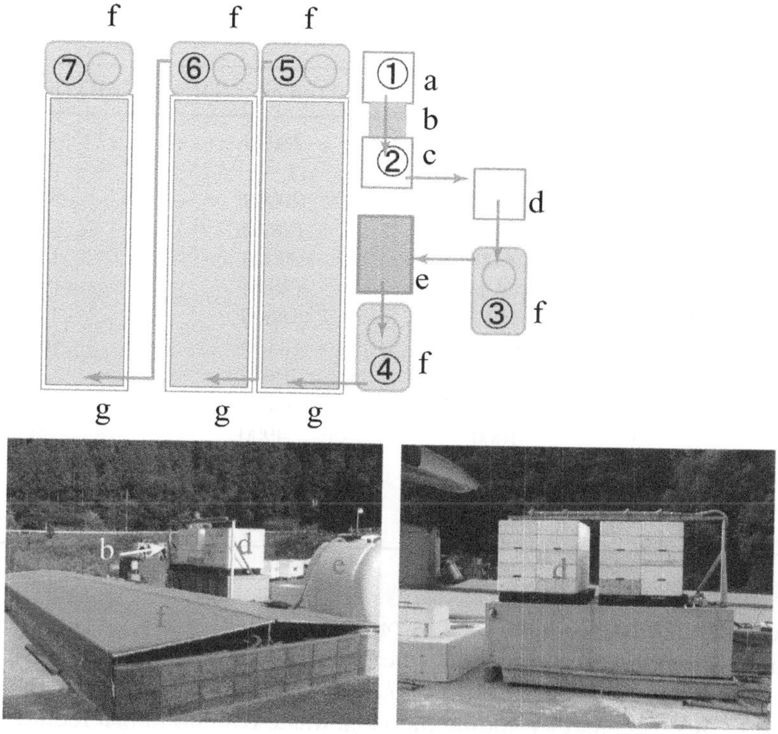

Figure 8.12. Large-scale wastewater purifying plant. a: Wastewater bath; b: solid–liquid separator; c: slurry bath; d: neutralization tank; e: filter with volcanic soil chamber; f: treated water tank; and g: slanted-soil chamber. ①–⑦: Sampling spots. Arrow shows flow of water.

constructed a large-scale wastewater purifying plant specified for yuzu wastewater (Figure 8.12). The efficiency of this system on the decontamination rate (DR) was checked. After 1 ton of yuzu wastewater was run, seven samples of treated water at each spot (1–7) were analyzed. The DR for 7 at the terminal stage was as follows: SS: 99.9%, BOD: 99.8%, and COD: 99.4%. It is concluded that this large-scale wastewater purifying system can effectively operate to treat yuzu suspended wastewater.

8.2.3 Practical Uses of Post-Distilled Yuzu Waste Residue

The post-distilled yuzu waste residue is barely decomposed by microorganisms, because it is highly acid and contains few nitrogenous compounds. The residue contains, on the other hand, a large amount of decomposable carbohydrates as a carbon source. If a suitable carbon–nitrogen ratio is accomplished by blending the waste slugs with cattle dung and poultry manure, the residue will be applicable to a compost material. Additionally, several *Lactobacillus* spp. were isolated from the post-distilled waste residue. Those *Lactobacillus* species will be possibly

TABLE 8.5. Qualities of treated wastewater at various stages and decontamination rates (DR) of treated wastewater to raw water

Sampling Ports	pH	SS (mg/L) (DR)	BOD (mg/L) (DR)	COD (mg/L) (DR)
①	3.5	34000 (—)	28000 (—)	43000 (—)
②	3.4	23000 (32.4)	20000 (28.6)	34000 (20.9)
③	6.5	9500 (72.1)	20000 (28.6)	16000 (62.8)
④	4.7	4500 (86.8.)	18000 (35.7)	17000 (60.5)
⑤	5.5	410 (98.8)	10000 (64.3)	3600 (91.6)
⑥	7.0	1000 (97.1)	4900 (82.5)	1000 (97.7)
⑦	8.9	41 (99.9)	56 (99.8)	240 (99.4)

used for commercial products such as pickled vegetables, soy sauces, fermented soybean pastes, *kimchi*, and other fermented foods. It was also demonstrated in farming of Japanese amberjack, *Seriola quinqueradiata*, that yuzu flavor was adhered to this fish meat by adding the yuzu waste residue to fish feed. This kind of fish is called *yuzu buri*, meaning Japanese amberjack with yuzu flavor. Recently, this aromatic fish is commercially produced in Japan.

8.2.4 Products of Yuzu Essential Oil

Yuzu essential oil is important not only for food flavoring and aromatherapy oil, but also for cosmetics and/or toilet goods such as hair treatments, bath soaps, shampoos, bath fragrant additives, and oil-blotting tissue manufactured by microencapsulation of yuzu oil. It is expected that the characteristically strong-impact yuzu aroma will be accepted worldwide in the future.

REFERENCES

Doss, R.P., Gould, S.J., Johnson, K.J.R., Flath, R.A., Kohnert, R.L. (1989). (*Z*)-Oxacyclotridec-10-en-2-one, an alfalfa weevil feeding deterrent from *Medicago rugosa*. *Phytochemistry* **28**: 3311–3315.

Eskin, N.A.M. (1979). *Plant pigments, flavors and textures: The chemistry and biochemistry of selected compounds*. New York: Academic Press, pp. 65–66.

Grant, G.T., Morris, E.R., Rees, D.A., Smith, P.J.C., Thom, D. (1973). Biological interactions between polysaccharides and divalent cations: The egg-box model. *FEBS Letters* **32**: 195–198.

Hatano, N., Yazaki, R., Asai, N. (2000). *Hajimeteno Funtai Gijutsu*. Tokyo: Kogyo Chosakai Publishing.

Hirose, N., Tsuge, H. (1989). Improved extraction method for Vitamin B_6 derivatives from biological materials with ultrasonication. *Vitamins* **63**: 627–633.

Japan External Trade Organization. (2008). Citrus (oranges, grapefruits, lemons). *JETRO Agro-trade Handbook*, pp. 72–79.

Japan Patent Office. (1999). Flavor and fragrance. *Collection of Flavor and Fragrance Technology*, No. 1.

Japan Patent Office. (2000). Flavor. *Collection of Flavor and Fragrance Technology*, No. 2.

Japan Patent Office. (2001). Fragrance. *Collection of Flavor and Fragrance Technology*, No. 3.

Kawakubo, S., Sasaki, K., Maruta, T., Suzuki, Y., Omukai, K. (2007). Field determination of leachable arsenic in soil by ultrasonic extraction–molybdenum blue colorimetry. *Journal of the Society of Inorganic Materials, Japan* **14**: 166–170.

Kimura, T., Sugahara, T., Fukuya, Y., Hiroko, S. (1996a). Effects of ultrasonication on water-extraction method for Rishiri-kombu soup stock. *Journal of Home Economics of Japan* **47**: 453–460.

Kimura, T., Sugahara, T., Fukuya, Y., Sasaki, H. (1996b). Effects of ultrasonication in heating extraction method on preparation of soup stock from Rishiri-kombu. *Journal of Cookery Science of Japan* **29**: 178–185.

Kimura, T., Sugahara, T., Fukuya, Y., Sasaki, H. (1997). Effects of ultrasonication on the preparation method for chicken-bone soup stock. *Journal of Home Economics of Japan* **48**: 153–160.

Kondo, T. (1987). New microencapsulation technology. Sogoh-Gijutsu-Center.

Lamb, H. (1993). *Hydrodynamics*. New York: Cambridge University Press, p. 599.

Lan-Phi, N.T., Minh-Tu, N.T., Nishiyama, C., Sawamura, M. (2006). Characterization of the odour volatiles in *Citrus aurantifolia* Persa lime oil from Vietnam. In: Bredie, W.L.P., Petersen, M.A. (eds.), *Flavour science: Recent advances and trends*. Amsterdam: Elsevier, pp. 193–196.

Lan-Phi, N.T., Shimamura, T., Ukeda, H., Sawamura, M. (2009). Chemical and aroma profiles of yuzu (*Citrus junos*) peel oils of different cultivars. *Food Chemistry* **115**: 1042–1047.

Lawrence, B.M. (2009). A preliminary report on the world production of some selected essential oils and countries. *Perfumer & Flavorist* **34**: 38–44.

Matukura, T., Hayashi, H., Orikoshi, E. (2008). Yeastseal (yeast capsule) series. *Foods and Food Ingredients Journal of Japan* **213**: 1061–1066.

Miyazawa, N., Tomita, N., Nakanishi, K., Ookubo, Y., Maeda, T. (2008). Study on the key aroma components of yuzu peel oil. *Annual Meeting of Japan Society for Bioscience, Biotechnology, and Agrochemistry*, Nagoya, Japan, p. 6.

Morris, E.R., Powell, D.A., Gidley, M.J., Rees, D.A. (1982). Conformations and interactions of pectins: I. Polymorphism between gel and solid states of calcium polygalacturonate. *Journal of Molecular Biology* **155**: 507–516.

Njoroge, S.M., Ukeda, H., Sawamura, M. (1996). Changes in the volatile composition of yuzu (*Citrus junos* Tanaka) cold-pressed oil during storage. *Journal of Agricultural and Food Chemistry* **44**: 550–556.

Powell, D.A., Morris, E.R., Gidley, M.J., Rees, D.A. (1982). Conformations and interactions of pectins: II. Influence of residue sequence on chain association in calcium pectate gels. *Journal of Molecular Biology* **155**: 517–531.

San-Ei Gen, F.F.I. (2006). JP 3885195; Microcapsules and Oral Constituent. Japan Kokai Tokkyo Koho; WO 2003/041509.

Sawamura, M. (2000). Volatile components of essential oil of the *Citrus* genus. In: Pandalai, S.G. (ed.), *Recent research developments in agricultural & food chemistry*. Trivandrum, India: Research Signpost, pp. 131–164.

Sawamura, M. (2005). Method for extraction of essential oils. Tokyo: Japan Kokai Tokkyo Koho, 3842794.

Sawamura, M., Song, H.S., Ozaki, K., Ishikawa, J., Ukeda, H. (1999). Inhibitory effects of citrus essential oils and their components on the formation of *N*-nitrosodimethylamine. *Journal of Agricultural and Food Chemistry* **47**: 4868–4872.

Song, H.S., Sawamura, M., Ito, T., Ukeda, H. (1999). Chemical compositions of the volatile part of yuzu (*Citrus junos* Tanaka) peel cold-pressed oils from Japan and Korea. *Flavour and Fragrance Journal* **14**: 383–389.

Sun, F., Littlejohn, D., Gibson, M.D. (1998). Ultrasonication extraction and solid phase extraction clean-up for determination of U.S. EPA 16 priority pollutant polycyclic aromatic hydrocarbons in soils by reversed-phase liquid chromatography with ultraviolet absorption detection. *Analytica Chimica Acta* **364**: 1–11.

Swingle, W.T. (1943). The botany of *Citrus* and its wide relatives. In: Webber, H.J., Bachelor, L.D. (eds.), *The citrus industry, vol. 1*. Berkeley, CA: University of California Press, pp. 190–430.

Tanaka, M. (2008). Application of microcapsules for food materials. *Foods and Food Ingredients Journal of Japan* **213**: 1072–1078.

Tho, I., Arne Sande, S., Kleinebudde, P. (2005). Cross-linking of amidated low-methoxylated pectin with calcium during extrusion/spheronisation: Effect on particle size and shape. *Chemical Engineering Science* **60**: 3899–3907.

Tsuchiya, M. (2008). World production of fruits 2001–2006, *Report of Japan Fruit Juice Association*, No. **598**, pp. 67–81.

Yoo, K.M., Lee, K.W., Park, J.B., Lee, H.J., Hwang, I.K. (2004). Variation in major antioxidants and total antioxidant activity of yuzu (*Citrus junos* Sieb. ex Tanaka) during maturation and between cultivars. *Journal of Agricultural and Food Chemistry* **52**: 5907–5913.

Yukawa, C., Iwabuchi, H. (1994). Study on the volatile components of yuzu (*Citrus junos* Sieb. ex T. Tanaka). *Japanese Journal of Food Chemistry* **1**: 46–49.

INDEX

Citrus Essential Oils: Flavor and Fragrance, Edited by Masayoshi Sawamura

Printed and bound by CPI Group (UK) Ltd, Croydon, CR0 4YY
16/09/2026
14963409-0006